AF697632

GENERAL PSYCHOLOGY SERIES
EDITORS
Arnold P. Goldstein, Syracuse University
Leonard Krasner, Stanford University & SUNY at Stony Brook

HANDBOOK OF PSYCHIATRIC REHABILITATION

(VOL. 166)

Titles of Related Interest

Goldstein/Hersen HANDBOOK OF PSYCHOLOGICAL ASSESSMENT, Second Edition

Hersen/Last HANDBOOK OF CHILD AND ADULT PSYCHOPATHOLOGY: A Longitudinal Perspective

Liberman/DeRisi/Mueser SOCIAL SKILLS TRAINING FOR PSYCHIATRIC PATIENTS

Matson/Mulick HANDBOOK OF MENTAL RETARDATION, Second Edition

Saigh POSTTRAUMATIC STRESS DISORDER: A Behavioral Approach to Assessment and Treatment

Van Hasselt/Strain/Hersen HANDBOOK OF DEVELOPMENTAL AND PHYSICAL DISABILITIES

WM
200
H236

HANDBOOK OF PSYCHIATRIC REHABILITATION

Edited by

ROBERT PAUL LIBERMAN, M.D.

UCLA School of Medicine,
Brentwood (Psychiatric) Division
of the West Los Angeles VA Medical Center,
Camarillo State Hospital

ALLYN AND BACON
Boston London Toronto Sydney Tokyo Singapore

Big Spring State Hospital

Copyright © 1992 by Allyn and Bacon
A Division of Simon & Schuster, Inc.
160 Gould Street
Needham Heights, MA 02194

All rights reserved. No part of the material protected by this copyright notice may be reproduced or utilized in any form or by any means, electronic or mechanical, including photocopying, recording, or by any information storage and retrieval system, without written permission from the copyright owner.

Printed in the United States of America

10 9 8 7 6 5 4 3 2 96 95 94 93 92

ISBN 0-205-14557-4

Library of Congress Cataloging-in-Publication Data

Handbook of psychiatric rehabilitation / edited by Robert Paul Liberman.
p. cm. — (general psychology series : 166)
Includes index.

1. Mentally ill—Rehabilitation. 2. Community mental health services. I. Liberman, Robert Paul, 1937–
[DNLM: 1. Community Psychiatry. 2. Psychotic Disorders--rehabilitation. WM 200 H236]
RC439.5.H36 1991
616.89′06—dc20
DNLM/DLC
for Library of Congress 90-14251
CIP

9 780205 145577 90000>

ISBN 0-205-14557-4
H45578

Dedicated to the hardy band of clinicians and researchers who know the wounds from battle with the scourge of serious mental disabilities, but who are revived by their constant search for more effective rehabilitation methods and the certainty that their work will be translated into better lives for the mentally ill, their families, and their caregivers.

CONTENTS

FOREWORD

Louis Jolyon West

The acceptance of mentally ill persons by the community, the relative tolerance of their deviant behaviors, and the devising of more or less useful activities for them have been characteristic of many "primitive" societies from antiquity to the present day. Furthermore, the cruelties of civilization toward its deviant individuals were not totally unmitigated during the premodern era; there were voices of reason to be heard from Hippocrates to Johannes Weyer to Benjamin Rush to Dorothea Dix. There were also commonsense undertakings by certain relatively enlightened communities even in the worst of times. One thinks of the tradition at Gheel, in Belgium, where since the 13th century mentally ill people have been placed with local families and where they are helped to learn useful occupations, often improving and sometimes recovering completely.

By and large, however, modern societies are exceedingly intolerant of social and behavioral deviance. Even when this deviance is caused by physical or mental debility, acceptance does not seem to come naturally or easily in these days of preoccupation with superficial images, quick fixes, and bottom lines. Laws intended to improve reasonable opportunity for the physically handicapped (e.g., ramps for wheelchairs, parking spaces for the handicapped, equal opportunity in employment) are only a recent nicety, and even today are far from adequate. The mentally disabled face even worse sociopolitical rejection and neglect. Our failure as a nation to deal humanely—even sensibly—with this problem is a scandal that unfortunately seems to shock precious few of those responsible for the making and carrying out of public policy.

Thus, at a time when the Western sense of morality—which underlay the development of moral treatment of the mentally ill in the 19th century—seems to have fallen into desuetude, this *Handbook of Psychiatric Rehabilitation* comes to us like a sunny day in midwinter. Professor Robert Paul Liberman and his colleagues have contributed enormously, not only to the enlightenment of those responsible for rehabilitation of chronic psychotic patients but also to the moral sensibility that requires us to labor in this vineyard. Their contributions demonstrate that such rehabilitation is the logical result of the integration of advances in biological psychiatry, psychological therapies (including individual, group, and family approaches), social methods of skills training, occupational therapy, and environmental maneuvers such as partial hospitalization, structured residential settings, specially designed programs in various industries, and the like.

The development of pharmacologic treatments for those with chronic mental illnesses has made it possible for many patients to return to society rather than to remain indefinitely hospitalized. However, medications alone have not ensured that these former patients will be able to get along outside of hospitals: to work, to relate well to others, to achieve some quality of life. That is why psychiatric rehabilitation has increasingly become recognized as an important extension of other more generally accepted forms of treatment. It is through rehabilitation that psychiatric patients acquire the tools needed to truly live rather than to merely exist outside the hospital.

Liberman, through his work as the director of UCLA's Clinical Research Center for Schizophrenia and Psychiatric Rehabilitation, at Camarillo State Hospital, and as chief of Rehabilitation at the UCLA-affiliated West Los Angeles Veterans Affairs Medical Center, Brentwood Division, has shown that chronic mentally ill patients can be helped significantly by treatments and special training methods that build and enhance coping and social skills. The methods designed and validated by him and his colleagues over the past 15 years have become cornerstones of their new, major component of care for the mentally ill and are well described in this book. Liberman's work has demonstrated that social skills can be learned in a generalizable and durable fashion and that such skills are protective against stress-induced relapse.

Under Liberman, the rehabilitation service for psychiatric patients at the West Los Angeles Veterans Affairs Medical Center has become a model for training programs in social skills, vocational restoration, and independent living. His interdisciplinary team of mental health and rehabilitation professionals serves as a national resource for clinicians and researchers. Furthermore, through the years his many publications, educational videotapes, and worldwide lectures and workshops have expanded his vision of proper extended care for the mentally ill to an appreciative international audience.

In this volume, Liberman has assembled state-of-the-art overviews of all aspects of psychiatric rehabilitation. The first chapter provides a thorough discussion of the philosophy and methods of psychiatric rehabilitation and places it in historical perspective. The second chapter summarizes the psychological principles that underlie various methods and interventions in the rehabilitation process. Subsequent chapters cover specific subjects relevant to a comprehensive approach to psychiatric rehabilitation. These topics include diagnosis and functional assessment, social skills training, the hospital inpatient model for social learning, the training-in-community-living model, sex and acquired immunodeficiency syndrome education programs, vocational rehabilitation, family intervention, case management, rehabilitation of elderly patients, and the effects of symptom-oriented treatments on employability of mental patients.

Liberman and his colleagues describe elements of rehabilitation with such clarity that they can be readily adapted to special situations by service agencies of various kinds. This makes the *Handbook of Psychiatric Rehabilitation* an immensely practical manual for caregivers representing many disciplines.

It should now be considered the definitive text in the field of psychiatric rehabilitation. It will bring new vigor and renewed hope to many clinicians, patients, and families. Ultimately, if logic and sensibility prevail, and humane morality rises again within the body politic, it may stir our society to a greater and more consistent effort on behalf of those whom fate has victimized with mental illness.

PREFACE

The heterogeneous symptoms, functional disabilities, and social role handicaps that make up long-term mental disorders such as schizophrenia pose a broad challenge to treatment and rehabilitation. Cognitive impairments that endure even during periods of symptom remission interfere with chronic mental patients' acquiring the coping skills required for community adaption. Moreover, the volatile and emotionally burdensome course of chronic mental disorders frequently robs patients of supportive family and social supports, thereby diminishing crucial buffers against stress. The stress-related, brain disorders that include schizophrenia, bipolar illness, and chronic depressive and obsessive-compulsive disorders cannot be "cured"; instead, like most chronic biomedical disorders, a rehabilitative emphasis must be developed that aims at a lifelong effort to build protection against the noxious effects of stressors superimposed upon psychobiological vulnerability.

An emerging technology of rehabilitation has been demonstrably protective against stress-induced relapse in persons with long-term mental illness. The technology includes a two-faceted approach: (a) building coping and social skills in afflicted individuals and their families and caregivers, and (b) creating prosthetic environments that confer social support and flexible levels of intervention and management of the illness through continuous treatment teams and rehabilitative venues. While psychotropic drugs form the cornerstone of treating chronic mental disorders—especially the positive symptoms—rehabilitation modalities can reduce or compensate for patients' social and occupational disability and handicaps. A research base is being built, driven by conceptual frameworks and hypotheses grown from scientific work in psychiatry and psychology, that offers promise to connect the biomedical with the psychosocial elements of a truly scientific approach to these disorders.

Psychiatric rehabilitation has been primarily associated with the care of persons with chronic mental disorders; however, psychiatric expertise in conceptualization and clinical intervention has also been applied to the rehabilitation of persons with chronic medical and surgical problems, such as in pain management, stroke, and cardiovascular rehabilitation. It would be advisable to restrict the term "psychiatric rehabilitation" to those disorders that are primarily the responsibility and within the purview of the discipline of psychiatry—namely the disorders listed in the *Diagnostic and Statistical Manual of Mental Disorders*, 3rd edition—revised and its subsequent editions, published by the American Psychiatric Association. There are numbers of books available to guide the professional interested in psychiatric and behavioral contributions to the rehabilitation of medical and surgical disorders. This *Handbook of Psychiatric Rehabilitation* is the first definitive and scholarly work devoted to the rehabilitation of the psychiatrically disabled.

To consolidate the current knowledge and technology in psychiatric rehabilitation, professionals in the field need to equip themselves with a common set of values, attitudes, terms, and goals that are based on the prevailing conceptual and research base. The *Handbook of Psychiatric Rehabilitation* provides the rehabilitation worker as well as students and administrators with a common set of assumptions and a current grasp of the state of the art in this field. The handbook should also help to improve the involvement and satisfaction of consumers and their advocates in rehabilitation by clarifying appropriate goals for services and making available knowledge on the most effective techniques. The handbook's focus on empirical measurement of outcomes and results of rehabilitation should also assist administrators and policymakers in their concern for cost effectiveness and accountability of rehabilitation services.

The *Handbook of Psychiatric Rehabilitation* includes a comprehensive account of the conceptual and historical development of the field of psychiatric rehabilitation, its roots in laboratory sciences that elucidate psychopathology, and the principle arenas in which skill building and prosthetic environments have been developed to equip mentally disabled persons and their caregivers with protection against the adverse effects of psychobiological vulnerability and socioenvironmental stressors. Chapters are written by scientist-practitioners who have had an abiding interest and clinical involvement in the particular areas that they address. The latest findings are reported and put into perspective in social skills training, family management and psychoeducation, vocational rehabilitation, geropsychiatric rehabilitation, case management, training in community living, social learning programs, and sex and acquired immunodeficiency syndrome education. Furthermore, the two cornerstones of clinical assessment preparatory to designing rehabilitation programs—evaluation of psychopathology and of functional behaviors—are delineated in chapters replete with clinical illustrations of methods for performing such assessment.

For whom is the handbook intended? To galvanize the field of psychiatric rehabilitation, an alliance or partnership is essential among disparate groups, many of whom have heretofore been walled off from each other and working in rival camps. Thus, the *Handbook of Psychiatric Rehabilitation* should be required reading for psychiatrists, clinical and counseling psychologists, rehabilitation counselors, vocational evaluators, occupational therapists, recreational and other rehabilitation therapists, social workers, psychiatric nurses, and the full array of students and trainees in these mental health and rehabilitation disciplines. In addition, administrators of psychiatric hospitals, community support programs, psychosocial rehabilitation programs, mental health clinics and centers, and vocational rehabilitation programs would clearly benefit from the overview of the field provided by the handbook. Because consumer involvement is so critical to the success of psychiatric rehabilitation, it is imperative that patients, clients, advocates, and family members also have access to the up-to-date information carried in the handbook.

If progress continues to be made by the field of psychiatric rehabilitation, a second edition of the *Handbook of Psychiatric Rehabilitation* will be needed in 5 years. The current edition can help to speed our way into the future as we learn more about disabling psychiatric disorders and devise more effective treatment techniques and service delivery methods.

Robert Paul Liberman
March 30, 1991

HANDBOOK OF PSYCHIATRIC REHABILITATION

CHAPTER 1

PRINCIPLES AND PRACTICE OF PSYCHIATRIC REHABILITATION

William A. Anthony
Robert Paul Liberman

The essential elements of a psychiatric rehabilitation approach have been hinted at for well over a century. Different elements of the psychiatric rehabilitation approach have periodically moved in and out of favor, highlighted almost serendipitously as the mental health field progressed through various developmental phases. Currently there is a consensus developing as to what constitutes the field of psychiatric rehabilitation. The overall goal of psychiatric rehabilitation is to assure that the person with a psychiatric disability can perform those physical, emotional, social, and intellectual skills needed to live, learn, and work in the community with the least amount of support necessary from agents of the helping professions (Anthony, 1979). The major methods by which this goal is accomplished involve either teaching persons the specific skills needed to function effectively or developing the community and environmental resources needed to support or strengthen their present levels of functioning (Anthony, Cohen, & Cohen, 1983; Livneh, 1984; Liberman & Evans, 1985).

The work of current researchers and practitioners will determine whether psychiatric rehabilitation becomes an evolving field of study and practice or merely a historical footnote. At present it seems that many mental health professionals recognize the need for rehabilitation interventions to complement existing treatment approaches (Anthony, 1977; Liberman & Foy, 1983). This recognition of need does not mean that psychiatric rehabilitation is a well-understood field of study. Because all types of mental

---

Parts of this chapter were reproduced from W. A. Anthony & R. P. Liberman, 1986, The Practice of Psychiatric Rehabilitation, in *Schizophrenia Bulletin, 12*, 542–559.

health disciplines practice psychiatric rehabilitation, and because relevant research and conceptual articles appear in a wide range of professional journals, psychiatric rehabilitation is a field that until recently has been difficult to define.

HISTORICAL DEVELOPMENT

The origins of the psychiatric rehabilitation field are rooted in several historical developments: (a) the moral therapy era, (b) the inclusion of the psychiatrically disabled in public-supported vocational rehabilitation programs, (c) the development of community mental health ideology, (d) the psychosocial rehabilitation center movement, and (e) the development of skills-training techniques as an effective mental health intervention.

Moral Therapy Era

The 19th century reformists for more humane care of the mentally ill aimed "to treat the patients as far as their condition would possibly admit, as if they were still in the enjoyment of the healthy exercise of their mental faculties . . . and to make their condition as comfortable as possible" (Bockoven, 1963, p. 16). Moral treatment stressed a comprehensive assessment of the psychiatrically disabled, examining the person's work, play, and social activities. For example, a chaplain at a British asylum recognized the importance of patients' reentry into social life "by obtaining for them a change of scene and air and assisting them to obtain suitable employment" (Hawkins, 1971, p. 107). Consistent with present-day rehabilitation practice, moral treatment recognized that structured activity can have therapeutic value. Today the goal of psychiatric rehabilitation practice is to have the person do something differently.

Vocational Rehabilitation Programs

While initial government programs for employment of the disabled, sparked by the end of World War I, focused on the physically handicapped, they did demonstrate that rehabilitation principles could be effectively implemented and won public support for rehabilitation as a societal responsibility. The 1943 amendments to the United States Vocational Rehabilitation Act extended financial support and vocational rehabilitation services to the psychiatrically disabled, with similar legislation appearing at the same time in England. These governmental actions provided legitimacy to the idea of training and rehabilitating people with psychiatric disabilities and grounded the practice of psychiatric rehabilitation in the vocational arena. Discovery of the capacity of the mentally retarded for gainful employment led to studies on the effects of psychiatric disability on work and to the introduction of paid industrial subcontract work in large mental hospitals (Carstairs, O'Connor, & Rawnsley, 1956; O'Connor & Tizard, 1956).

The last 3 decades have seen the scope of rehabilitation move beyond a singular concern with vocational functioning to additional arenas of social and community functioning; however, vocational activity has remained a preeminent ingredient in current rehabilitation practices (Beard, Propst, & Malamud, 1982; Grob, 1983). Lamb (1982) has written that "work therapy geared to the capability of the individual patient should be a cornerstone of community treatment of the long-term patient" (p. 176).

Community Mental Health

In the late 1950s and early 1960s, the legislation that established community-based treatment for the mentally ill and retarded endorsed the parity between physical and psychiatric disorders and their treatment. Mental illness and retardation no longer merited removal from society to large institutions; thus, the British Mental Health Act of 1959 supported "forms of training and social services which can be given without bringing patients into hospital as inpatients or which make it possible to discharge them from hospital sooner" (Royal Commission on the Law Relating to Mental Illness &

Mental Deficiency, 1954–1957, p. 76). A new basic assumption prevailed—namely, people with major mental illness should be helped to maintain themselves in the community in as normal a manner as possible. Unfortunately, community mental health centers (CMHCs) failed to provide the comprehensive services needed by the severely psychiatrically disabled (Braun, Kochanski, Shapiro, et al., 1981) who were not a high-priority population for the CMHCs, perhaps because their interdisciplinary staff members lacked techniques for effective work with chronic psychotics (Liberman, King, & DeRisi, 1976).

The deinstitutionalization movement, which accompanied the opening of the CMHCs, fostered an appreciation of the value of work training in the preparation of patients for resettlement in the community. Psychiatrists were forced to match their view of the patient's abilities and disabilities against the realities of adaptation in the "real world." Studies were carried out in industrial therapy programs that showed the benefits and hazards of work for the mentally ill, changed the attitudes of citizens and professionals about the employability of mentally ill persons, and led to job placement programs (Bennett, 1983).

Consistent with modern concepts of rehabilitation are those additional elements of community mental health ideology—accessibility to and comprehensiveness of services and continuity of care. The emphasis on treating patients in proximity to their natural families and work settings has now been extended by the initiative of the National Institute of Mental Health for community support programs, a move that has encouraged state and local investments in a spectrum of services for the mentally ill. In turn, this has meant an infusion of key operating principles for psychiatric rehabilitation, including case management, coordination, and advocacy with a variety of agencies capable of meeting the full range of needs of persons with severe psychiatric disabilities as well as involvement of patients and relatives in self-help and assertive outreach.

Instead of expending great effort on reversing the socially disabling effects of institutionalism, community-based rehabilitation has focused on the somewhat different problems of young adults with severe psychiatric disability, many of whom have spent only brief episodes in mental hospitals. Such individuals demonstrate severe handicaps in social adaptation and often resist engagement in professional services; moreover, their deficits, while less extensive than those of the older institutionalized patient, are marked by instability, intercurrent crises, and sensitivity to stress. Thus, even though many CMHC personnel seemed to be preoccupied by primary prevention for the not-yet ill, and enamored of intensive verbal therapy for the not-yet chronic, some of the innovations of the CMHC initiative became very much a part of the psychiatric rehabilitation field.

Psychosocial Rehabilitation Centers

The realization that severely and persistently mentally ill persons would rarely experience a full return of psychosocial functioning in the community led to a movement emphasizing accommodation of the needs of these persons in sustaining some semblance of normality. With mental health professionals' neglect of the mentally ill, nonprofessionals and patients themselves initiated psychosocial self-help clubs located in cities where the mentally ill congregated in large numbers. The early clubs, such as Fountain House and Horizon House, were founded by groups of ex-patients for the purpose of mutual aid and support. These early social clubs gave birth to comprehensive, multiservice psychosocial rehabilitation centers such as Thresholds in Chicago; the Social Rehabilitation Center in Fairfax, Virginia; Center Club in Boston; Fellowship House in Miami; Hill House in Cleveland; and Portals House in Los Angeles. The psychosocial centers assist patients to deal with their real-life problems by providing opportunities for acceptable role performance and successful mutually interdependent relationships with others, by buffering stressors, and by making available a range of housing and employment options. From the beginning, these centers have emphasized (a) strategies to help people cope with the environment rather than succumb to it, (b) health induction rather than symptom reduction, and (c) belief in the potential productivity of the most severely psychiatrically disabled client (Beard, Propst, & Malamud, 1982).

Psychosocial centers have not valued the development of therapeutic insight (Dincin, 1981). Their orientation has been on reality factors rather than intrapsychic factors, and on improving the person's ability to do something in a specific environment, even in the presence of residual disability (Lamb, 1982).

Psychosocial centers have played a significant role in the development of the psychiatric rehabilitation field. Their influence in the foreseeable future should be even greater since Fountain House has been conducting a training program to assist CMHCs and other types of mental health settings to establish rehabilitation services based on the psychosocial center model. In a 5-year period, individuals from agencies located in 38 states, the District of Columbia, Sweden, and Canada have been trained. During that time the number of rehabilitation programs has increased from 18 to 148. As the number of psychosocial rehabilitation centers continues to grow, this serves to ensure the presence of settings in which future research can be conducted and new rehabilitation techniques tested.

Skills Training

The most recent development in shaping psychiatric rehabilitation has been the introduction of skills-training methods derived from social learning principles, human resource development training, and vocational rehabilitation. Effective coping with life stressors requires skills to promote problem solving, engage others in successful affiliative and instrumental relationships, mobilize supportive networks, and engage in work. Rehabilitation techniques that use active-directive learning principles—behavioral practice and role-playing, social and tangible reinforcement, shaping, coaching, and prompting, and generalization activities—strengthen an individual's problem-solving capacities and confer protection against exacerbations of psychiatric symptoms (Cohen, Ridley, & Cohen, 1983; Wallace & Liberman, 1985).

Skills training has been found effective in group and individual therapy, family therapy, milieu therapy, and vocational settings (Anthony, Howell, & Danley, 1984; Eisenberg & Cole, 1986; Liberman, DeRisi, & Mueser, 1989). The point of teaching interpersonal skills is to improve the individual's ability to master the challenges and problems inherent in daily life. It is assumed that, within genetic and constitutional constraints, each patient tries to do his or her best, so that the problem lies not in resistance or lack of motivation but in a deficit of some sort. The source of deficit is regarded as less important than using remedial training methods to enhance the individual's ability to cope. Successful coping leads to attainment of social and emotional goals that define competence and adjustment. While skills-training approaches have shown much promise and empirical efficacy (Carkhuff, 1982, 1983; Paul & Lentz, 1977), they have been adopted by practitioners very slowly because of the demanding competencies required of those who seek to do such training (Backer, Liberman, & Kuehnel, 1986; Cohen, Danley, & Nemec, 1986).

CONCEPTUAL FRAMEWORK FOR REHABILITATION

Within the last several decades, a consensus has developed about what constitutes a conceptual model for rehabilitation and its underlying philosophy as well as what constitutes appropriate rehabilitation practice. As revealed in Table 1.1, the conceptual model was introduced by leaders in physical

Table 1.1. Stages in the Rehabilitation of Chronic Mental Patients, with Examples of the Elements of Each

STAGE	DEFINITION	EXAMPLE	INTERVENTION
Pathology	Lesions or abnormalities in the central nervous system caused by agents or processes responsible for the etiology and maintenance of the biobehavioral disorder	Brain tumors or infections etiologically linked to psychotic symptoms	Laboratory and radiographic tests
Impairment	Any loss or abnormality of psychological, physiological, or anatomical structure or function (resulting from underlying pathology)	Positive and negative symptoms of schizophrenia (delusions, anhedonia)	Syndromal diagnosis, pharmacotherapy, hospitalization
Disability	Any restriction or lack (resulting from an impairment) of ability to perform an activity in the manner or within the range considered normal for a human being	Deficient social skills	Functional assessment, skills training, social support
Handicap	A disadvantage for a given individual (resulting from an impairment or a disability) that limits or prevents the fulfillment of a role that is normal (depending on age, sex, social, cultural factors) for that individual	Unemployment, homelessness	National and State vocational rehabilitation policies; community support programs

medicine and rehabilitation and later extended to the mental health disciplines. Both physically and psychiatrically disabled persons exhibit disability in social function; handicaps in role performance; needs for a wide range of services, often for a long period of time; and frequent failure to experience total recovery. Rehabilitation of patients with psychiatric disorders, as with physical illnesses, begins when the pathology and impairments of the acute state stabilize. In cardiac rehabilitation, intervention begins after the myocardial infarction and its associated pain and stress have resolved. Similarly, rehabilitation for a person with schizophrenia begins when the acute and florid psychotic symptoms recede or stabilize. Even if symptoms persist, rehabilitation can proceed within the limits of the individual's capability to respond to training and supportive interventions. The focus of the rehabilitation practitioner is on remediating disabilities and compensation for handicaps (Frey, 1984; Wood, 1980).

The pathology in schizophrenia is still poorly understood, although brain-imaging techniques are revealing intriguing leads for understanding structural and functional abnormalities in certain brain regions. Symptoms such as delusions, hallucinations, and thought disorder are the impairments of schizophrenia. These impairments can impede an individual's ability to perform certain skills and activities which, in turn, can limit the fulfillment of social and vocational roles.

In view of the intrusion of symptoms of major mental disorders—delusions, hallucinations, depression, and anxiety—on the cognitive and interpersonal capabilities of afflicted individuals, it is not surprising that such impairments lead to significant disability and handicap. For example, unemployment has been found to be as high as 70%

or higher in the severely mentally disabled (Anthony, 1979; Goldstrom & Manderscheid, 1982). Unemployment is a prime index of handicap since the demands of work in modern society accentuate the deficits, deviance, and stigma of mental patients. Employment rates following hospital discharge range between 10% and 30%, and only 10% to 15% of patients sustain their employment 1 to 5 years after discharge, with more recent studies revealing lower rates (Anthony, Buell, Sharratt, & Althoff, 1972; Anthony, Howell, & Danley, 1984; Liberman, DeRisi, & Mueser, 1989). Difficulties in work tolerance, endurance, following instruction, cooperating with co-workers and supervisors, problem solving, task orientation, sustained concentration, and ability to accept criticism and ask for assistance are all examples of disabilities that are caused by symptomatic and cognitive impairments and that lead to significant handicap.

Thus, the impairments, disabilities, and handicaps of persons with psychiatric disorders are related to their psychiatric symptoms and to their vocational and social deficits. Symptomatic and functional problems exist on a continuum. For example, the nature of the illness can influence the severity and chronicity of the symptoms and social dysfunctions. Individuals with schizophrenia generally are more impaired and disabled than those with affective or anxiety disorders (Coryell & Tsuang, 1982; Harrow, Grinker, & Silverstein, 1978; Weinberger & Kleinman, 1986). Within any one type of disorder, however, symptomatic and social-vocational course and outcomes vary considerably, both for different individuals and for the same individual over time (Liberman, 1982a). Moreover, there are not always high correlations among the major dimensions of outcome of severe mental disorders: for example, social functioning may be adequate even in the face of poor vocational functioning and persisting symptoms (Anthony, 1979; Strauss & Carpenter, 1981). Alternately, symptoms may persist but still permit adequate job adjustment (Anthony & Buell, 1974; Anthony & Jansen, 1984). The variability in the manifestations of major mental disorders is one of the most salient features of these disorders and can best be understood and studied through the interplay of vulnerability, stress, coping, and competence factors.

Stress-Vulnerability-Protective Factors

The vulnerability-stress-coping-competence model of major mental disorders explains the onset, course, and outcome of symptoms and social functioning as a complex interaction among biological, environmental, and behavioral factors (Liberman, 1982b; Nuechterlein & Dawson, 1984) and is congruent with the rehabilitation conceptualization. Psychobiological vulnerability may result in psychotic symptoms when stressful life events of ambient tensions in the family or work setting overwhelm coping skills.

Vulnerability and stressors, as shown in Figure 1.1, are moderated in their impact on impairment, disability, and handicap by the presence and action of protective and potentiating factors. Prime among protective factors are coping and competence exercised by individuals, families, natural support systems, and professional treatment. Examples of protective factors include rehabilitation programs that offer skill building, social support, or transitional employment. Coping and competence can be attributes of the individual or of the social environment. From this point of view, an exacerbation or relapse of schizophrenic symptoms that accompanied abuse of street drugs (e.g., PCP, amphetamines) would result from this stressful action of these drugs on the individual's underlying biological diathesis for schizophrenia. In like manner, stressful life events (e.g., loss of a trusted therapist or discharge from long-term hospitalization) that overwhelm the protective effects of medication, personal coping, and social support can also lead to symptomatic exacerbation. Even in the absence of a time-limited stressor, vulnerable individuals can succumb to ambient

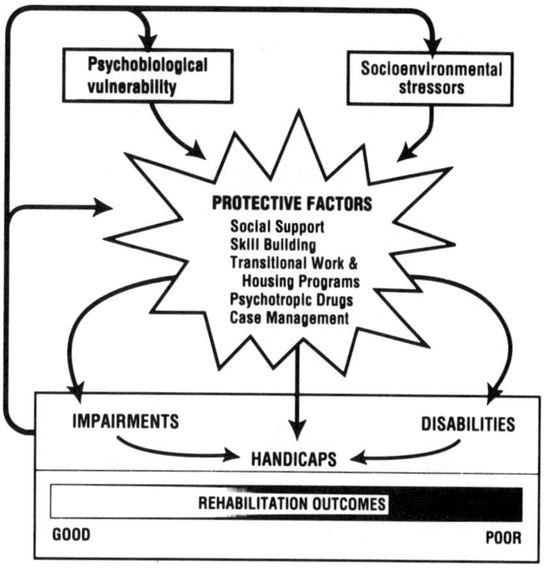

Figure 1.1. Factors affecting mental disorders. In the "Stress-Vulnerability-Coping-Competence" model of serious mental disorders, the symptoms and basic cognitive and emotional deficits of the disorder (impairments), associated social and vocational disabilities, and social role handicaps are affected by the underlying psychobiological vulnerability combined by stressors such as family tension or drugs of abuse. Protective factors that can promote afflicted individuals' coping and competence in dealing with stress include psychotropic medications and social skills training. Protective factors act through strengthening individual vulnerable individuals' capacity to cope with socioenvironmental stressors and reduce morbidity and disability of the disorder.

levels of challenge, tension, or conflict in their environment if they lack the protection conferred by medication, coping abilities, and social support.

The vulnerability-stress-coping-competence odel highlights the role of specific psychosocial interventions in developing personal and familial coping skills, and interpersonal and vocational competence as protective factors in the course of mental disorders. Psychosocial protective factors buffer the impact of potentiators and stressors, and thereby reduce the probability of symptomatic relapse. Socially learned coping helps individuals to satisfy their instrumental and social-emotional needs by meeting the challenges and solving the problems of everyday life. Coping and competence protect an individual with a given level of vulnerability to schizophrenia from stressful life events and ambient levels of environmental tension. At any level of psychopathology, coping can reduce the social, occupation, and self-care impairments that are associated with the disorder.

The model also encourages investigators to design optimal psychopharmacological interventions to modify the effect of psychobiological vulnerability factors. For example, antipsychotic medication serves as a personal protective factor against biological vulnerability; it thereby decreases relapse rates and improves the course of schizophrenic disorders. Antipsychotic medication also raises the threshold at which environmental potentiators and stressors precipitate psychotic symptoms in an individual with a given level of vulnerability to schizophrenic episodes (Leff, Hirsch, & Gaind, 1973; Vaughn & Leff, 1976; Vaughn, Snyder, Freeman, et al., 1982). However, the modulation of biological vulnerability by antipsychotic medication cannot fully remediate a vulnerable individual's susceptibility to relapse when faced with severe stressors, loss of social support, or diminution in personal problem-solving skills. Even with reliable ingestion of neuroleptics, for example, upwards of 30% to 40% of schizophrenic patients relapse within a year (Carkhuff, 1983; Paul & Lentz, 1977).

In this vulnerability-stress-coping-competence model, the appearance or exacerbation of characteristic schizophrenic symptoms and associated disabilities may occur in susceptible individuals when

- underlying psychobiological vulnerability factors are triggered, which is more likely in the absence of optimal antipsychotic medication

- stressful life events intervene that exceed the individual's coping skills and competencies in social and instrumental roles
- the social support network weakens or diminishes
- coping and problem-solving skills atrophy as a result of disuse, reinforcement of the sick role, or loss of motivation

Impairment, Disability, and Handicap

From the point of view of rehabilitation professionals, the psychobiological abnormalities in the nervous system that produce deficiencies in cognitive, attentional, and autonomic functions, and in regulation of arousal and information processing, represent the active pathology or disease state. The neurosciences are just beginning to develop instruments and techniques that can sensitively measure these abnormalities. However, they can be inferred through assessment of impairments that presumably index the more basic disturbances in brain function.

While impairments in physical rehabilitation include vision or hearing loss, reduced range of motion in an extremity, and loss of strength in a muscle group, psychiatric impairments can include thought disorder and speech incoherence, delusions, hallucinations, anxiety, depression, loss of concentration or memory, distractibility, and apathy and anhedonia. Thus, psychiatric symptoms and cognitive-emotional deficits are both correlates of the course and outcome of psychiatric illnesses and of the pathological processes in the nervous system. Presumably these impairments are somewhat specific for each of the major mental disorders and vary with the severity of the underlying psychobiological vulnerability. The specificity of the impairments enables diagnosticians to categorize psychiatric disorders reliably (e.g., *Diagnostic and Statistical Manual of Mental Disorders*, 3rd ed, revised [DSM-III-R]); however, there is considerable overlap among disorders as evidenced by the presence of delusions and hallucinations in a variety of psychotic disorders (Pfohl & Andreasen, 1986).

When functional limitations imposed by psychiatric impairments result in decrements in the ability to perform certain activities, the individual is said to have a disability. Disabilities are defined as inability or limitation to perform tasks expected of an individual within a social environment. Among individuals with severe psychiatric disorders such as schizophrenia, disabilities include poor self-care skills (e.g., cooking, cleaning, grooming, and care of teeth), social withdrawal and seclusiveness, abandonment of family responsibilities, and work incapacity. DSM-III-R (American Psychiatric Association, 1980) has highlighted the importance of these disabilities by including them as criteria for many diagnosable psychiatric conditions. To be diagnosed as having schizophrenia, for example, a patient must not only experience the characteristic symptoms of thought disorder, delusions, and hallucinations; he or she must also evince a "deterioration from a previous level of functioning in such areas as work, social relations, and self-care" (American Psychiatric Association, 1980, p. 189).

The disabilities shown by persons with psychiatric disorders are influenced by the same protective and risk factors that influence the appearance, exacerbation, and remission of symptoms or impairments. Thus, correlations between symptoms and disabilities would be expected; however, not every impairment results in a disability. Furthermore, similar patterns of disability can result from different disorders and impairments. Persons with mental retardation or affective disorders may have the same profile of disabilities as those with schizophrenia. Social and vocational disabilities form a major cluster of behaviors that both reflect and influence the course and outcome of a psychiatric disorder.

Research data substantiate a consistent relationship between a person's abilities and vocational outcome. For example, in every study in which work adjustment skills were assessed, they were found to be significantly related to future work performance (Anthony & Jansen, 1984). Similar to these data on work adjustment skills, rating of interpersonal or social skills has been found to predict vocational performance even though social functioning was measured differently in the various studies (Anthony, Cohen, & Cohen, 1984).

A final element in the rehabilitation model is handicap, which occurs when disabilities place the individual at a disadvantage relative to others in society. This can occur through stigma and discrimination, as when employers are reluctant to hire persons with mental illnesses. Handicap also occurs because society does not provide settings in which mentally ill persons can find accommodation and compensation for their impairments and disabilities. Wheelchairs and ramps have enabled paraplegics to overcome their impairments and disabilities to find renumerative work and fulfilling recreation; hence, their handicaps are compensated for. Because mentally ill persons require special social environments to compensate for their problems, overcoming their handicaps is much more difficult. Long-term institutional care in state and county mental hospitals was formerly society's method of dealing with the impairments and disabilities of psychiatric patients; unfortunately, institutionalization also created its own set of secondary disabilities and handicaps. That society has not yet succeeded in compensating for the impairments and disabilities of psychiatric patients is reflected in the extraordinarily high rates of unemployment and homelessness among this population (Anthony, Cohen, & Vitalo, 1978; Koegel, 1988).

REHABILITATION INTERVENTIONS

The conceptual framework elucidated above, joined with the rehabilitation view of disability, provides a coherent set of strategies for rehabilitation interventions with the psychiatrically disabled. The clinical practice of psychiatric rehabilitation, just like its counterpart in physical rehabilitation, comprises two intervention strategies: (a) patient skill development and (b) environmental resource development. In developing these intervention techniques, psychiatric rehabilitation practice is guided by the basic philosophy of rehabilitation; that is, disabled persons need skills and environmental supports to fulfill the role demands of various living, learning, and working environments. The assumption of clinical rehabilitation is that if psychiatrically disabled persons' skills and/or the supports in their immediate environment are augmented, they will be more able to perform those activities necessary to function in specific roles of their choice. In other words, interventions designed to lessen or compensate for the disability are assumed to lead to a decrease in the handicap.

Multidimensional Treatment

Psychiatric treatment and rehabilitation can be visualized with the help of the diagram shown in Figure 1.2. One dimension of the cube is the stage of schizophrenia; this indicates the nature and severity of symptoms, from early signs through a full psychotic episode to remission or chronic illness. The second dimension consists of treatment and rehabilitation techniques—drug therapy, family and cognitive therapies, social skills training, and vocational rehabilitation. The third dimension is support programs aimed at minimizing residual handicaps; these include family support, social service entitlements, case management, and psychosocial clubs. Thinking about schizophrenia in this way allows us to match treatment, rehabilitation, and support programs with specific impairments, disabilities, and handicaps.

Antipsychotic medication and social skills training, both included in the second dimension of the cube, are mutually reinforcing; patients can be taught to recognize their symptoms early and cooperate with the psychiatrist in beginning drug treatment. At

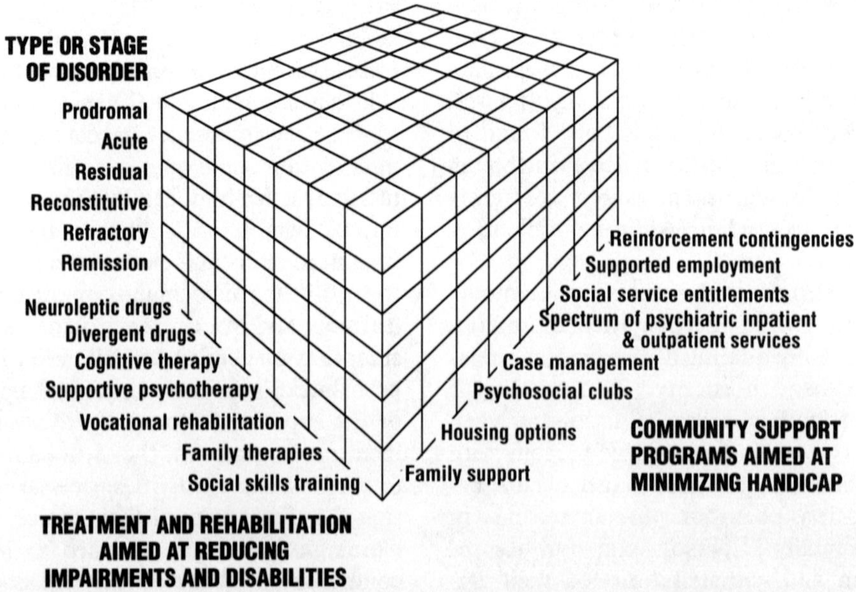

Figure 1.2. The "complex cube" of psychiatric rehabilitation. Rehabilitation interventions are displayed along the horizontal axis of this three-dimensional diagram. Specific interventions should be keyed to the stage or type of disorder and its level of severity, which are displayed along the vertical axis. In addition, rehabilitation interventions must be offered within the context of available and accessible supportive programs for community living, which are displayed along the third dimension of the diagram.

Brentwood Veterans Administration Hospital a program for teaching social and living skills includes a symptom self-management module in which patients are taught to identify and respond to their own specific warning signals of relapse. Patients who do not have periods of remission learn to keep persistent symptoms from interfering too much with daily life. Patients are also shown how to reduce stress by living more healthful lives—for example, by refusing alcohol and street drugs. In teaching this system, a training manual, videotapes, and a patient workbook are used.

Patients learn how to discuss warning signals with their physicians and relatives, to describe the signals and monitor them periodically by completing a check list, to enlist relatives in identifying an impending relapse, to request help from relatives and friends, and to cope with denial. They are also encouraged to communicate with eye contact and to learn audible speech.

These skills are taught in several ways. Patients are first motivated to participate by being shown clearly the value of what is to be taught. They watch a videotape in which actors play the parts of patients; then they model the skills that are the subject of the lesson. Videotapes are used to capture attention and to compensate for the cognitive deficits common in patients with schizophrenia. The videotape is followed by a question-and-answer session to ensure that patients are absorbing the information. Then they practice the skills by role-playing.

A series of problem-solving exercises are also used. In the first of these, patients are taught how to mobilize the resources necessary to use the skills they are learning. Problems include using the telephone, making an appointment, and arranging for transportation to see the doctor. In a second series of exercises, patients are taught how to cope with obstacles to using these skills—for example, what to do after arriving at a clinic to discuss signs of relapse and finding that the doctor has been called away for an emergency. Eventually the scene of training must shift from the clinic, hospital, or doctor's office to the patient's natural environment. Patients are asked to complete homework assignments in which they use the skills independently, and booster sessions help them maintain the skills.

These methods can be used to teach instrumental survival skills (money management, medication management, finding and maintaining a job, personal care and hygiene) and affiliative skills (friendship, dating, conversation, family communication). The program must be individualized, and patients must be allowed to set their own goals as much as possible. This training can now be provided by psychiatrists or other mental health professionals as an individual, family, or group psychotherapy service reimbursable by insurance. It is usually offered along with medication and social support (the third dimensions of the cube).

Interventions begin with a comprehensive medical-psychiatric diagnosis and a functional and resource assessment. This enables mental health and rehabilitation professionals to describe individuals by diagnostic disorder, level of behavioral functioning, and amount of environmental supports, key to identifying their impairments and disabilities. Identification of impairments and disabilities permits the mental health and rehabilitation practitioner to prioritize problems, formulate specific goals, and organize and implement treatment and rehabilitation plans. Medical-psychiatric diagnosis and a functional and resource assessment are necessary to match patients to drug and psychosocial treatments and rehabilitation programs that will be effective (Taylor, Liberman, & Agras, 1982). Furthermore, knowing the patient's diagnosis aids the clinician in providing the patient and family members with a reasonable prognosis and in determining the degree to which environmental versus remedial skills training can be provided to overcome handicaps.

Reduction of Impairments

Rehabilitation intervention with psychiatric patients requires reduction or elimination of the symptomatic and cognitive impairments that interfere with social and vocational performance. Intervention for reducing impairments is fortunately available from psychopharmacology. The past 20 years have seen major accomplishments in both treatment and prevention of morbidity from psychopathology through the use of antipsychotic, antidepressant, and anxiolytic drugs. Note that these psychotropic drugs are not panaceas. Even when taken regularly, they are frequently able only to reduce rather than abolish symptoms, and delay rather than prevent relapse. Psychotropic drugs are also associated with unpleasant side effects which at times can interfere with skills-training activities. However, they are usually helpful in reducing impairments to the point at which psychosocial strategies can be used effectively to remediate disabilities and handicap.

While a patient's symptoms and syndromal diagnosis clearly impair social and vocational performance, as is highlighted by the mixed symptomatic and functional criteria in DSM-III-R, the remitting and exacerbating nature of most major mental disorders obscures the relationship between psychopathology at time A and behavioral functioning at time B. The changing character of the symptomatic impairments of psychiatric disorders with the passage of time accounts for the insubstantial correlations often found between psychopathology measured during an acute episode and future work performance (Anthony & Jansen, 1984).

The disappointing failure of research studies to find correlations between impairments and disabilities might be a result of their having been conducted in an era preceding the availability of objective and reliable instruments for eliciting and rating psychopathology. Research using the standardization in diagnosis brought about by DSM-III-R has yielded studies that suggest a stronger relationship between syndromes and long-term outcome (Kendell, Brockington, & Leff, 1979; Knesevich, Zalcman, & Clayton, 1983; Lewine, Fogg, & Meltzer, 1983; Tsuang, Woolson, & Fleming, 1979). For example, when the severity of psychopathology is compounded by a patient's having multiple diagnoses, vocational outcomes are significantly worse. This was exemplified in a study of patients with drug abuse, some of whom had concomitant psychotic symptoms as well. A majority of individuals with both substance abuse and chronic psychotic symptoms did poorly in their occupational efforts; in fact, their vocational status was as impaired as that of patients suffering from chronic schizophrenia (Perkins, Simpson, & Tsuang, 1986).

Remediation of Disabilities Through Skills Training

Once a patient has benefited optimally from psychotropic drugs and the therapeutic effects of brief hospitalization, rehabilitation strategies use skills training to remediate disabilities in social, family, and vocational functioning. Skills training as a principle strategy in psychiatric rehabilitation starts from the assumption that many patients will suffer persisting disabilities despite the best efforts at pharmacotherapy and hospitalization. A relatively new field, training of social and vocational skills has relevance for a wide variety of psychiatric patients and for the professionals who serve them.

The psychiatric disorders with the greatest chronicity—schizophrenia, major depression, and organic syndromes—are those most in need of a skills-training focus. While appropriate drug treatment significantly reduces symptoms in most persons suffering from schizophrenia and mood disorders, many patients are refractory to drugs and others experience continuing social and vocational handicaps even with symptomatic improvement. The negative or deficit symptoms of schizophrenia, for example, pose a largely unanswered challenge to the pharmacopeia. Social withdrawal, apathy, energy, slovenliness, and anhedonia do not respond as well to neuroleptic drugs as do hallucinations, delusions, and thought disorder. Neither do drugs teach life and coping skills, except indirectly through removal or reduction of symptoms. Most schizophrenic persons need to learn or relearn social and personal skills for surviving in the community. Skills training can begin immediately after the stabilization of an acute episode or exacerbation of a psychiatric disorder, both of which usually result in the loss of social and role functioning.

Because the goals of rehabilitation center on adjustment to everyday life, it is vital for the schizophrenic individual to participate maximally in the choice of objectives and in the learning process. Comprehensive rehabilitation involves assessment, training, and modification of living environments in those areas relevant to personal and community life—self-care, including medication and symptom management; family relations; peer and friendship relations; avocational and employment pursuits; money management and consumerism; residential living; recreational activities; transportation; food preparation; and choice and use of public agencies. Specific goal setting, within these generic areas, should actively involve the patient, his or her family, and significant others.

Skills training has been viewed as an effective way of increasing the coping and competence of mental patients (Anthony, 1979; Liberman, Falloon, & Wallace, 1984; Wallace et al., 1980). Several sources of empirical data recommend skills training to improve patients' competence and coping ability. Many studies have highlighted the importance of premorbid and postmorbid social competence as a predictor of outcome in major psychiatric disorders (Buell & Anthony, 1976; Presly, Grubb, & Semple, 1982). This finding suggests that social-skills training might improve the long-term prognosis by upgrading the postmorbid social competence of chronic patients. Second, the magnitude of deficits in social and living skills has been well documented in chronic psychiatric patients. In one study major functional deficits in social and personal areas were found in over 50% of a sample of chronic psychiatric patients (Sylph, Ross, & Kedward, 1977). Two studies of schizophrenic patients found that both discharge and remission rates were significantly higher among patients who had higher levels of living and social skills (Farkas, Rogers, & Thurer, 1986; Linn, Klett, & Caffey, 1980). In another large-scale study comparing depressed patients and normal individuals, social introversion and interpersonal dependency were the most significant premorbid personal characteristics associated with the patient sample (Hirschfeld, Klerman, Clayton, et al., 1983).

Moreover, accounts of well-controlled and efficacious training programs to enhance social, vocational, and living skills have appeared in the recent scientific literature (Falloon, Boyd, & McGill, 1984; Jacobs, Kardashian, Kreinbring, Ponder, & Simpson, 1984; Kelly & Lamparski, 1985; Monti, Corriveau, & Curran, 1982; Monti, et al., 1979; Nelson & Cone, 1979). The learning of social and living skills is often facilitated by the concurrent administration of appropriate types and doses of psychotropic drugs; therefore, it is important for rehabilitation practitioners using skills-training methods to work in close liaison with medical psychiatric practitioners who prescribe psychotropic drugs. Judicious administration of psychotropic drugs reduces cognitive and symptomatic impairments, enabling patients to attend to learning stimuli and to engage actively in skills-training procedures (Wallace et al., 1980).

In 1974, Anthony and Margules published a review that concluded that "persons with a psychiatric disability can in fact learn useful skills" (p. 102). Specifically, the studies reviewed at that time and again 10 years later (Anthony, Cohen, & Cohen, 1984) showed that psychiatrically disabled persons could learn a variety of self-care, social-interpersonal, and intellectual skills. An example is training programs that have had an impact on the psychiatrically disabled person's skills in a variety of areas, including personal hygiene, cooking, use of public transportation, use of recreational facilities, physical fitness, interpersonal skills, self-control skills, job-interviewing skills, family relationship skills, money management, job-seeking and work-adjustment skills (Anthony, 1979; Falloon, Doane, & Pederson, 1985; Wallace & Liberman, 1985).

In many of these studies, psychiatrically disabled persons who were long-term inpatients with a lengthy history of symptomatic behavior were successfully trained. For example, in a longitudinal, follow-through study of over 200 chronic psychotic patients who were involved in an intensive rehabilitation program as part of their discharge from Vermont State Hospital in the late 1950s, approximately two-thirds were functioning in a near-normal fashion in social and vocational roles 20 years later in the community (Harding & Brooks, 1984). It has now become accepted that psychiatrically disabled persons can learn skills and that chronicity and symptomatology may qualify but do not prevent the learning of skills. The results of these studies are thus seen as supportive of a psychiatric rehabilitation approach, with its emphasis on assessing and increasing psychiatrically disabled persons' skills.

Social and vocational skills training uses procedures based on principles of human learning to teach specific interpersonal skills and to promote the generalization and maintenance of these skills. The training procedures have been empirically tested and "packaged" for ready access by practitioners.

While many psychosocial programs bill themselves as offering social-skills training, it is important to distinguish between nonspecific group activities that engage patients in socialization and methods that deliberately and systematically use behavioral learning techniques in a structured approach to skills building (Farkas, Cohen, & Nemec, 1986). While socialization activities can lead to acquisition of skills through incidental learning during spontaneous social interactions, they do not harness social learning and reinforcement techniques that may be required to promote the acquisition, generalization, and durability of skills needed in interpersonal situations (Liberman, King, DeRisi, & McCann, 1975). The learning disabilities experienced by many persons with prolonged psychiatric disorders require the use of highly directive behavioral techniques for training in social skills. Most psychiatrically disabled individuals have attentional and information-processing deficits. They show hyperarousal or underarousal in psychophysiological testing, and they experience overstimulation from emotional stressors or even from therapy sessions that are not carefully structured and modulated. These individuals often fail to be motivated by the customary forms of social and tangible rewards available in traditional therapy. In addition, they may lack conversational ability, a basic building block for social competence. Persons with schizophrenia, in particular, are deficient in social initiative and perception, and they have difficulty generating alternatives for coping with everyday problems such as missing a bus, making an appointment, or getting help with bothersome drug side effects. They tend to make less eye contact, have more verbal dysfluencies, and use less vocal intonation, all of which may impair social learning (Liberman, Falloon, & Wallace, 1984).

Skills-training procedures must be tailored to the needs of the individual patient, as patients present different constellations of social abilities and deficiencies. Moreover, a comprehensive assessment of personal and community resources that can be tapped for promoting the learning of skills should be a prelude to goal setting and skills training (Cohen, Ridley, & Cohen, 1983).

Several training models are presently available to the clinician. Longest in use is a treatment package for training skills that includes specific, goal-oriented instructions to the patient, the therapist's modeling appropriate use of the skills, the patient's role-playing interpersonal situations, and the therapist's reinforcing and providing corrective feedback to the patient (Cohen, Danley, & Nemec, 1986; Liberman, King, DeRisi, & McCann, 1975). Recently, training within an information-processing framework has been shown to be effective for patients capable of learning problem-solving strategies (Foy, Wallace, & Liberman, 1983; Medication Management Module, 1986). Disabled individuals are taught to improve their perception of information in immediate interpersonal situations, process that information to choose a response, and send a response back to the other person. However, both of these approaches are ineffective for patients with severe attentional deficiencies. A model using attention focusing procedures that simplify the learning of complex skills has been effective in training conversational skills in some seriously regressed, chronic psychiatric patients (Liberman, Massel, Mosk, et al., 1985).

Remediating Disabilities Through Environmental Support

When restoration of social and vocational functioning through skills training is limited by continuing deficits or refractory symptoms, rehabilitation strategies aim at helping the individual compensate for the disability by (a) locating living, learning, and working environments that can accommodate the residual deficits and symptoms; and (b) adjusting the individual's and family's expectations to a level of functioning that is realistically attainable. Thus, environmental modification and supportive-prosthetic social and vocational environments are complementary approaches to skills training in the reconstruction of social roles for patients with severe and chronic psychiatric disorders.

Environmental interventions attempt to provide the patient with supportive persons, supportive settings, or both. A support person might reduce a person's disability and handicap through a number of different roles (e.g., advocate, companion, counselor, and adviser). Attempts at making the setting more supportive focus on the programs or resources within the environment rather than on support persons per se (e.g., sheltered work and living settings, and special discharge programs). The distinction between supportive persons and supportive settings simply highlights the different ways in which environmental modifications occur. In practice, these modifications often occur simultaneously.

The main identifying feature of both types of supportive interventions, as distinguished from skill-development interventions, is that they do not attempt to change the patient's behavior systematically and directly. Rather, the attempt is simply to support and accommodate the patient's present level of functioning. Several studies have clearly demonstrated the positive impact on patient outcome of a support person (Katkin, Ginsburg, Rifkin, & Scott, 1971; Katkin, Zimmerman, Rosenthal, & Ginsburg, 1975). For example, one project used citizens from the discharged patient's rural neighborhood to function as supportive case workers. Over a 12-month period, inpatient days were decreased by as much as 92% (Cannady, 1982).

Witheridge, Dincin, and Appleby (1982) have reported on the use of a support team for psychiatrically disabled individuals at high risk for readmission. Working out of the patients' homes and neighborhoods, this team attempted to develop an individualized support system for each patient. Of the original 50 participants, 41 remained in the program. One-year follow-up data indicated that average days hospitalized per year decreased from 98.1 to 36.6. Even better results were obtained in a similar program that has been a model for assertive outreach and advocacy for chronic mentally ill persons (Stein & Test, 1978). This model program, named variously Training in Community Living or Program for Assertive Community Treatment is fully described in Chapter 7.

Stickney, Hall, and Gardner (1980) investigated the effects of introducing both a support person and a more supportive environment, separately and in combination, at the time of the patient's hospital discharge. They studied the impact of four predischarge formats, which differed in level of personal and environmental support. The goal of the discharge plan was to increase use of the CMHC and to decrease recidivism for 400 patients discharged from a state mental hospital. The results of the study demonstrated the impact of increasing personal and environmental support on patient compliance with referral and 1-year hospital recidivism rates. With minimal support, the respective referral compliance and recidivism percentages were 22% and 68%; with increased personal support, 36% and 39%; with increased environmental support, 68% and 31%; and with both increased personal and environmental support, 75% and 28%. Thus, whenever an added element of support was introduced, the referral compliance percentage increased and the recidivism rate decreased.

Other workers have reported results from an environmental intervention study based directly on the principles of psychiatric rehabilitation (Ballantyne, 1983; Wasylenski, Goering, Lancee, Ballantyne, & Farkas, 1985). Community rehabilitation workers were trained to provide interpersonal support and case management to patients being discharged from the hospital. Compared to a matched group of patients receiving traditional discharge planning and aftercare, patients in the experimental group were discharged an average of 21 days sooner and participated in approximately twice as many aftercare services. Patient perception of the program indicated high levels of involvement and satisfaction. At 6-month follow-up, over 75% of the patients were still involved in the program; 87% reported "feeling understood"; and 88% reported "feeling like a partner" in the rehabilitation planning process. In addition, there were significant differences in instrumental role functioning as student, worker, or homemaker.

Weinman and Kleiner (1978) compared the effectiveness of community-based "en-

Big Spring State Hospital

ablers" with two hospital-based conditions: social-environmental therapy and traditional hospital treatment. The enablers' major roles were to assist their patients in coping with community life and escort them to various community resources. Personal support proved superior to each of the hospital-based treatment approaches in recidivism, patient self-esteem, and patient instrumental and role performance.

Supportive interventions, operationalized initially in psychosocial rehabilitation centers have now been implemented in a number of different living, learning, and working environments. A recent review of the research on vocational programs suggests the importance of the support dimension in the working area. Bond and Boyer (1988) reported that of those 10 empirical studies that used paid employment, including transitional and sheltered, as an outcome criterion, eight studies reported positive results.

The last decade has seen vocational programming, consistent with the philosophy and principles of rehabilitation in general, moving toward the concept of ongoing job support (Bond, 1987). *Supported employment* is the term used to describe a vocational intervention characterized by permanent competitive employment, in integrated settings, with on-and-off job-site support for as long and as intensively as one needs it. The concept of supported employment originated in the field of mental retardation and has been extended, albeit with programmatic differences, to those with psychiatric disabilities (Anthony & Blanch, 1987). The only published supported employment research to date compared successful and nonsuccessful supported employment participants. While the successfully employed persons were more likely to have become disabled prior to age 19, no differences between the two groups were found in severity of symptomatology, diagnosis, and functioning in other life contexts (Trotter, Minkoff, Harrison, & Hoops, 1988). Similar to *supported work* is the concept of *supported learning* for those adults who wish to pursue postsecondary education or training. Just as individuals who wish to work may need support in their job attempts, so might individuals who wish to attend postsecondary school or training programs need support for their attempts to enter or reenter the learning environment (Unger, 1989; Unger & Anthony, 1989; Unger, Danley, Kohn, & Hutchinson, 1987). When such support is available, evidence suggests that substantial vocational and educational improvement can occur, as was the case for a group of severely mentally ill adults who took part in the university-based rehabilitation program. Also of interest, the attrition rate was only 30% over the 16-month program, a figure considerably below the 1-year attrition rates of over 50% in other treatment or rehabilitation programs (Stanton et al., 1984; Unger & Anthony, 1989).

Another outcome area in which ongoing support is needed is housing. The concept of supported housing has been advanced to replace the continuum model in which patients moved to more independent housing settings. In contrast, the supported housing model supports psychiatrically disabled persons in choosing, getting and/or keeping normal, permanent housing (Blanch, Carling, & Ridgway, 1988). Medders and Colman (1985) evaluated the Assisted Independent Living Program in San Francisco in which staff serve as hired consultants to groups of patients who form their own households, find their own living situation, determine their own household routines, and hire and fire staff. Initial program results indicated a substantial reduction in days of hospitalization. However, no research has been done on other patient outcomes or on the specific aspects of this innovative program that are most important to its success.

Overcoming Handicap

In addition to clinical rehabilitation interventions of skill and support development, psychiatrically disabled persons can be helped to overcome their handicaps through societal rehabilitation initiatives (Anthony, 1972). Societal rehabilitation is designed to change the system in which psychiatrically disabled persons must function. Unlike clinical rehabilitation, its focus is neither on the skills of specific psychiatrically disabled individuals nor on their unique environments. Rather, the focus is on system changes that can help many psychiatrically disabled persons overcome their handicaps. Examples of this type of system intervention are the Targeted Job Tax Credit legislation, changes in the length of the trial work period in the Social Security Disability program, and the development of a European-type quota system for the employment of disabled workers. The importance of these system-type interventions cannot be overemphasized. Obstacles in overcoming a handicap may be more a function of a nonaccommodating and discriminating social and economic system than of the person's impairment and disability.

Clinical and societal rehabilitation are not mutually exclusive. As a matter of fact, the 1973 amendments to the Vocational Rehabilitation Act recognized the value of societal rehabilitation efforts. The amendments established the principle of affirmative action by contractors who do business with the federal government and also attempted to establish the government as a model employer with respect to architectural access.

The National Institute of Mental Health Community Support System (CSS) is an example of a system-level response to the difficulties encountered by persons with a psychiatric disability. CSS incorporates both clinical and societal rehabilitation (Turner & TenHoor, 1978). The Community Support System initiative includes the components of a broader context or system in which psychiatric rehabilitation interventions should be provided, as illustrated by the third dimension of Figure 1.2.

Several attempts have been made to evaluate the impact of CSS programming introduced through state and federal legislation and funding (Bond, 1987). For example, a historical analysis of hospitalization rates in Oregon (Hammaker, 1983) showed a period of backsliding and lack of coordination in services in the late 1970s, no real changes during a period of statewide CSS planning (1977–1979), and a dramatic decrease in hospital bed-day use when funding and monitoring of CSS services actually began (1980–1982). Similarly, Lannon and associates (Lannon, Banks, & Morrissey, 1988) demonstrated improvement or maintenance of high levels of community tenure for older CSS clients in New York state, although there was no improvement for younger clients.

Another CSS initiative is the core service agency or lead agency concept, as well as various case management models. In case management, specific pools of high risk or high demand patients are directly assigned to a specific individual, team, or organization who are responsible for delivering and coordinating necessary treatment and rehabilitation. While not all studies of case management have reported positive results (Franklin, Solovitz, Mason, Clemons, & Miller, 1987) most evaluations of this approach have demonstrated the effectiveness of case management teams who assume responsibility for providing or coordinating all needed services for a specific group of clients (Bond, Miller, Krumweid, & Ward, 1988; Bond, Witheridge, Wasmer, et al., 1988; Brekke & Test, 1987; Field & Yegge, 1982; Test, Knoedler, & Allness, 1985). These studies suggest that assignment of responsibility for specific clients can reduce dropout rates, lead to allocation of more time to more disabled patients, and reduce hospitalization (Bond, 1987). The specific factors that lead to success are still uncertain and there is some question about the translation of case management into formats that can reliably yield clinical improvements in symptoms and social and occupational functioning. One major challenge for future evaluation and research is to determine whether the addition of skills training to the competencies of case managers might improve the rehabilitation outcomes of clients and reduce their need for supportive services (Grusky et al., 1987; Liberman & Mueser, 1989; Test, Knoedler, & Allness, 1985).

INTEGRATING REHABILITATION STRATEGIES

In view of the pervasive impairments, disabilities, and handicaps of most persons with chronic mental disorders, a combined approach to psychiatric rehabilitation employing skills training and environmental modification strategies is most often required. As the following case vignettes illustrate, the rehabilitation practitioner or team needs to integrate skills training, social support, and governmental incentives and regulations to bring about optimal outcomes.

Case Examples

Case 1

Larry, 28 years old, had been living the life of a hermit for over 4 years, in a rundown trailer behind his parents' rural home. He showed clear signs of schizophrenia—inappropriate laughter, talking to "his voices," fears that others were making fun of him or would hurt him, and inability to concentrate to the point that he had given up his previous interests in reading, surfing, guitar playing, and watching television. Nonetheless, he refused all efforts by his parents to obtain treatment and denied that he was ill.

His parents were counseled to make visits to a psychiatrist even without Larry's participation, making it clear to him that they were suffering from his illness and needed help for their own stress. This action rapidly led to his acceding to psychiatric consultation and agreeing to try antipsychotic medication. Within 3 months, his symptoms had receded and he was able to consider rehabilitation. With his impairments controlled, he demonstrated an ability to work in a simulated work capacity assessment and was referred to a transitional center where he could make stepwise progress toward independent apartment living and a job. Obtaining Social Security Supplemental Income made it possible for him to pay for this rehabilitation which overcame his handicap of social isolation and potential for homelessness.

He participated in social-skills training to remediate his disabilities in communication and self-assertion. His psychiatrist used skills-training modules to teach Larry medication self-management and symptom self-management, the latter a systematic program aimed at giving patients the capacity to identify their early warning signals of relapse and to cope with persistent symptoms. He became more tolerant of socializing as his verbal and nonverbal communication skills improved and he even started dating a young woman, an arena of life that he had abandoned over 8 years before. After 2 years in the transitional rehabilitation center, he was living with a roommate in an apartment. He graduated from a training program in welding, obtaining a remunerative position, which permitted him to leave the Social Security disability rolls. Interventions aimed at his impairments, disabilities, and handicaps all combined to bring about a favorable rehabilitation outcome.

Case 2

A 30-year-old male with a 15-year history of being in and out of private and state psychiatric hospitals decided he would like to get a job in the community after being in a psychosocial work adjustment program for 1 year. He did not have a good work history; 6 months was the longest he had ever been able to hold a job. Using the targeted job tax credit legislation as an incentive to the employer, the psychiatric rehabilitation team was able to find this disabled person a job working in a video repair shop, employment that was consistent with the patient's interests and talents. To keep his job at the repair shop, the patient needed to learn the skills of taking orders from authority figures, such as showing understanding of what others said and expressing his own thoughts and feelings to others. These social perception and expressive skills were learned in a series of social skills-training sessions. The team also made the environment more supportive to the patient by educating the employer to the patient's needs and obtained employer agreement to reduce the initial work load until the disabled person became comfortable with the new environment.

Combined Services Work Best

In general, all available interventions are used in combination—psychotropic medication, partial and full hospitalization, case management, skills training, social self-help clubs, and environmental support initiative—to achieve the maximum degree of adaptation that is feasible. The emphasis on each type of intervention varies with the nature of the disorder, the premorbid level of competence of the patient, and the phase of illness.

Historically, psychiatric treatment has developed effective interventions aimed at the patient's impairments. Somatic treatments in particular have been increasingly successful in alleviating the signs and symptoms of psychopathology. Antipsychotic and antidepressant medications minimize the signs and symptoms of illness, while rehabilitation interventions maximize coping efforts, adaptation, and personal strengths (Leitner & Dragow, 1972). Both approaches are essential in a complementary strategy to optimize patients' course and outcome of their disorders. Eliminating or suppressing impairments does not lead automatically to more functional behaviors. Likewise, a decrease in disability does not always lead to reductions in impairment. Note that a chronic or severe impairment (e.g., diabetes, schizophrenia, and stroke) does not always result in chronic disability or handicap. What the impairment does is increase the risk of chronic disability and handicap (Anthony, 1988, 1982).

Because effective rehabilitation typically includes more than one type of rehabilitation intervention, often different types of agencies are involved in the rehabilitation effort. The needs of persons with psychiatric disabilities are numerous and often cut across the functions of different agencies. Several studies conducted at the Boston University Center for Psychiatric Rehabilitation have found patients' vocational outcome to be correlated with the degree of integration between vocational rehabilitation services and mental health services the patient receives (Dellario, 1985; Rogers, Anthony, & Danley, 1989).

Psychiatric Rehabilitation Process

With the emerging consensus that major psychiatric disorders are stress-linked biomedical disorders, rehabilitation approaches have grown out of eclectic and empirical traditions emphasizing the development of patients' skills or supportive environments for coping with the enduring disabilities and handicaps of illnesses such as schizophrenia and mood disorders. Psychiatric rehabilitation uses assessment and intervention techniques based on such orientations as social learning and behavior therapy (Carkhuff, 1983; Liberman & Evans, 1985; Liberman & Foy, 1983), client-centered therapy (Rogers, 1957), human resource development (Carkhuff, 1972, 1983), and lifespan developmental psychology (Pepper, 1985; Strauss & Carpenter, 1981).

The psychiatrically disabled person must be involved as much as possible in setting rehabilitation goals—a process that necessitates the development of a trusting, mutually respectful, and empathic relationship with service providers. The preferred mode of intervention combines judicious and rational psychopharmacology with an educational approach that trains patients directly in the knowledge and skills they need to function in society. "Teaching as Treatment" (Carkhuff, 1972) is supplemented by interventions in the person's immediate environment, in the community support system, and at the societal level. An operational philosophy defining the scope of psychosocial rehabilitation has recently been issued by the National Institute of Mental Health (Stockdill, 1985).

> "Psychosocial rehabilitation" refers to a spectrum of programs for persons with long-term, severe psychiatric disabilities. The goal is to improve the quality of life for these individuals by assisting them to assume responsibility over their lives and to function as actively and independently in society as possible. The programs are designed to both strengthen the individual's skills and to develop the environmental supports necessary to sustain the individual in the community.
>
> Major services, which may be offered on a continuum, should be coordinated with those offered by other agencies providing psychiatric as well as the broad array of human services. The specific services include opportunities to meet social/recreational needs, vocational training and job placement, rehabilitative residential services, training the skills of daily and community living, and case management services. In addition, some psychosocial rehabilitation programs include patient assessment and goal-planning activities, educational programs, and family support activities.
>
> The services, which the individual may need to use on a short-term basis or indefinitely to achieve or maintain community adjustment, are provided in the context of a supportive, normalizing environment in the community. They are offered in a manner that emphasizes the "personhood" rather than the "patienthood" of the individual; that maximizes the individual's responsibility, control and feelings of self-worth, and that encourages patient and family "ownership" in the rehabilitation process. (p. 2)

The rehabilitation process encompasses three overlapping stages that recur for as long as the patient requires professional services (Anthony, Cohen, & Cohen, 1983). Assessment at the symptomatic, functional, and resource levels unites the patient and professional in a collaborative planning phase. Through diagnostic and assessment interviews, inventories, informants, historical data, role plays, and direct behavioral observation, the assessment yields information about the psychiatrically disabled person's current deficits, psychopathology, skills, and supports as well as the skill level demanded by the living, learning, or working environments in which the patient wishes to function.

The assessment information enables the rehabilitation practitioner to work with the patient and family member in the planning phase to develop a rehabilitation plan that specifies how the person or the person's environment must change to achieve the goals of rehabilitation. With respect to changes in the person, the plan develops the skill steps the person needs to raise his or her level of functioning to the level required by the environment. With respect to changes in the person's environment, a sequential plan describes what and how the necessary coordination, advocacy, and modifications are to be made. The rehabilitation plan also identifies the persons (e.g., practitioner, patient, agency, and family member) responsible for implementing the various parts of the plan.

In the intervention phase, the rehabilitation plan is implemented to increase the person's skills and to make the environment more supportive of the person's functioning. These interventions can lead to the achievement of the rehabilitation goals, first identified during the assessment phase. Repeated and regular monitoring of the change process informs all concerned about goal attainment, provides data for quality assurance, and enables clinical decisions to be made about continuation or change of interventions and goals.

Psychiatric rehabilitation is the recovery of social and instrumental role functioning to the fullest extent possible through learning procedures and environmental supports. When restoration of functioning is limited by continuing deficits and symptoms, rehabilitation efforts aim at helping the individual (a) acquire living, learning, and working environments that are compensatory; and (b) adjust to the level of functioning that is realistically attainable. Because of the limitations of currently available training methods, patients with more chronically disabling disorders, such as schizophrenia or organic brain disorders, may be unable to reestablish specific impaired or lost skills. In such cases, alternate compensatory skills and environments, such as learning to function in sheltered employment and residential settings, would be the focus of rehabilitative efforts.

With chronic psychiatric disorders, some amount of continuing symptoms and residual impairment makes necessary the acceptance of disability and the identification of new, attainable goals. Learning how to cope with symptoms, manage medication, and utilize professional resources when necessary become important targets for rehabilitation. When deficits preclude gainful employment, the patient and family need assistance in generating alternative types of meaningful activity, social contacts, and daily structure. While persisting symptoms may limit the level of functional engagement in life, the reciprocal also holds—namely, the more that rehabilitation improves the patient's social and role performance, the more likely it is that symptoms will be displaced or held in check. The goals of rehabilitation professionals are to sustain symptomatic improvement over the long haul; establish or reestablish interpersonal and independent living skills; and help the individual reach a satisfactory quality of life.

Comprehensive rehabilitation involves assessment, training, and modification of environments in areas relevant to personal and community life. Professionals contributing to psychiatric rehabilitation include psychologists, vocational rehabilitation counselors, occupational therapists, recreational therapists, nurses, social workers, psychiatrists, and mental health paraprofessionals. The professionals are careful not to overlook the natural caregivers in the patient's living environment—for example, peers, relatives, and operators of board-and-care homes.

DISSEMINATION OF PSYCHIATRIC REHABILITATION

The psychiatric rehabilitation approach is anchored in a rehabilitation philosophy, based on a set of empirical facts, articulated by a comprehensive process, and grounded in observable, programmatic interventions and practitioner skills. As a result, it is increasingly possible to provide training and consultation in psychiatric rehabilitation so that more practitioners become skilled in the use of efficacious techniques and more programs become rehabilitation oriented.

Becoming an expert in the field of psychiatric rehabilitation is not something one does overnight. It is *not* something one automatically acquires when hired to "do rehabilitation." At the University of California at Los Angeles (UCLA) Clinical Research Center for Schizophrenia and Psychiatric Rehabilitation, two decades of experience in training a wide spectrum of mental health professionals have led to the conclusion that three to six months of intensive, supervised and competency-based training—using an experiential, apprenticeship model—is required for trainees to acquire mastery and confidence in using skills-development methods of rehabilitation.

The recent development of modules for training mentally disabled individuals in the full array of community adaptation skills has offered practitioners a readily learned user-friendly treatment package that vastly reduces the time and effort required to become proficient in skills-training modalities (see Chapter 3 for an example of a module for teaching symptom self-management skills).

In the past, people were neither trained nor educated in psychiatric rehabilitation (Anthony, Cohen, & Farkas, 1987). Rather they learned their skills on the job, in psychosocial rehabilitation centers, or under the tutelage of mentors who pioneered methods of behavior therapy for the seriously mentally disabled. Now, however, the popularity of the field has increased and more and more people are engaged in psychiatric rehabilitation in settings as diverse as community mental health centers, psychiatric hospitals, community residential programs, vocational programs, day treatment and partial-care centers, and social clubs. As a result the need for technical assistance, staff training, and consultation has grown exponentially.

During the last decade, the Center for Psychiatric Rehabilitation at Boston University has carried out over 100 major technical assistance projects throughout the United States and Canada. Elements of the Center's technical assistance approach have been evaluated during that time span. The earliest data were collected on a materials development and training project. Anthony et al., (1980) wrote six books and an accompanying training manual designed to teach specific skills of psychiatric rehabilitation practice. A 150-hour training program based on these six training books was provided to practicing mental health and vocational rehabilitation practitioners and rehabilitation counseling interns. The evaluations of the training indicated that these psychiatric rehabilitation skills could be successfully learned and measured, and that trainees considered these skills to be important in the performance of their jobs. The results also suggested that clients of practitioners who scored high on written assessments of these skills were more likely to report feeling understood and involved, and to have been taught new skills (Rehabilitation Research Brief, 1980).

A later study examined the impact on patients of case managers trained in many of these rehabilitation skills (Goering, Wasylenski, Farkas, Lancee, & Ballantyne, 1988). Outcome data collected at a 2-year follow-up indicated that the patients served by trained case managers outperformed a matched control group on measures of instrumental role functioning, independent housing status, occupational status, and social isolation. Rogers, Anthony, and Danley (1989) trained vocational rehabilitation counselors and mental health practitioners from the same county in some of these psychiatric rehabilitation skills in a project designed to foster interagency collaboration between vocational rehabilitation and mental health agencies. Results over a 4-year period showed significant positive changes in the percentages of patients referred for services who were subsequently rehabilitated into competitive employment.

Concurrent with the studies of the impact on patients of practitioner training was a study of the impact of training and consultation strategies on practitioner and program changes. For example, staff members from mental health agencies were trained to be trainers in psychiatric rehabilitation. These newly trained trainers then trained practitioners in their own agencies. Evaluation of this "training-of-trainers" strategy suggested that mental health workers in these agencies were able to acquire and apply the skills of psychiatric rehabilitation. The training strategy also appeared to be effective in helping the agencies adapt the philosophy, principles, and skills of psychiatric rehabilitation (Rogers, Cohen, Danley, Hutchinson, & Anthony, 1986). Similar results were achieved in a training and dissemination program carried out by the UCLA Clinical Research Center which involved over 40 community mental health centers nationwide (Liberman, Eckman, Kuehnel, Rosenstein, & Kuehnel, 1982).

In addition to developing and researching a strategy for training practitioners and trainers, the Boston University Center for Psychiatric Rehabilitation has developed and evaluated a consultation technology designed to change an agency's program toward a rehabilitation approach. Implementation of the consultant technology typically results in changes in the agency's physical environment, funding, daily operation, staffing, mission, program structure, and record keeping (Anthony, Cohen, & Farkas, 1987).

The essential characteristics of a psychiatric rehabilitation program have been defined (Anthony, Cohen, & Farkas, 1982; Liberman & Evans, 1985; Liberman & Foy, 1983) and a technology to measure a program's compatibility with these ideal characteristics has been created and field tested (Farkas & Anthony, 1989). Similar to the training-of-trainers strategy for practitioner training, a strategy for training consultants was developed and evaluated. Fishbein (1988) reports on one state's efforts to assess the quality of the psychiatric rehabilitation services provided in the state's 55 partial-care programs and to implement the psychiatric rehabilitation approach broadly throughout the state's existing partial-care programs. In this project, program consultants received training in psychiatric rehabilitation consultation technology (Farkas & Anthony, 1989). Results suggested that "partial-care programs can comprehensively adopt the psychiatric rehabilitation approach if they are provided with in-depth technical assistance in the core psychiatric rehabilitation principles and practices" (Fishbein, 1988).

The other type of setting which needs technical assistance is university training programs, which have been notoriously slow in offering a psychiatric rehabilitation curriculum (Anthony, Cohen, & Farkas, in press). In order to develop a technical assistance capacity for preservice settings, a graduate-level curriculum in psychiatric rehabilitation was first developed and evaluated at Boston University. Program evaluation data indicated that the students' skill levels increased significantly; follow-up surveys of the program's graduates indicated that after graduation only 12% of the respondents chose to work with a population other than the severely psychiatrically disabled; 88% of the respondents reported that the program had been "very helpful" in their work after graduation (Farkas, O'Brien, & Nemec, 1988). Based on the experiences gained in implementing this graduate program, the Center for Psychiatric Rehabilitation is currently developing and field-testing, in six universities around the country, a strategy designed to disseminate to other preservice programs the psychiatric rehabilitation curriculum developed at Boston University.

At the UCLA Clinical Research Center for Schizophrenia and Psychiatric Rehabilitation, a curriculum has been designed for graduate students, interns, and residents in the core mental health and rehabilitation disciplines. The curriculum includes a practical textbook (Liberman, 1987) replete with case examples and learning exercises, a demonstration video cassette that displays the comprehensive approach to psychiatric rehabilitation, and an instructor's syllabus or course outline. This curriculum has been evaluated in various settings (Kuehnel & Liberman, 1990) and has been employed in the teaching of psychiatric residents, psychology interns, and occupational therapy students.

CONCLUSIONS

There are many patients who for the foreseeable future will remain relatively refractory to skills training and environmental support programs aimed at independent living and full employment. Such individuals can still benefit, however, from rehabilitation. It is possible to improve social adjustment, role performance, and autonomy and quality of life even within the limited opportunities provided by a mental hospital or residential care facility in the community.

Research conducted by a large number of investigators in the United States and Europe supports the following conclusions:

1. Severely psychiatrically disabled persons can learn skills.
2. The psychiatrically disabled person's skills are positively related to measures of rehabilitation outcome.

3. Skill-development interventions improve the psychiatrically disabled person's rehabilitation outcome.
4. Environmental resource development improves the psychiatrically disabled person's rehabilitation outcome.

In our attempts to conceptualize psychiatric rehabilitation, the "key and lock" analogy might be apt. While it is desirable to maximize an individual's social and instrumental role functioning through training and reeducative procedures, persistent deficits are likely to plague the patient, the family, and the rehabilitation team. Endeavors to upgrade the patient's repertoire of skills hone the "key," but it is often necessary to modify the "lock"—the patient's environment. Recent interventions aimed at modification of the family environment have led to dramatic reductions in relapse, exacerbation, and rehospitalization of patients with schizophrenia (see chapter 9, Family Management). Other examples of environmental prostheses are sheltered workshops, transitional and supported employment, halfway houses, and psychosocial clubs.

Guiding the rehabilitation profession is

- optimism that desirable change is possible if principles of human learning can be harnessed to the needs of the patient
- belief that motivation for change can come from special arrangements of the patient's rehabilitation and natural environments, as well as from within the patient
- confidence that by building upon the patient's assets and interests, including supportive treatment and family environments, even small improvements can lead to significant functional changes and can uplift the patient's quality of life

Principles of rehabilitation have the potential to tie researchers and professionals engaged in psychiatric rehabilitation into a cohesive, empirically based field. Rehabilitation practice has taken root in a variety of settings, including mental health centers and clinics, mental hospitals, general hospitals, psychosocial centers, and community support programs. More than ever before, psychiatric rehabilitation is perceived as a legitimate and credible field of practice, education, and research; as complementary to the existing fields of psychiatric treatment; and as a necessary component of mental health system planning and policy making.

REFERENCES

American Psychiatric Association (1980). *Diagnostic and statistical manual of mental disorders* (3rd ed.). Washington, DC: Author.

Anthony, W. A. (1972). Societal rehabilitation: Changing society's attitudes toward the physically and mentally disabled. *Rehabilitation Psychology, 19*, 117–126.

Anthony, W. A. (1977). Psychological rehabilitation: A concept in need of a method. *American Psychologist, 32*, 658–662.

Anthony, W. A. (1979). *Principles of psychiatric rehabilitation*. Baltimore, MD: University Park Press.

Anthony, W. A. (1982). Explaining "psychiatric rehabilitation" by an analogy to "physical rehabilitation." *Psychosocial Rehabilitation Journal, 5*, 61–65.

Anthony, W. A. (1988). A rehabilitation model for rehabilitating the psychiatrically disabled. *Rehabilitation Counseling Bulletin, 24*, 6–21.

Anthony, W. A., & Blanch, A. (1987). Supported employment for persons who are psychiatrically disabled: An historical and conceptual perspective. *Psychosocial Rehabilitation Journal, 11*, 5–23.

Anthony, W. A., & Blanch, A. (1989). Research on community support services: What have we learned? *Psychosocial Rehabilitation Journal, 12*(3), 55–81.

Anthony, W. A., Buell, G. J., Sharratt, S., & Althoff, M. E. (1972). Efficacy of psychiatric rehabilitation. *Psychological Bulletin, 78*, 447–456.

Anthony, W. A., & Buell, G. J. (1974). Predicting psychiatric rehabilitation outcome using demographic characteristics: A replication. *Journal of Counseling Psychology, 21*, 421–422.

Anthony, W. A., Cohen, M., & Cohen, B.

(1983). The philosophy, treatment process and principles of the psychiatric rehabilitation approach. *New Directions in Mental Health, 17*, 67–79.

Anthony, W. A., Cohen, M. R., & Cohen, B. (1984). Psychiatric rehabilitation. In J. Talbott (Ed.), *The chronic mental patient: Five years later* (pp. 213-252). New York: Grune & Stratton.

Anthony, W. A., Cohen, M., & Farkas, M. (1982). A psychiatric rehabilitation treatment program: Can I recognize one if I see one? *Community Mental Health Journal, 18*, 83–96.

Anthony, W. A., Cohen, M., & Farkas, M. (1987). Training and technical assistance in psychiatric rehabilitation. In A. Meyerson (Ed.), *Psychiatric disability: Clinical, administrative and legal aspects*. Washington, DC: American Psychiatric Association Press.

Anthony, W. A., Cohen, M., & Farkas, M. (in press). Professional pre-service training for working with the long-term mentally ill. *Community Mental Health Journal*.

Anthony, W. A., Cohen, M., Pierce, R., Cohen, B. F., Spanid, L., & Vitalo, R. (1980). *Psychiatric rehabilitation practice series: Books 1–6*. Baltimore, MD: University Park Press.

Anthony, W. A., Cohen, M. R., & Vitalo, R. (1978). The measurement of rehabilitation outcome. *Schizophrenia Bulletin, 4*, 365–383.

Anthony, W. A., Howell, J., & Danley, K. (1984). The vocational rehabilitation of the psychiatrically disabled. In M. Mirabi (Ed.), *The chronically mentally ill: Research and services* (pp. 215–237). New York: SP Medical & Scientific Books.

Anthony, W. A., & Jansen, M. (1984). Predicting the vocational capacity of the chronically mentally ill: Research and policy implications. *American Psychologist, 39*, 537–544.

Anthony, W. A., & Margules, A. (1974). Toward improving the efficacy of psychiatric rehabilitation: A skills training approach. *Rehabilitation Psychology, 21*, 101–105.

Backer, T. E., Liberman, R. P., & Kuehnel, T. G. (1986). Dissemination and adoption of innovative psychosocial interventions. *Journal of Consulting & Clinical Psychology, 54*, 111–118.

Ballantyne, R. (1983). Community rehabilitation services: A new approach to aftercare. *Network, 3*, 4–6.

Beard, J. H., Propst, R. N., & Malamud, T. J. (1982). The Fountain House model of psychiatric rehabilitation. *Psychosocial Rehabilitation Journal, 5*, 47–59.

Bennett, D. H. (1983). The historical development of rehabilitation services. In F. N. Watts & D. H. Bennett (Eds.), *Theory and practice of psychiatric rehabilitation* (pp. 15–42). New York: Wiley.

Blanch, A., Carling, P., & Ridgway, P. (1988). Normal housing with specialized supports: A psychiatric rehabilitation approach to living in the community. *Rehabilitation Psychology, 33*, 47–55.

Bockoven, J. S. (1963). *Moral treatment in American psychiatry*. New York: Springer.

Bond, G. (1987). Supported work as a modification of the transitional employment model for clients with psychiatric disabilities. *Psychosocial Rehabilitation Journal, 11*, 55–73.

Bond, G. R., & Boyer, S. L. (1988). The evaluation of vocational programs for the mentally ill: A review. In J. A. Ciardiello & M. D. Bell (Eds.), *Vocational rehabilitation of persons with prolonged mental illness*. Baltimore, MD: Johns Hopkins Press, pp. 231-263.

Bond, G. R., Miller, L. D., Krumweid, R. D., & Ward, R. S. (1988). Assertive case management in three DMHCs: A controlled study. *Hospital and Community Psychiatry, 39*, 411–418.

Bond, G. R., Witheridge, T. F., Wasmer, D., Dincin, J., McRae, S. A., Mayes, J., & Ward, R. S. (1988). *Short-term assertive outreach and service coordination: A comparison of two crisis housing alternatives to a psychiatric hospitalization*. (Manuscript submitted for publication).

Braun, P., Kochanski, G., Shapiro, R., Greenberg, S., Gudeman, J. E., Johnson, S., & Shore, M. F. (1981). Overview: Deinstitutionalization of psychiatric patients. *American Journal of Psychiatry, 131*, 736-749.

Brekke, J. S., & Test, M. A. (1987). An empirical analysis of services delivered in a model community support program. *Psychosocial Rehabilitation Journal, 10*(4), 51–62.

Buell, G. J., & Anthony, W. A. (1976). The relationship between patient demographic characteristics and psychiatric rehabilitation outcome. *Community Mental Health Journal, 11*, 208–214.

Cannady, D. (1982). Chronics and cleaning ladies. *Psychosocial Rehabilitation Journal, 5*, 13–16.

Carkhuff, R. R. (1972). New directions in training for helping professionals: Towards a technology for human and community resource development. *The Counseling Psychologist, 3*, 12–20.

Carkhuff, R. R. (1983). *Interpersonal skills and human productivity*. Amherst, MA: Human Resource Development Press.

Carstairs, G. M., O'Connor, N., & Rawnsley, K. (1956). Organization of a hospital workshop for chronic psychotic patients. *British Journal of Preventive and Social Medicine, 10*, 136–140.

Cohen, M. R., Danley, K., & Nemec, P. (1986). *Psychiatric rehabilitation trainer packages: Direct skills teaching*. Boston, MA: Center for Psychiatric Rehabilitation, Boston University.

Cohen, B. F., Ridley, D., & Cohen, M. R. (1983). Teaching skills to severely psychiatrically disabled persons. In H. A. Marlowe (Ed.), *Developing competence* (pp. 96–115). Tampa, FL: University of South Florida Press.

Coryell, W. H., & Tsuang, M. T. (1982). Schizophreniform disorder: Comparisons with schizophrenia and affective disorder. *Archives of General Psychiatry, 39*, 66–69.

Dellario, D. J. (1985). The relationship between mental health, vocational rehabilitation, interagency functioning, and outcome of psychiatrically disabled persons. *Rehabilitation Counseling Bulletin, 28*, 167–171.

Dincin, J. (1981). A community agency model. In J. A. Talbot (Ed.), *The chronic mentally ill* (pp. 212–226). New York: Human Sciences Press.

Eisenberg, M. G., & Cole, H. (1986). A behavioral approach to job seeking for psychiatrically impaired persons. *Journal of Rehabilitation*, April/May/June, 46–49.

Falloon, I. R. H., Boyd, J., & McGill, C. (1984). *Family care of schizophrenia*. New York: Guilford Press.

Falloon, I. R. H., Doane, J. A., & Pederson, J. (1985). Family versus individual management in prevention of morbidity of schizophrenia: III. Family functioning. *Archives of General Psychiatry, 42*, 887–896.

Farkas, M., & Anthony, W. A. (Eds.) (1989). *Psychiatric rehabilitation programs: Putting therapy into practice*. Baltimore, MD: Johns Hopkins Press.

Farkas, M., Cohen, M. R., & Nemec, P. (1986). *Psychiatric rehabilitation programs: Putting concepts into practice?* Boston, MA: Center for Psychiatric Rehabilitation, Boston University.

Farkas, M., O'Brien, W. F., & Nemec, P. (1988). A graduate level curriculum in psychiatric rehabilitation: Filling a need. *Psychosocial Rehabilitation Journal, 12*, 53–66.

Farkas, M., Rogers, S., & Thurer, S. (1986). *Rehabilitation outcome for the recently deinstitutionalized client: The ones we left behind*. Boston, MA: Center for Psychiatric Rehabilitation, Boston University.

Field, G., & Yegge, L. (1982). A client outcome study of a community support demonstration project. *Psychosocial Rehabilitation Journal, 6* (2), 15–22.

Fishbein, S. M. (1988). Partial care as a vehicle for rehabilitation of individuals with severe psychiatric disability. *Rehabilitation Psychology, 33*, 57–64.

Foy, D. W., Wallace, C. J., & Liberman, R. P. (1983). Advances in social skills training for chronic mental patients. In K. D. Craig & R. J. McMahon (Eds.), *Advances in clinical behavior therapy* (pp. 153–172). New York: Brunner/Mazel.

Franklin, J. L., Solovitz, B., Mason, M., Clemons, J. R., & Miller, G. E. (1987). An evaluation of case management. *American Journal of Public Health, 77*, 674–678.

Frey, W. D. (1984). Functional assessment in the 80's: A conceptual enigma, a technical challenge. In A. Halpern & M. Fuhrer (Eds.), *Functional assessment in rehabilitation* (pp. 11–43). New York: Brooke Publishing.

Goering, P. N., Wasylenski, D. A., Farkas, M., Lancee, W. J., & Ballantyne, R. (1988). What difference does case management make? *Hospital and Community Psychiatry, 39*, 282–286.

Goldstrom, I., & Manderscheid, R. (1982). The chronically mentally ill: A descriptive analysis from the uniform client data instrument. *Community Support Services Journal, 2*, 4–9.

Grob, S. (1983). Psychosocial rehabilitation centers: Old wine in a new bottle. In I. Barofsky & R. Budson (Eds.), *The chronic psychiatric patient in the community* (pp. 265–280). Jamaica, NY: SP Medical and Scientific Books.

Grusky, O., Tiernay, K., Anspach, R., Dans, D., Holstein, J., Unruh, D., & Vandewater, S. (1987). Descriptive evaluation of community support programs. *International Journal of Mental Health, 15*(4), 26–43.

Hammaker, R. (1983). A client outcome evaluation of the statewide implementation of community support services. *Psychosocial Rehabilitation Journal, 7*(1), 2–10.

Harding, C. M., & Brooks, G. W. (1984). Life assessment of a cohort of chronic schizophrenics discharged 20 years ago. In I. S. Mednick, S. M. Harway, & K. Finello (Eds.), *The handbook of longitudinal research* (pp. 375–393). New York: Praeger Press.

Harrow, M., Grinker, R. R., & Silverstein, M. L. (1978). Is modern-day schizophrenic outcome still negative? *American Journal of Psychiatry, 135*, 1156–1162.

Hawkins, H. (1971). A plea for convalescent homes in connection with asylums for the insane poor. *Journal of Mental Science, 17*, 107–116.

Hirschfeld, R. M. A., Klerman, G. L., Clayton, P. J., et al. (1983). Assessing personality: Effects of the depressive state on trait measurement. *American Journal of Psychiatry, 140*, 695–699.

Jacobs, H. E., Kardashian, S., Kreinbring, R. K., Ponder, R., & Simpson, A. R. (1984). A skills-oriented model for facilitating employment among psychiatrically disabled persons. *Rehabilitation Counseling Bulletin, 28*, 87–96.

Katkin, S., Ginsburg, M., Rifkin, J. J., & Scott, R. (1971). Effectiveness of female volunteers in the treatment of outpatients. *Journal of Counseling Psychology, 18*, 97–100.

Katkin, S., Zimmerman, U., Rosenthal, T., & Ginsberg, M. (1975). Using volunteer therapists to reduce hospital readmissions. *Hospital & Community Psychiatry, 26*, 151–153.

Kelly, J. A., & Lamparski, D. M. (1985). Outpatient treatment of schizophrenics: Social skills and problem-solving training. In M. Hersen & A. S. Bellack (Eds.), *Handbook of clinical behavior therapy with adults* (pp. 485–508). New York: Plenum Press.

Kendell, R. E., Brockington, I. F., & Leff, J. P. (1979). Prognostic implications of six alternative definitions of schizophrenia. *Archives of General Psychiatry, 36*, 25–31.

Knesevich, J. W., Zalcman, S. J., & Clayton, P. J. (1983). Six year follow-up of patients with carefully diagnosed good- and poor-prognosis schizophrenia. *American Journal of Psychiatry, 140*, 1507–1510.

Koegel, P. (1991). Understanding homelessness: An ethnographic approach. In R. Jahiel (Ed.), *Homelessness: A prevention-oriented approach.* Baltimore: John Hopkins University Press.

Kuehnel, T. G., & Liberman, R. P. (1990). Competency-based training of psychiatric practitioners in the rehabilitation of chronic mental disorders. In H. Lefley & D. Johnson (Eds.), *Mental health professionals and families of the mentally ill.* Washington, DC: American Psychiatric Press.

Lamb, H. R. (1982). *Treating the long-term mentally ill.* San Francisco: Jossey-Bass.

Lannon, P. B., Banks, S. M., & Morrissey, J. P. (1988). Community tenure patterns of the New York State CSS population: A longitudinal impact assessment. *Psychosocial Rehabilitation Journal, 11*(4), 47–60.

Leff, J. P., Hirsch, S. R., & Gaind, R. (1973). Life events and maintenance therapy in schizophrenic relapse. *British Journal of Psychiatry, 123*, 659–668.

Leitner, L., & Drasgow, J. (1972, July–August). Battling recidivism. *Journal of Rehabilitation*, 29–31.

Lewine, R. M., Fogg, L., & Meltzer, H. Y. (1983). Assessment of negative and positive symptoms in schizophrenia. *Schizophrenia Bulletin, 9*, 968–976.

Liberman, R. P. (1982a). Social factors in schizophrenia. In L. Grinspoon (Ed.), *The American Psychiatric Association annual review* (pp. 97–111). Washington, DC: American Psychiatric Press.

Liberman, R. P. (1982b). What is schizophrenia? *Schizophrenia Bulletin, 8*, 435–437.

Liberman, R. P. (Ed.). (1987). *Psychiatric rehabilitation of chronic mental patients.* Washington, DC: American Psychiatric Press.

Liberman, R. P., DeRisi, W. J., & Mueser, K. T. (1989). *Social skills training for psychiatric patients.* Elmsford, NY: Pergamon Press.

Liberman, R. P., Eckman, T., Kuehnel, T. G., Rosenstein, J., & Kuehnel, J. (1982). Dissemination of new behavioral therapy programs to community mental health centers. *American Journal of Psychiatry, 139*, 224–226.

Liberman, R. P., & Evans, C. C. (1985). Behavioral rehabilitation for chronic mental patients. *Journal of Clinical Psychopharmacology, 5*, 8S–14S.

Liberman, R. P., Falloon, I. R. H., & Wallace, C. J. (1984). Drug-psychosocial interventions in the treatment of schizophrenia. In M. Mirabi (Ed.), *The chronically mentally ill: Research and services* (pp. 175–212). New York: SP Medical & Scientific Books.

Liberman, R. P., & Foy, D. W. (1983). Psychiatric rehabilitation for chronic mental patients. *Psychiatric Annals, 13*, 539–545.

Liberman, R. P., King, L. W., DeRisi, W. J., & McCann, M. (1975). *Personal effectiveness: Guiding people to assert themselves and improve their social skills*. Champaign, IL: Research Press.

Liberman, R. P., King, L. W., & DeRisi, W. J. (1976). Behavior analysis and therapy in community mental health. In H. Leitenberg (Ed.), *Handbook of behavior analysis and modification* (pp. 566–603). Englewood Cliffs, NJ: Prentice-Hall.

Liberman, R. P., Massel, H. K., Mosk, M., et al. (1985). Social skills training for chronic mental patients. *Hospital & Community Psychiatry, 36*, 396–403.

Liberman, R. P., & Mueser, K. T. (1989). Psychosocial therapies for schizophrenia. In H. I. Kaplan & B. J. Sadock (Eds.), *Comprehensive textbook of psychiatry* (5th ed., pp. 792–896). Baltimore, MD: Williams and Wilkins.

Linn, M. W., Klett, C. J., & Caffey, E. M. (1980). Foster home characteristics and psychiatric patient outcome. *Archives of General Psychiatry, 41*, 157–161.

Livneh, H. (1984). Psychiatric rehabilitation: A dialogue with Bill Anthony. *Journal of Counseling and Development, 63*, 86–90.

Medders, N. M., & Colman, A. D. (1985). The assisted independent living program: A new model for community care. *Psychiatry Annals, 15*, 667–672.

Medication Management Module. (1986). *A skills training program to teach patients reliable use of antipsychotic drugs* (plus five other modules in the Social & Independent Living Skills series). Available from the Camarillo-UCLA Research Center, Box A, Camarillo, CA 93011.

Monti, P. M., Corriveau, S. P., & Curran, J. P. (1982). Social skills training for psychiatric patients: Treatment and outcome. In J. P. Curran & P. M. Monti (Eds.), *Social skills training: A practical handbook for assessment and treatment* (pp. 185–223). New York: Guilford Press.

Monti, P. M., Fink, E., Norman, W., Curran, J. P., Hayes, S., & Caldwell, A. (1979). The effects of social skills training groups and social skills bibliotherapy with psychiatric patients. *Journal of Consulting and Clinical Psychology, 47*, 189–191.

Nelson, G. L., & Cone, J. D. (1979). Multiple baseline analysis of token economy for psychiatric inpatients. *Journal of Applied Behavior Analysis, 12*, 255–271.

Nuechterlein, K., & Dawson, M. (1984). A heuristic vulnerability/stress model of schizophrenic episodes. *Schizophrenia Bulletin, 10*, 300–312.

O'Connor, R. N., & Tizard, J. (1956). *The social problems of mental deficiency*. London: Pergamon Press.

Paul, G. L., & Lentz, R. (1977). *Psychosocial treatment of chronic mental patients*. Cambridge, MA: Harvard University Press.

Pepper, B. (1985). The young adult chronic patient: Population overview. *Journal of Clinical Psychopharmacology, 5*, 5S–8S.

Perkins, K. A., Simpson, J. C., & Tsuang, M. T. (1986). Ten year follow-up of drug abusers with acute or chronic psychosis. *Hospital and Community Psychiatry, 37*, 481–484.

Pfohl, B., & Andreasen, N. C. (1986). Schizophrenia: Diagnosis and classification. In A. J. Frances & R. F. Hales (Eds.), *Psychiatry update: The American Psychiatric Association annual review* (Vol. 5, pp. 7–24). Washington, DC: American Psychiatric Press.

Presly, A. J., Grubb, A. B., & Semple, D. (1982). Predictors of successful rehabilitation in long-stay patients. *Acta Psychiatrica Scandinavica, 66*, 83–88.

Rehabilitation Research Brief. (1980). *A skills training approach in psychiatric rehabilitation*. Washington, DC: National Institute of Handicapped Research.

Rogers, C. R. (1957). The necessary and sufficient conditions of therapeutic personality change. *Journal of Consulting and Clinical Psychology, 21*, 95–107.

Rogers, E. S., Anthony, W. A., & Danley, K. (1989). The impact of interagency collaboration on system and client outcome. *Rehabilitation Counseling Bulletin, 33*(2), 100–109.

Rogers, E. S., Cohen, B. F., Danley, K. S., Hutchinson, D., & Anthony, W. A. (1986). Training mental health workers in psychiatric rehabilitation. *Schizophrenia Bulletin, 12*, 709–719.

Royal Commission on the *Law relating to mental illness and mental deficiency 1954–1957*. (1957). London: Her Majesty's Stationery Office.

Stanton, A. H., Gunderson, J. G., Knapp, P. H., Frank, A. F., Vannicelli, M. O., Schnitzer, R., & Rosenthal, R. (1984). Effects of psychotherapy on schizophrenia: I. Design and implementation of a controlled study. *Schizophrenia Bulletin, 10*, 520-563.

Stein, L. I., & Test, M. A. (1978). *Alternatives to mental hospital treatment*. New York: Plenum Press.

Stickney, S. K., Hall, R. L., & Gardner, E. R. (1980). The effect of referral procedures on aftercare compliance. *Hospital & Community Psychiatry, 31*, 567-569.

Stockdill, J. (1985). *Definition of psychosocial rehabilitation*. Technical Assistance Transmittal No. 1-NIMH Office of State & Community Liaison to State Mental Health Directors. Rockville, MD: National Institute of Mental Health.

Strauss, J. S., & Carpenter, W. T., Jr. (1981). *Schizophrenia*. New York: Plenum Press.

Sylph, J. A., Ross, H. E., & Kedward, H. B. (1977). Social disability in chronic psychiatric patients. *American Journal of Psychiatry, 134*, 1391-1394.

Taylor, C. B., Liberman, R. P., & Agras, W. S. (1982). Treatment evaluation and behavior therapy. In J. Lewis & G. Usdin (Eds.), *Treatment planning in psychiatry* (pp. 151-224). Washington, DC: American Psychiatric Press.

Test, M. A., Knoedler, W. H., & Allness, D. J. (1985). The long-term treatment of young schizophrenics in a community support program. In L. I. Stein & M. A. Test (Eds.), *The training in community living model: A decade of experience* (New Directions for Mental Health Services No. 26). San Francisco: Jossey-Bass.

Trotter, S., Minkoff, K., Harrison, K., & Hoops, J. (1988). Supported work: An innovative approach to the vocational rehabilitation of persons who are psychiatrically disabled. *Rehabilitation Psychology, 33*, 27-36.

Tsuang, M. T., Woolson, R. F., & Fleming, J. A. (1979). Long term outcome of major psychoses. *Archives of General Psychiatry, 36*, 1295-1301.

Turner, J., & TenHoor, W. (1978). The NIMH Community Support Program: Pilot approach to a needed social reform. *Schizophrenia Bulletin, 4*, 319-348.

Unger, K. V. (1989). Rehabilitation through education: Rethinking the context. In M. Farkas & W. Anthony (Eds.), *Psychiatric rehabilitation program services: Putting theory into practice*. Baltimore, MD: Johns Hopkins University Press.

Unger, K. V., & Anthony, W. (1989). *Psychiatric rehabilitation for young adults in a university setting*. Unpublished manuscript, Boston University, Boston, MA.

Unger, K. V., Danley, K. S., Kohn, L., & Hutchinson, D. (1987). Rehabilitation through education: A university-based continuing education program for young adults with psychiatric disabilities on a university campus. *Psychosocial Rehabilitation Journal, 10*, 35-49.

Vaughn, C. E., & Leff, J. P. (1976). The measurement of expressed emotion in the families of psychiatric patients. *British Journal of Social and Clinical Psychology, 15*, 157-165.

Vaughn, C. E., Snyder, K. S., Freeman, W., Jones, S., & Falloon, I. R. H. (1982). Family factors in schizophrenic relapse: A replication. *Schizophrenia Bulletin, 8*, 425-426.

Wallace, C. J., & Liberman, R. P. (1985). Social skills training for patients with schizophrenia: A controlled clinical trial. *Psychiatry Research, 15*, 239-247.

Wallace, C. J., Nelson, C. J., Liberman, R. P., Aitchison, R. A., Lukoff, D., Elder, J. T., & Ferris, C. (1980). A review and critique of social skills training with schizophrenic patients. *Schizophrenia Bulletin, 6*, 42-63.

Wasylenski, D. A., Goering, P. N., Lancee, W. J., Ballantyne, R., & Farkas, M. D. (1985). Impact of a case manager program on psychiatric aftercare. *Journal of Nervous and Mental Disease, 173*, 303-308.

Weinberger, D. R., & Kleinman, J. E. (1986). Observations on the brain in schizophrenia. In A. J. Frances & R. E. Hales (Eds.), *Psychiatry update: The American Psychiatric Association annual review* (pp. 42-67). Washington, DC: American Psychiatric Press.

Weinman, B., & Kleiner, F. J. (1978). The impact of community living and community member intervention on the adjustment of the chronic psychiatric patient. In L. I. Stein & M. A. Test (Eds.), *Alternatives to mental hospital treatment* (pp. 139-159). New York: Plenum Press.

Witheridge, T. F., Dincin, J., & Appleby, L. (1982). Working with the most frequent recidivists: A total team approach to assertive resource management. *Psychosocial Rehabilitation Journal, 5*, 9-11.

Wood, P. H. N. (1980). Appreciating the consequences of disease—The classification of impairments, disability, and handicaps. *The WHO Chronicle, 34*, 376-380.

CHAPTER 2

FROM LABORATORY TO CLINIC: PSYCHOLOGICAL METHODS AND PRINCIPLES IN PSYCHIATRIC REHABILITATION

Will Spaulding
Mary Sullivan

The principles, methods, and technologies of clinical psychology can be useful in psychiatric rehabilitation. Clinical psychology has always been involved with assessment of individual differences in basic psychological processes; that is, in psychophysiological functioning, attention, learning, thinking, and reasoning. In the subfield of experimental psychopathology, this involvement has focused on abnormalities and deficits that are characteristic of schizophrenia and other severe psychiatric disorders. Traditionally, the goals of assessing these characteristics have been to evaluate their relevance to psychiatric diagnosis and to learn something about the etiology of the disorders. The advent of psychiatric rehabilitation provides a new frame of reference for clinical psychology and experimental psychopathology—to assess individual psychological differences for their relevance to formulating rehabilitation goals, to evaluate those differences as potential assets or obstacles, and to apply an understanding of the psychological characteristics of severe psychiatric disorders to skill training and other rehabilitation technologies.

Functional assessment and skill training are key aspects of psychiatric rehabilitation (Liberman & Anthony, 1986). However, purely functional assessment and the skill training strategy it engenders neglects what is known about the basic psychological processes that underlie psychiatric disorders, especially schizophrenia (Liberman, Nuechterlein, & Wallace, 1982). Furthermore, even groups of patients who are homogeneous with respect to psychiatric diagnosis are

This chapter was funded in part by a Research and Development contract granted to Will Spaulding by Lincoln Regional Center, Nebraska Department of Institutions.

known to be heterogeneous with respect to basic psychological functioning. Therefore, there can be great variability in patients' ability to benefit from generic intervention procedures. However effective the skill-training approach, a hypothesis worth examining is that assessment and training procedures that are sensitive to patients' individual differences in basic psychological processes will be more effective than procedures that are insensitive to those differences.

Application of methods from the experimental psychopathology laboratory may also provide more fine-grained measures of treatment outcome and rehabilitation progress. For example, both pharmacological and skill-training interventions rely on measures of observable behavior as indices of treatment response. Such behaviors are in many cases far down a causal chain from the actual neurobiological locus of treatment action. They are also observed long after the crucial treatment effect occurs, and they are influenced by many confounding environmental factors. Laboratory measurement of changes in more molecular or basic psychological functions may provide earlier and more accurate prediction of the eventual strength and significance of the treatment effect.

The literatures of clinical psychology, experimental psychopathology, and psychiatric rehabilitation are ripe for cross-fertilization. This chapter presents a collection of the principles, methods, and technologies that such a cross-fertilization can produce. The focus will be on applications from the experimental psychopathology of schizophrenia. Schizophrenia is the diagnosis of the plurality of patients in need of psychiatric rehabilitation, and it has been a nosological keystone in psychopathology research. It is important to note, however, that no specific psychological deficit has been found to be unique to schizophrenia. Other psychotic or severely disordered patients can have the deficits found in patients with schizophrenia. Moreover, within the category of schizophrenia, patients have different constellations of deficits. Thus, the applications that follow from the experimental study of schizophrenia are not necessarily limited to patients with schizophrenia. Further, such applications may require adjustment and tailoring because of individual differences among patients within the schizophrenia spectrum. The current state of our knowledge demands that clinical applications be evaluated empirically on a case-by-case basis.

Cross-fertilization of clinical psychology, experimental psychopathology, and psychiatric rehabilitation yields products that fall into three general categories:

1. concepts and principles that form a conceptual framework for assessment and treatment strategies;
2. measurement methods that form an assessment repertoire;
3. intervention methods that form a treatment armamentarium.

In the next section of this chapter a set of concepts and principles will be discussed which give organization and direction to application of clinical and laboratory methods. In the subsequent sections this organization will be followed as specific assessment and intervention methods are described.

PRINCIPLES AND CONCEPTS

Two main ideas in the psychopathology of schizophrenia organize its application to psychiatric rehabilitation. These are *pervasiveness of expression* and the *diathesis-stress model* of etiology and course of illness.

Pervasiveness of Expression

The idea of pervasiveness in schizophrenia represents a convergence of several models of psychopathology. In ego psychology, schizophrenia has been conceptualized as severe deficits across a range of ego functions (Bellak, Hurvich, & Gediman, 1973).

In biomedical models schizophrenic symptoms and disabilities can be seen as a final common pathway at social-behavioral levels of functioning with tributaries extending to neurophysiological abnormalities (Strauss & Carpenter, 1981). In behavioral psychopathology, schizophrenia represents deficits across a variety of response systems (Adams, Doster, & Calhoun, 1977) or across levels of functioning (Spaulding, 1986). Models based on general systems theory (Scheflin, 1981) and models of human occupation (Kielhofner, Burke, & Igi, 1982) describe disorganization of adaptive subsystems. Key to all these models is the concept of "levels of functioning"; that is, the idea that molar social behavior represents the integration of specific processes that operate at more molecular psychophysiological, perceptual, attentional, and cognitive levels. From this perspective, schizophrenia can be characterized by deficits at all these levels. Although there is agreement that deficits are pervasively distributed in schizophrenia, the causal relationships among deficits are incompletely understood.

One implication of the pervasiveness principle is that skill-training interventions that address relatively molar levels of function (e.g., performing the role of worker or family member) may rely on the integrity of more molecular functions (e.g., attending to instructions and other communications, appropriately interpreting novel situations, appreciating the value of acquiring better role performance). If the more molecular functions are faulty, and this is not taken into account, the intervention may fail. Similarly, relatively molar deficits may compromise more molecular interventions. For example, *motivation* is a complex, molar set of processes that includes the ability to attribute value to activities, conceptualize the future, delay gratification, and other abilities. If the patient is unmotivated (i.e., lacks the ability to engage the molar processes associated with motivation) to learn new molecular skills, then skill training will probably fail.

This principle is applied intuitively by most clinicians experienced with severely disordered patients. For example, the decision not to include a patient in group therapy while acutely psychotic, or to maintain an antipsychotic drug regimen during job training, implies an appreciation of the effects of molecular deficits on molar interventions. However, intuitive application is often not good enough. There are many molecular deficits that may potentially interfere with molar performance, and even the most experienced clinician cannot hope to identify them all without systematic assessment. One of the important purposes of laboratory assessment of basic psychological functioning should therefore be to identify molecular deficits that could compromise skill acquisition and other more molar aspects of rehabilitation progress.

The pervasiveness principle also raises the question of whether treatments can be applied to reduce or eliminate molecular-level deficits that indirectly impair molar functioning. Antipsychotic drug effects are clearly an example of this in that action at the neurochemical level produces improvements in social functioning. It may also be that specific psychological deficits, once identified, can be reduced or eliminated by psychosocial interventions, thereby improving more molar functioning. There is reason to believe that at least some patients can benefit from such interventions, as the following discussion will show. However, most of the evidence comes from small-scale clinical studies and case reports, and there is inconsistency in the degree to which molecular changes generalize to molar levels of functioning.

Diathesis-Stress Model

Virtually all contemporary theories of schizophrenia hypothesize a diathesis-stress model of etiology and course of illness. Like pervasiveness, the idea of diathesis-stress represents the convergence of a diversity of theory and data (Cromwell & Spaulding, 1978; Liberman, Nuechterlein, & Wallace,

1982; Meehl, 1962; Nuechterlein & Dawson, 1984a; Zubin & Spring, 1977). The diathesis-stress view includes two interacting etiological factors: (a) A diathesis, or vulnerability, is a deficit that exists before the onset of illness, predisposes a person to the illness and endures over time, even during periods of remission. (b) Stress is an environmental event or series of events that place a demand on the person. Stress interacts with the diathesis, either at a particular time or cumulatively, to precipitate illness episodes. A corollary of the stress-diathesis concept is that schizophrenia exists in at least two phases. In one, a vulnerable state exists, represented by a particular pattern of enduring deficits. In the second phase, these predisposing deficits interact with stress to produce the illness state, represented by characteristic symptoms, associated disabilities, and even more psychological impairments.

For application in psychiatric rehabilitation the diathesis-stress view can be elaborated into a four-phase model of the course of schizophrenia. In the first, or vulnerability phase, there are no symptoms of schizophrenia but there is a constellation of relatively subtle deficits in basic psychological functioning, many of which can be detected only by laboratory methods. These deficits are of great interest in etiological research and they may prove relevant to primary prevention, but they typically would not be relevant to rehabilitation.

The second or prodromal phase is the period that precedes psychosis and appearance of the characteristic symptoms of schizophrenia. In the prodromal phase nonpsychotic and prepsychotic symptoms begin to appear, and the vulnerability-linked basic deficits may become more severe. The prodromal phase is the least completely understood phase of schizophrenia and is especially difficult to study with laboratory methods. Recent findings (Herz, 1986) suggest that prodromal symptoms can be clinically recognized and that intervention during this phase can sometimes avert recurrence of acute psychosis. Further study of prodromal phenomena in the psychopathology laboratory may identify measures that are even more sensitive to impending psychosis than clinical symptoms, or that indicate alternative interventions to prevent psychosis most reliably. Laboratory methods may also prove useful for evaluating the prodromal phase in patients who have not had an acute psychotic phase before. The clinical interview methods that predict relapse in patients who are known to have had previous psychotic episodes would be ineffective for patients who have not had previous episodes. Traditional psychological measures such as the Rorschach test have been used to evaluate "incipient schizophrenia" for many years, and validity research (Johnston & Holtzman, 1979) suggests they may actually be effective for this particular purpose.

In the acute psychotic stage of schizophrenia most of the basic psychological functions that can be measured in the laboratory are severely impaired, whether or not they are abnormal in the vulnerability or prodromal phases. Some measures are very sensitive to remission of the acute stage and may therefore be useful in evaluating acute-phase treatment. For example, normalization of some basic psychological functions predates the observable clinical effects of antipsychotic drugs (Spohn, Lacoursiere, Thompson, & Coyne, 1977) that may take as long as several weeks to appear. For some patients, use of laboratory measures could reduce the time required to find the optimal antipsychotic agent. Some psychological intervention techniques, especially those that address the psychophysiological level of functioning, may be useful during the acute phase.

The fourth or residual stage of schizophrenia follows remission of acute psychotic symptoms. It is characterized by continued peculiarities of cognition, effect, and behavior, which may persist for years. Neurological "soft signs," negative symptoms and neuropsychological impairments, as well as other abnormalities in basic psychological functions, are common in this phase. It is in the residual phase that most of the skill-training components of psychiatric rehabilitation are mobilized, and so assessment and treatment of psychological deficits that could compromise skill training are particularly important. Also, the deficits that appear in the residual phase can function as vulnerability factors that militate for relapse, just as similar deficits militate for initial onset in the vulnerability phase. Identification and correction of old and new vulnerability factors in the residual stage thus can affect the future course of the illness, independent of other rehabilitation interventions.

After the initial onset and remission of the acute phase of schizophrenia, the patient may continue to cycle between prodromal, acute, and residual phases for the rest of his or her life. The phases of the illness, and the disruptions of basic psychological functioning that accompany those phases, should be taken into account when one is planning and implementing rehabilitation programs. Systematic assessment of basic deficits as they change from phase to phase can inform the rehabilitation plan, and sometimes successful remediation of deficits can facilitate rehabilitation progress and admit new possibilities.

ASSESSMENT AND TREATMENT APPLICATIONS

In keeping with the principle of pervasiveness of expression, the discussion of specific assessment and treatment applications will be organized according to the levels of functioning they address. In keeping with the diathesis-stress model, the relevance of specific methods to particular phases of the disorder will be discussed within each level of functioning.

Psychophysiological Level of Functioning

It has long been known that psychophysiological abnormalities are associated with the symptomatology and etiology of schizophrenia (Dawson & Nuechterlein, 1984). For example, in the vulnerability phase, an electrodermal response that does not habituate to repeated evoking stimuli has been associated in some studies with eventual onset of schizophrenia among children at risk for the disorder (although some studies have failed to find this relationship and it remains controversial). In the acute and residual phases, patients show a pattern of either hyperarousal or hypoarousal. The former is characterized by high resting baseline levels of autonomic activity, high frequency of spontaneous sympathetic discharges (responses not associated with any observable evoking stimulus), more intense responses to stimuli, absence of habituation to repeated stimuli, infrequent electroencephalogram (EEG) alpha activity, faster than normal alpha-blocking (disruption of the alpha wave by an unexpected stimulus), and abnormal relationships between stimulus and response intensities. Hypoarousal is associated with low resting baselines and an absence of responsivity. Recently, preliminary longitudinal studies (Dawson, Nuechterlein, & Schell, 1989) suggest that changes in patients' psychophysiological activity are associated with schizophrenic relapse.

The specific role of psychophysiological arousal in schizophrenia has been the subject of much discussion, and there are probably several different roles. One theory (Storms & Broen, 1969), inspired by Hullian learning theory, includes a hypothesis that the behavioral and cognitive disorganization associated with the acute phase is the result of extremely high arousal bringing about the collapse of *response hierarchies*. Response hierarchies are the learned and conditioned patterns of overt and covert responses that give behavior its order and organization. When high arousal causes response hierarchies to collapse, behavior becomes disorganized. When arousal moderates, the hierarchies reorganize, but the new organization may be abnormal or maladaptive. Thus psychiatric symptoms can be understood as either the direct result of response hierarchy collapse or the result of maladaptive symptom-producing reorganization. An alternative (but not necessarily incompatible) theory (Dawson & Nuechterlein, 1984) holds that high arousal temporarily reduces *cognitive capacity*, the resources available for processing information in the central nervous system (CNS), and thereby produces psychological impairment.

Arousal is now thought to be an extremely complex phenomenon. The central and peripheral arousal associated with psychosis may or may not be analogous to the more moderate fluctuations of arousal characteristic of everyday life. In psychiatric disorders there may be an abnormal degree of independence between arousal subsystems that normally work in concert. In schizophrenia there may be several different types of arousal abnormality. Antipsychotic drugs clearly have an arousal-reducing effect, but it is unknown whether this effect is responsible for other cognitive and behavioral drug effects. Nevertheless, it is clear that arousal-reducing drugs and nonpharmacological techniques for reducing arousal, such as limiting sensory input (Azima & Kramer, 1956; Reitman & Cleveland, 1964), relaxation training (Zeisset, 1968), and providing a highly structured but nonarousing milieu (Carpenter, McGlashan, & Strauss, 1977), have a beneficial effect on acute and residual psychotic symptoms.

Arousal Reduction

Relaxation training has become a popular modality for a diversity of psychiatric patients, including those with severe and chronic disorders. A case supervised by the senior author illustrates the impact of a simple relaxation intervention:

The patient was a 26-year-old man with a long history of schizophrenia, psychiatric hospitalization, and failures in rehabilitative efforts. Even when optimally medicated, he was visibly tense and anxious. His arousal became more pronounced in minimally stressful social interactions. His social behavior was punctuated in such situations by frequent tantrums which sometimes included threats, physical assaults, and incoherence. He saw himself as a hopeless case, out of control of himself and his environment, a belief shared by mental health providers and relatives.

The patient was taught standard relaxation techniques. He responded unusually well and reported practicing the exercises even more frequently than prescribed. He came to see the exercises as one acceptable thing he could do to "feel good." He also readily accepted a suggestion that his success with the exercises showed he was potentially more in control than he had believed. His self-esteem and motivation to participate in rehabilitation activities improved accordingly. He began to perceive correctly that he was more effective in interpersonal interactions when not extremely aroused. His improved social performance had a significant impact on clinicians, who became more willing to work with him and tolerate his other behavioral deficits.

Desensitization techniques incorporate relaxation training and use conditioning principles to reduce fear, anxiety, or anger. The result is a reduction of psychophysiological arousal in the presence of stimuli that previously elicited those emotions. In patients with phobias and other anxiety disorders, desensitization effects are usually relatively specific: a fear and/or avoidance response in a specific stimulus situation is reduced or eliminated. In schizophrenic patients, desensitization effects may be more generalized. Slade (1972) used systematic desensitization to a series of family scenes (e.g., talking to mother, arguing with father) with a hallucinating patient and found improvements in self-rated mood measures as well as a reduction in hallucinations. Similar results have been achieved with a variety of related techniques, including in vivo desensitization (Alumbaugh, 1971), implosive therapy (Hogan, 1970), and induced anxiety (Cockshott, 1971; Friedberg, 1969).

Systematic desensitization is not always successful with patients with pervasive disorders (Serber & Nelson, 1971). Techniques that require attention and cooperation may be difficult for such patients. Attention and/or motivation may be deficient, so preliminary interventions or compensatory strategies may be necessary.

Biofeedback may prove to be a useful adjunct to arousal-reducing techniques in schizophrenics. Although biofeedback does not significantly add to the effects of relaxation training in less severely disordered patients (Budzynski, 1977), it appears to be more important with lower functioning patients (Small, Giganti, & Steinberg, 1978). A recent report (Schneider & Pope, 1982) raises the intriguing possibility that biofeedback can produce changes in patients' EEG analogous to those produced by antipsychotic drugs. Further research may confirm that specific psychophysiological abnormalities associated with the etiology of schizophrenia can be mitigated with psychological interventions.

Self-Regulation Skill Training

Recently the cross-fertilization of clinical psychophysiology and experimental psychopathology with skill-training approaches in psychiatric rehabilitation has led to the concept of training *self-regulation skills*. The idea is that vulnerability to onset or relapse of schizophrenia includes deficient abilities to manage optimally the stress of everyday life. Improved ability to manage stress, especially to self-regulate the psychophysiological functions involved in the stress response, should lead to decreased vulnerability. Also, because of reduced stress and anxiety associated with everyday events, compliance and cooperation with other rehabilitation activities should improve.

In a systematic attempt to use a stress management training package with patients with schizophrenia (Lukoff, Wallace, Liberman, & Burke, 1986), therapists combined daily yoga, exercise, meditation, positive imaging, and stress education in a "holistic health" program. After 9 weeks of treatment the treated group displayed at least as great and possibly greater improvement on a variety of measures of psychopathology as did a comparable group trained in social skills, while the social-skills group showed greater improvement in social functioning. All subjects in this study were also treated with antipsychotic medication and a "token economy."

In a recent study in our laboratory (Spaulding, Wyss, Littrell, & Sullivan, 1988) we studied the effects of a self-regulation training program on patients' biochemical stress responses. The focus was on cortisol, a hormone that is normally secreted in response to stressful situations. In normal people, systemic cortisol levels are higher under stress. Cortisol levels even discriminate between situations that are truly stressful (i.e., the person experiences negative affect and finds the situation aversive) and those that are challenging (i.e., the situation may be equally complex or dangerous, but the person experiences positive affect and exhilaration) (Dienstbier, 1989). We found that before self-regulation training, patients showed abnormally weak cortisol responses to stressful conditions. This is consistent with previous findings with very chronic schizophrenic patients. Presumably, they have lost their ability to mobilize the biochemical stress response. This could also be related to the autonomic hypoarousal often seen in such patients, which has been hypothesized to represent a self-protective reaction against hyperarousal. After 10 weeks of self-regulation training, which consisted of relaxation training, biofeedback, and a skill-training group focused on emotional functioning, the patients' high-stress cortisol levels had risen and their response profiles looked more similar to those of normal subjects (See Figure 2.1).

The results of this study suggest that the response of pervasively disordered patients to self-regulation training and related psychophysiological interventions may be more

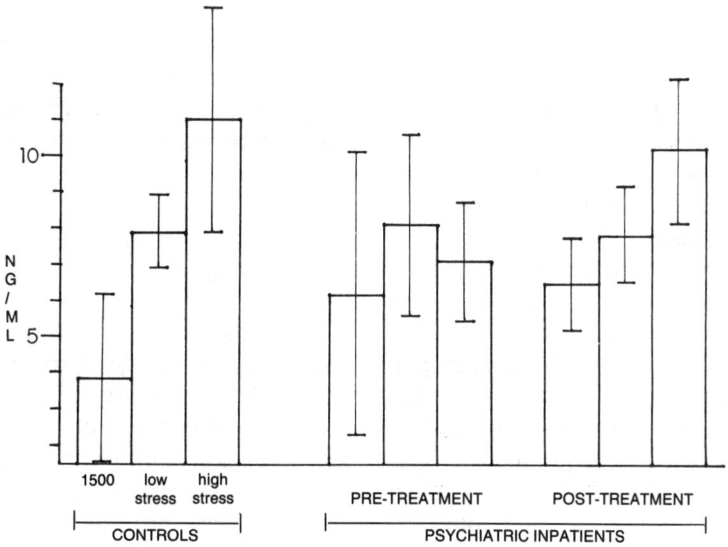

Figure 2.1. Salivary cortisol levels (ng/mL) of normal controls compared with pre- and posttreatment levels of psychiatric inpatients, collected at a standard time of day (1500 hours) and under low- and high-stress conditions. There is a significant difference between the standard and the stress samples in normals ($t = 2.4$, $p < .03$ for standard vs. low stress; $t = 3.8$, $p < .002$ for standard vs. high stress) not found in the inpatients. After treatment the inpatients' profile more resembled the controls', although the controls' high-stress level had increased ($t = 2.7$, $p < .02$).

than simply a reduction of arousal. Also, the intercorrelations between measures suggested that there are at least two different types or dimensions of self-regulation deficits. The first kind of deficit is characterized by high systemic cortisol in high-stress and low-stress situations, poor personal and social functioning, and independence from subjective distress or psychophysiological activation. The second kind of deficit is characterized by high levels of subjective distress and psychophysiological arousal, high cortisol only in high-stress situations, and independence from personal and social functioning. Further research may support the hypothesis that there are different types of self-regulation problems among pervasively disordered patients. These different deficits will probably require different kinds of compensatory skill training for optimal effect. If so, clinical and laboratory assessment of psychophysiological, cognitive, and behavioral aspects of self-regulation will be important.

Attentional Level of Functioning

Attention is one of the most difficult and changing concepts in psychology. In popular terminology, we usually think of attention as the subset of perceptions, images, and thoughts that occupy our conscious awareness at any given point in time. William James referred to the "center stage" of our conscious mind. We can shift our attention to change the particular things that are on center stage. This ability is usually taken for granted—we can hardly imagine being without it.

Kraepelin and Bleuler saw the value of applying the idea of attention to schizophrenia. Attentional disorder was one of Bleuler's "five A's" that described the cardinal features of the illness. That patients with schizophrenia have problems in attention is perhaps one of the most universally acknowledged facts of psychiatry. However, as experimental psychology evolved in the 20th century, it became more and more evident that the concept of attention as described by William James simply could not account for the complexity of phenomena observed in the laboratory. Accordingly, the applicability of the concept to schizophrenia came under scrutiny and has remained under intensive study for decades.

Today attention is understood to be a broad category of mental abilities. The boundary between attention and other psychological functions is seldom clear. In psychopathology, severe psychiatric disorders have been found to be associated with many specific abnormalities that fall into the general category of *attentional deficits*. Whether these deficits represent true attentional abnormalities or whether they are artifacts of other abnormalities of arousal, affect, perception, or thought is always debatable. Fortunately, the theoretical disputes do not have to be fully resolved before principles of attention and methods for measuring and modifying it can be applied clinically.

A number of the attentional deficits found in actively psychotic patients with schizophrenia can also be found in remitted patients, children at risk, and even in the nondisordered relatives of patients (Nuechterlein & Dawson, 1984b). It is widely hypothesized that these are at least *markers* of biopsychological vulnerabilities that predispose people to the illness, and in some cases the attentional abnormality may represent the vulnerability itself. As with psychophysiological vulnerability markers, the clinical implications of attentional abnormalities in the vulnerability phase are probably limited to prevention strategies.

In the acute phase most of the vulnerability-linked attentional abnormalities become more severe, and new abnormalities appear. The hierarchy collapse model, among others, has been used to account for this. As the acute phase abates, all the attentional deficits may not disappear or return to previous levels of severity. In the residual phase there may be attentional deficits that are as severe as those in the acute phase. Needless to say, these deficits can have a devastating effect on the patient's personal and social functioning, and on acquisition of skills in rehabilitation activities.

Modifying Attentional Functioning

Over the years there have been a number of reports of success in modifying and even normalizing some of the attentional deficits found in the acute or residual phases of schizophrenia. Originally, these were incidental observations made in the course of laboratory procedures intended to shed more light on the nature of the deficits (Kaplan, 1975; Karras, 1962; McAllister, 1970). Later, especially as interest grew in the clinical technology of cognitive behavior therapy, more explicit attempts were made to identify and correct specific attentional problems.

Meichenbaum and Cameron (1973) developed a method for strengthening attentional functioning that emphasizes use of self-instructions during task performance. Patients were taught to "talk to themselves," first vocally and later covertly, while performing attention-demanding tasks. Self-talk included instructions to keep attention focused on the tasks and to resist distraction; it also included self-reinforcing statements. Effects appeared in such diverse areas as psychiatric status, psychomotor performance, projective test performance, and interview behavior. Subsequent studies of self-instructional training with pervasively disordered patients yielded mixed results. In a review of these studies, Bentall, Higson, and Lowe (Adams, Brantley, Malatesta, & Turkat, 1981) conclude that the bulk of the evidence supports its efficacy, provided the self-instructional set is highly individualized, constructed after a careful idiographic assessment of each patient's attentional and cognitive difficulties.

Since self-instructional sets address a diversity of attentional and cognitive functions, the specific nature or role of attentional changes in self-instructional training cannot be determined. Cueing increases use of normal processes; it does not necessarily repair dysfunctional ones. Increased use of those processes may also (in the terminology of the response hierarchy model) help reorganize hierarchies in the attentional response system. Whatever the case, self-instructional training does improve patients' attentional performance and this facilitates performance at behavioral and social levels (Bentall, Higson, & Lowe, 1987).

Attentional deficits were more directly treated in a patient with schizophrenia in a case reported by Adams, Brantley, Malatesta, and Turkat (1981). In this treatment, several laboratory "distractibility" tasks from experimental psychopathology research were adapted for clinical use. The tasks were treated as exercises rather than tests, although they also yielded longitudinal measures of the patient's performance. Among other things, the patient practiced attending to recorded conversations while ignoring visual, auditory, or conversational distractions. Memory recall under distraction conditions was also practiced. The patient's performance on the laboratory measures improved with practice. At termination and 6-month follow-up, the patient also showed reduced thought disorder, increased social effectiveness, and improved mood.

In a case supervised by the senior author, the effectiveness of the above procedure was replicated:

The patient was a 25-year-old mother of one who was undergoing a stressful separation from her husband. She had been found by friends huddled in a closet with her child. She complained of hearing "the voice of the devil," and believed the devil was after the child. Before referring herself for psychiatric services, she underwent an "exorcism" at the suggestion of friends who belonged to a fundamentalist religious group. She reported later that the "exorcism" had relieved her of the belief that the devil was about to take her child, but the voices continued unabated and she still experienced extreme anxiety.

When first seen for psychiatric services, the patient met DSM-III criteria for paranoid schizophrenia. She was put on a low-dose regimen of haloperidol. She reported the drug improved her sleep cycle, blunted her anxiety, and diminished the voices somewhat. She also reported the content of the voices had changed from deprecation and threats to "just voices." However, even after the haloperidol was titrated to a point of optimal drug response, the voices were still a significant problem. She reported she could sometimes engage in stressful activities, which for her included ordinary tasks of daily living such as shopping or paying bills, but usually the voices became too intrusive and distracting for her to continue. To supplement the drug therapy an attentional training procedure was adapted from the "dichotic listening" paradigm (Wishner & Wahl, 1974) of experimental psychopathology. The patient practiced "shadowing" tape-recorded readings (repeating the recorded words aloud as they played) while a distraction tape also played. After only two sessions of the training procedure the patient was able to perform the task without error (errors on this task are "intrusions," or speaking distractor words instead of target words, and "disruptions," or losing the flow of the shadowed words). She reported she was able to ignore her hallucinated voices the same way she could ignore the distraction tape. She was instructed to use this disattention tactic whenever the voices became intrusive. The patient reported success in in vivo situations, and showed continuing improvement in her ability to perform activities that had previously been disrupted by hallucinations. Over the course of 4 months the haloperidol was gradually reduced and finally discontinued without a return of psychotic symptoms. At a 1-year follow-up she had experienced no relapses and had not required further drug therapy.

While these case reports suggest that attentional interventions have therapeutic potential, it should be noted that these anecdotal results were obtained with patients who were not chronic and who had relatively good social and personal functioning even while experiencing psychotic symptoms. A recent exploratory study in our laboratory (Stuve, 1988) tested the limits of attentional-level treatment with seven chronic institutionalized patients with poor personal and social functioning and severely deficient performance on a battery of attentional and cognitive tests (Spaulding, Garbin, & Dras, 1989). Five had a diagnosis of schizophrenia. One had an organic personality disorder, and one had been variously diagnosed as having schizophrenia, schizoaffective disorder, and atypical psychosis.

Each subject was given a preliminary performance assessment with a commercially available package of "video games" that were designed for cognitive rehabilitation of people with brain injury (Bracy, n.d.). From a set of 10 games, all of which put fairly specific demands on attentional functioning, a subset of games was chosen for each patient. The game selection criteria were that the patient could understand and engage in the game but could perform only at a deficient level. Thereafter each subject practiced the subset of games in 30-minute sessions 2 to 4 times per week, over an 8-week period. Instructions to practice for task improvement and a brief demonstration of each game were provided at the beginning of each session, but coaching and other interactions were otherwise avoided. The subjects were paid $1.00 at the end of each session regardless of their performance level.

The subjects' responses to this procedure were complex and individually unique. One subject "topped out" (reached an errorless performance level and stayed there) on one task. Six of the subjects showed improvement on various combinations of one to five tasks. There were several instances of no change, with one of the subjects showing no change on four out of five tasks. One subject improved on one task but deteriorated on three. Two subjects showed a trade-off change (one aspect of performance improved while another aspect deteriorated, such as a trade-off of speed for accuracy), each on a different task. On only one of the tasks, a simple visual scanning task, was there improvement by every subject who practiced the game. A more complex visual scanning task was too difficult for all but one of the subjects and he deteriorated with practice.

To construct a different view of the results, task improvement or deterioration was then broken down according to categories of performance; whether the change was in a hit rate, a false alarm rate, a response latency, or an error rate. Both improvement and deterioration occurred in all performance categories, with the exception of false alarm rate, where no subject deteriorated by showing more false alarms with practice. (This is complementary to the well-known laboratory finding that patients with chronic schizophrenia generally have an abnormally conservative response bias; i.e., they tend to commit fewer than normal false alarms in signal detection tasks.)

An important question in this and any other molecular-level treatment is whether improvements are general or specific. If the subjects' improvement (or deterioration) is general, one would expect high correlations between performance changes on paired tasks. If improvement is specific to one attentional process, these correlations are expected to be low. In this study, the subjects are heterogeneous with respect to specificity. Four had few significantly correlated task pairs, indicating a pattern of task-specific change. In three subjects at least half of the pairings were significantly correlated, indicating a more generalized pattern of change.

Finally, we attempted to identify possible molar-level generalization of attentional performance and response to the video game program. The subjects were rank-ordered for overall performance and for amount of improvement on the games they had practiced. Next they were rank-ordered for their scores on the Nurses Observational Scale for Inpatient Evaluation (NOSIE-30) (Honigfeld, Gillis, & Klett, 1966). The NOSIE-30 is a behavioral-observational instrument collected from ward staff on a weekly basis. It is a measure of impairments in personal and social functioning that has been used for many years in studies of severely impaired psychiatric patients. There were large and significant correlations between the NOSIE-30 and overall performance ($r = .82$; $p < .05$) and between the NOSIE-30 and amount of attentional improvement ($r = .86$; $p < .05$).

Taken together, the results of this pilot study suggest two important caveats for attentional treatment. First, the well-known heterogeneity of patients' attentional deficits extends to their response to attentional training. Each subject in this study showed a unique pattern of change. Some showed widespread improvement, some improved on some tasks but not on others, and one showed widespread deterioration. This complements the previously discussed conclusion about self-instructional training—that individualization of training may be a crucial factor. Second, there appears to be a close relationship between severity of attentional impairment, capacity to improve attentional functioning, and social-behavioral functioning. The most social-behaviorally impaired patients tend to be the ones who have the most severe attentional impairments, and they are the ones who improve the least or even deteriorate in attentional treatment.

There is clearly more research to be done on the effects of attentional treatment, especially in the most severely impaired patients. One area of inquiry that shows promise is the combination of attentional treatment with measures of electrophysiological brain activity (EEG). Clinicians have known for some time that patients with schizophrenia and other severe disorders have abnormal EEG patterns (Ellingson, 1954). Some of these abnormalities are in evoked potentials, which are the brain's response to specific laboratory stimuli (Shagass, Ornitz, Sutton, & Tueting, 1978). Recently a Japanese research group has produced evidence that abnormal evoked potentials in patients with schizophrenia can be somewhat normalized by attentional training procedures (Fukuda et al., 1989). Laboratory evaluation and training of brain activity as well as molecular attentional functioning may yield advances in cognitive therapy for schizophrenia.

Attention and Work Skills

Even if patients' attentional functioning can be modified in laboratory tasks, questions remain about whether attentional improvements can really have an impact on progress in rehabilitation. An exploratory study in our laboratory examined the role of attentional functioning in a work-skills training situation.

One aspect of attentional functioning that has particular relevance to work skills is continuous performance, the ability to maintain continuous attention and activity on a task. Individuals who cannot maintain continuous performance for more than a few minutes are poor candidates for vocational training of any kind. Continuous performance of work tasks is a relatively molar function, requiring vigilance, resistance to distraction, and repetitive use of instructions held in short-term memory. Severely disordered patients have deficits in all these specific functions and they are notoriously poor at continuous work performance. Little is known, however, about how continuous work performance might be improved through therapy that addresses primarily attentional functioning.

Nine subjects were selected for study from a pool of 136 psychiatric inpatients. The nine selected were not distinct from the others with respect to quality or severity of symptoms or chronicity, but they were the worst of the pool on a simple laboratory measure of work-related attention, the Continuous Work Performance Test (CWPT). The CWPT consists of several paper manipulation tasks: folding, cutting, stapling, unstapling, and sorting. Only one task is used in a single work session; the tasks are rotated across sessions to avoid monotony. The CWPT lasts for as long as the patient continuously performs the task (up to 30 minutes), and the score is simply the number of minutes the trainee performs the task without becoming distracted or otherwise stopping work. All nine of the patients selected for special training had CWPT scores of less than 5 minutes.

Training sessions were held three times per week, 30 minutes per session. A CWPT goal was set at the beginning of each session, with a therapist/trainer prompting maintenance of attention and providing encouragement, performance feedback, and praise for effort. The ultimate goal of the training was to achieve a CWPT score of 30 minutes for five consecutive sessions. At that point the trainee graduated to a more advanced training regimen involving increasingly complex tasks.

Of the original nine patients, seven reached the criterion for graduation and continued to progress in the subsequent stages of vocational training. One reached the criterion after 4 weeks of training but suffered a severe psychotic relapse shortly thereafter and was transferred to a more intensive care ward. The ninth patient showed a steady clinical deterioration over an 8-month period and finally had to be transferred. Despite her deteriorating condition, she did manage to increase her CWPT score from 5 to 10 minutes in 8 months.

Although there was no direct evidence that the work performance training contributed to the two relapses, this is a possibility that must always be considered in psychiatric rehabilitation. It is fairly clear that patients with schizophrenia are put at risk for psychotic relapse by some psychosocial interventions if they are not protected by an antipsychotic drug regime (Schooler & Spohn, 1982). Even for patients on drugs, relapse and clinical deterioration can occur spontaneously, even in low-stress environments. Both of the patients who relapsed in this study were taking antipsychotic drugs, but the possibility remains that they were overstimulated by the work performance training and other activities in their rehabilitation programs.

The process of the seven successful trainees is shown in Figure 2.2. Their CWPT scores are shown along with their NOSIE-30 scores so that their workshop performance can be compared with their global psychiatric status. Inspection of Figure 2.2 reveals that the seven patients all showed different longitudinal responses to the continuous work performance training. The amount of training required to reach criterion varied from 4 weeks, or 12 sessions, to 84 weeks. Five of the subjects showed a net improvement in NOSIE-30 ratings during the training period. In two of those, there was a relatively parallel, monotonic increase in both NOSIE-30 and CWPT. For these two, the hypothesis that CWPT improvement was secondary to general improvement in psychiatric status rather than a specific training effect cannot be ruled out. For subject 6, however, the work training was the only new intervention, introduced after his NOSIE-30 baseline had been stable for at least 10 months. It is more likely that for subject 6 the training produced a generalized change in clinical status. The other three subjects who had a net NOSIE-30 increase (subjects 1, 2, and 3) showed relatively steady CWPT improvement while their NOSIE-30 scores showed nonmonotonic fluctuations. For these three patients, CWPT progress does not appear to be correlated with improvement in symptoms or other areas of social and personal functioning. This is reminiscent of findings from longitudinal follow-up studies on schizophrenia (Strauss & Carpenter, 1981) that there is usually more change within various dimensions of work, symptoms, and social functioning than there is across such dimensions.

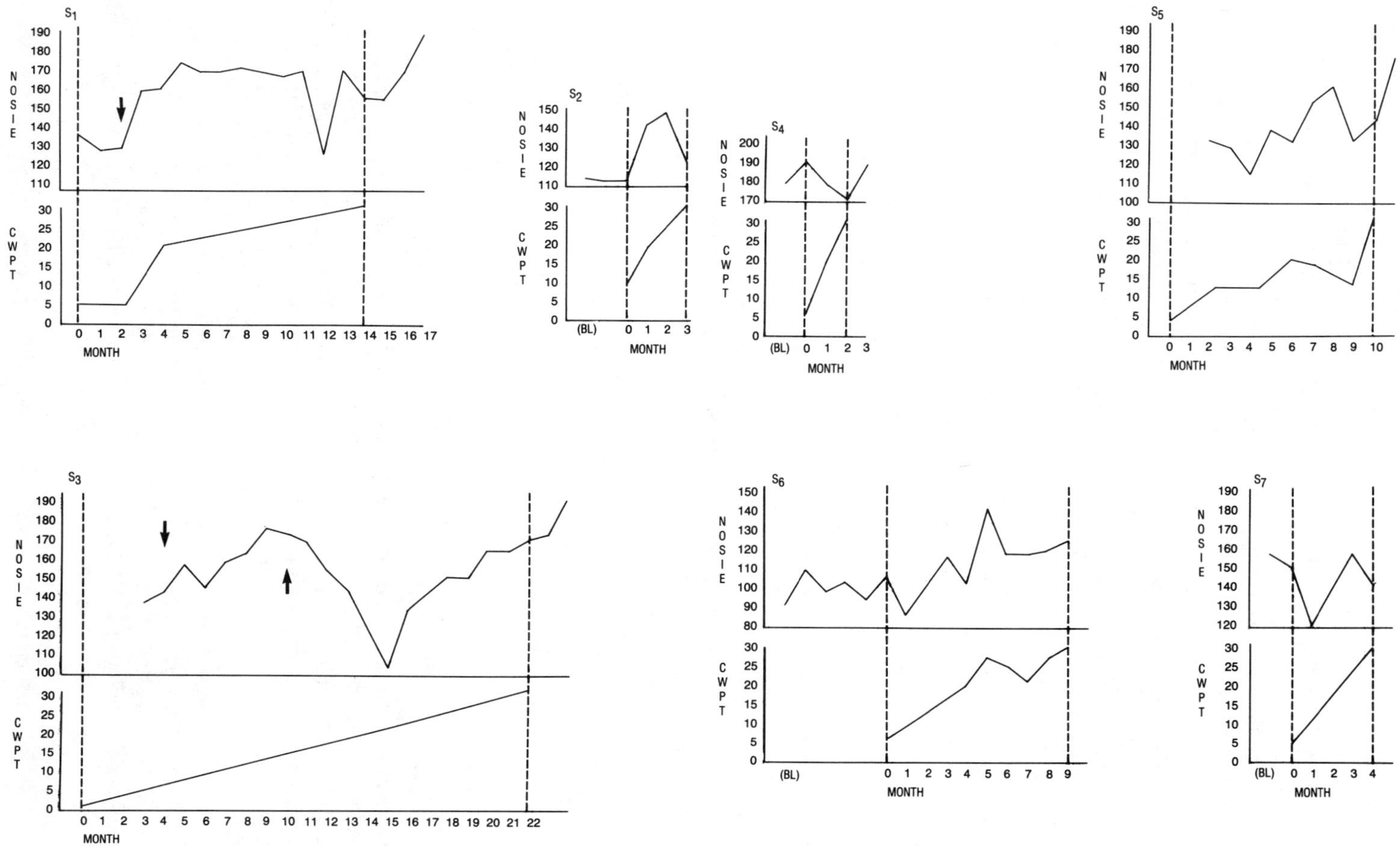

Figure 2.2. Progress of 7 patients on the Continuous Work Performance Task (CWPT), with concomitant scores on the Total Assets Scale of the Nurses Observational Scale for Inpatient Evaluation (NOSIE). Arrows indicate introduction of behavior modification program for subject 1 (S_1), neuroleptic drug titration for subject 3 (S_3).

In interpreting these results, it is important for one to consider that continuous work performance is influenced by learning and motivation as well as attention. This is evident in many studies showing that application of operant conditioning principles can produce remarkable improvement in continuous work performance in impaired populations (Rusch, Martin, & White, 1985). In fact, in the CWPT study, subject 1 showed the pronounced effect of a behavior modification program introduced after the beginning of attentional training. Token economy programming, a specific application of operant conditioning, has been validated in psychiatric rehabilitation for over 25 years (Glynn & Mueser, 1986). A number of related techniques are useful for suppressing symptoms and improving social functioning (Wong, Massel, Mosk, & Liberman, 1986). Operant conditioning is helpful for patients because they have lost their ability to respond to stimuli that are not temporally or conceptually immediate to their behavior (Salzinger, 1984). The direct, simplified and immediate behavior-consequence relationships which token economies provide compensate for this lost ability. Presumably, the ability is lost in the first place because of impairments in molecular functions that process stimuli and organize responses. Repair of these functions should therefore reduce the need for behavior-consequence immediacy and hence for operant control of behavior. More effective remediation of the psychophysiological, attentional, and cognitive dysfunctions of schizophrenia should increase the efficiency of operant conditioning for patients having schizophrenia and related disorders.

The pilot study on continuous work performance demonstrates four important points: (a) laboratory measures detected relevant psychological deficits in patients whose clinical status may not distinguish them from patients without the deficits; (b) the attentional deficits associated with continuous work performance were improved through psychosocial intervention; (c) patients showed individualized responses to treatment; and (d) improvement of the psychological deficit was associated with improvement of clinical status in some patients but not others. All of these findings point to the value of continued research and development of laboratory measurement of psychological functioning for selecting and sequencing skill-training interventions and for evaluating progress and outcome.

Attention and Social Skills

Another area of rehabilitation in which attentional deficits are particularly relevant is social-skills training (SST). As mentioned earlier, investigators in this area have expressed concern that some of schizophrenia's most significant characteristics are not addressed in skill training (Liberman, Nuechterlein, & Wallace, 1982). Attentional deficits are assumed to be limiting factors in social-skill acquisition in a group setting. In a test of the effects of an attentional training procedure on performance in a five-patient SST group, subjects' daily performance during SST sessions was assessed through observational scoring of videotapes and quizzes administered at the end of each session (Shuart, 1985). The rating scales were designed to assess observable behavior associated with task-oriented attentiveness, such as alert posture and eye contact. The quizzes assessed subjects' assimilation and retention of material presented and rehearsed in the SST session. After an initial baseline period, subjects received two sessions per week of either an attention-enhancing self-instructional training regimen similar to that developed by Meichenbaum and Cameron (1973) or a placebo procedure (semistructured conversation about the group sessions).

Attentional functioning showed a significant treatment effect. On the post–SST-session quizzes four of the five subjects showed an improvement over placebo/baseline when the attentional training was introduced. There was a significant rank order correlation ($r = .90$, $p < .05$) between absolute level of quiz performance at the end of the study and number of actual attentional training sessions (the latter was different for each subject). Observational ratings of attentional behavior made from videotapes of the SST sessions also showed significant improvement, although the effect was not strong enough to differentiate it from placebo effects.

Cognitive Level of Functioning

Cognition is a generic term that has been used to describe various aspects of psychological functioning. Sometimes it is used to describe the entire range of mental activity, but we will use it to refer specifically to the relatively molar psychological processes involved with concept formation, reasoning, and problem solving.

As with attentional deficits, cognitive deficits have long been associated with schizophrenia and other severe psychiatric disorders. Peculiarities of thought such as "magical thinking" are associated with proneness to psychosis (Fujioka & Chapman, 1984). Individuals with schizoid or schizotypal personality characteristics have difficulty with concept manipulation and problem solving (Spaulding, Garbin, & Dras, 1990). Relatives of schizophrenic patients show abnormalities on measures of thought disorder (Johnston & Holtzman, 1979). Cognitive abnormalities may therefore be vulnerabilities or prodromal symptoms. However, most of what is known about cognitive impairments is associated with the acute or residual phases, wherein many specific abnormalities have been described.

In application to psychiatric rehabilitation, it is most useful to consider first the cognitive requirements of specific rehabilitation activities, and then assess whether the patient can meet those cognitive requirements. If not, further cognitive assessment and treatment may be helpful.

Content-Oriented Interventions

Cognitive measures and interventions fall into two subcategories, process-oriented and content-oriented. Content-oriented interventions aim to change the content of key thought processes. Often they focus on attributions or beliefs about the self, such as one's ability to be successful or one's current level of personal and social functioning. Well-known techniques for modifying cognitive content have been developed to treat depression (Beck, 1976). Schizophrenic patients often have depressive syndromes and related attributional patterns, but it is not known whether they would also respond to such treatments.

Social-skills training can include cognitive content components that address more typically schizophrenic attributions. In one case study (Adams, Brantley, Malatesta, & Turkat, 1981) the patient was prone to attribute unsuccessful social interactions to persecutory intentions of other people. As the patient's social skills improved, these failures were reinterpreted as a result of formerly deficient skills. Successful interactions began to occur as a result of the improved skills, and this further reduced attributions of persecutory intent.

Patients' attributions about their own psychophysiological and perceptual experiences can be an important factor in determining how disabling those experiences are. For example, a patient with auditory hallucinations may believe that they are the result of a brain disorder, or may believe that they are the voice of Satan. The attributional difference could have a significant impact on how much the hallucinations interfere in rehabilitation activities. Johnson, Ross, and Mastria (1977) report a case in which misattributions of proprioceptive sensations produced the "delusional" belief that the patient was having sex with a supernatural "warm form." Observation revealed that the patient was generating the sensations himself. In a primarily didactic intervention, the patient was counseled to accept masturbation as normal and acceptable, and thus to understand his mysterious orgasms. This reformulation eliminated his delusional belief.

Various strategies for modifying patients' attributions are described by Valins and Nisbett (1971). Case reports of attributional modification using behavior therapy techniques for schizophrenic patients are described by Wong, Massel, Mosk, and Liberman (1986).

Self-instructional sets such as those developed by Meichenbaum and Cameron (1973) also include modification of cognitive content. In addition to cues for maintaining attention, the sets include self-reinforcing comments and reassurances against frustration when failure occurs. These are presumably elements in most people's self-instructional sets, albeit unconscious or taken for granted.

Process-Oriented Interventions

A relatively molar cognitive process is that described by the ego-psychological term *reality testing* (Bellak, Hurvich, & Gediman, 1973). Reality testing is a complex collection of cognitive activities that include sampling perceptual data, comparing it with information in memory, and devising plans to resolve discrepancies. Delusions and hallucinations can often be understood as the result of faulty reality testing, especially when perceptual data are distorted by psychophysiological or attentional impairments. Shemburg and Leventhal (1972) described several cases wherein symptoms were suppressed by procedures intended to encourage better reality testing. In one example a patient reported seeing blood flowing under the door into the therapy room. The therapist said loudly and firmly, "There is no blood there," and went to the door and put his hand on the floor, and then had the patient do the same. The patient was relieved and the therapist continued by discussing with her other ways of discriminating the real from the unreal. Specific therapeutic effects using objective laboratory measures of reality testing have not been studied, however, because precise measures of the component processes have not been developed.

Recently Johnson (1988) has developed a more highly operationalized cognitive model of reality testing, which she calls *reality monitoring*. Reality monitoring is a collection of cognitive skills by which a person selects information from memory, discriminates the sources of memory information, and uses the information to interpret ongoing events. Unlike the original concept of reality testing, the specific process of reality monitoring can be separately measured. The reality monitoring model may provide the laboratory measures prerequisite to assessment and treatment of patients who misinterpret or misattribute perceptual and memory information.

Another relatively molar cognitive process is *problem solving*, formalized by D'Zurilla and Goldfried (1974) as a five-stage process of problem recognition, analysis, solution generation, solution selection, and outcome evaluation. Therapeutic procedures to improve the problem solving of several patient populations, including chronic psychiatric patients, were developed by Spivack, Platt, and Shure (1976) and Wallace (1982). A variety of less severely disturbed patients also benefit from problem-solving therapy, which suggests that many people never completely learn this cognitive skill in the first place. In persons with schizophrenia the therapeutic effect may therefore be partially due to their learning a new cognitive skill. In addition, the highly formalized procedures of problem-solving therapy provide structure that could help reorganize a patient's collapsed cognitive response hierarchy. At any rate, outcome research is beginning to appear that suggests that a problem-solving approach enhances the effectiveness of social skills training (Wallace & Liberman, 1985).

There is probably considerable potential in quantitatively assessing performance in each stage of the problem-solving process and tailoring treatment accordingly. Instruments for clinically assessing the components of problem solving in severely disordered psychiatric patients are being developed and their properties investigated. A package of assessment and training materials for problem-solving skills in chronic psychiatric patients has been developed and partially validated by the Clinical Research Center for Schizophrenia at UCLA (Eckman, Donahoe, Liberman, & Marder, 1989; Donahoe, n.d a, n.d. b).

A more molecular cognitive process known to be deficient in many psychiatric patients is the formation of concepts. Two recent reports (Summerfield, Alphs, Wagman, Funderburk, & Strauss, 1989; Green, Ganzell, Satz, & Vaclav, 1990) suggest that psychological interventions can improve schizophrenic patients' performance on the Wisconsin Card Sorting Test (Lezak, 1983), a task that requires apprehension and manipulation of abstract concepts. Even patients whose cognitive functioning is grossly intact may have problems with concept *modulation*, the process of discarding a conceptual scheme when it is no longer useful and constructing a new one. This type of deficit appears to be particularly relevant to social cognition, as it is associated with hostility, belligerence, and persecutory beliefs (Spaulding, 1978) (although it also appears in many patients without such characteristics). It may be due to a particular style of processing information wherein new perceptual data are rejected in favor of memory data (Magaro, 1984). This tendency may in turn be a self-protective reaction to past psychotic experiences or the result of a maladaptively reorganized cognitive response hierarchy. A case study illustrates the clinical potential of modifying a concept modulation deficit in social cognition:

The patient was a 23-year-old man with chronic schizophrenia. After living for about 2 years in a supervised residential setting, he had made no rehabilitative progress, and his life had been punctuated by frequent altercations with service personnel and other patients. He had been denied admission to a residential psychosocial program because of his belligerent behavior and hostile demeanor.

The patient had been on a stable antipsychotic drug regimen for 12 months. His history indicated that drugs were necessary to control more florid psychotic symptoms. He was compliant with his drug regime and was judged to be optimally medicated. As part of a systematic assessment procedure, the patient was administered a battery of psychomotor, attentional, and cognitive tests (Spaulding, Garbin, & Dras, 1990). The patient was within normal limits in simple reaction time, backward masking performance, span of apprehension, distraction effects and redundancy effects in the reaction time task, vigilance, and size estimation. He showed an isolated deficit on a version of the Wisconsin Card Sorting Task. His difficulty was a tendency to adopt a particular scheme and perserveratively continue to use it long after the task demands had changed.

The laboratory data suggested that the patient had a specific conceptual deficit that was preventing him from using his reasonably good social repertoire in stressful situations. The nature of the deficit was hypothesized to be a tendency to schematize a situation rapidly, and then perseverate with that schema despite changes in the situation. The quality of the patient's attributional behavior in social situations suggested that he used a stereotypic conceptualization of all interactions—that the other person was trying in some way to take advantage of him. He was able to understand interactions in a better perspective when not in the situation, but this did not help when he was actively engaged.

An exercise was designed to increase his ability to reconceptualize a social situation rapidly, enabling him to reject his stereotype. For 10 therapy sessions, the patient was asked to generate alternative schematizations, first to inkblots and then to Thematic Apperception Test (TAT) cards. That is, he was instructed to generate as many different percepts (to the inkblots) or stories (to the TAT cards) as he could to a single stimulus. He found this extremely difficult, especially with the TAT cards. Gradually, however, he gained an ability to generate three to four stories for each card without bizarre or perseverative elements in subsequent stories. One particular card caused him extraordinary difficulty. He reported that it reminded him of an incident in his past that was still upsetting. Even after responding well to two or three cards, he could generate only one morbid scenario for the problem card. This experience served to demonstrate to the patient that his problem could be exacerbated by stressful situations. The conceptual exercise was accompanied by counseling about the importance of conceptual flexibility, especially in social situations.

After the end of the 10 exercise sessions, he was retested with the initial assessment battery. His previous conceptual deficit was normalized. He continued to receive regular counseling about social interactions, as he had before the exercises. In the following weeks, residential staff reported a positive change in his demeanor and attitudes. This was corroborated by an improvement in weekly NOSIE-30 ratings, particularly on the irritability subscale. At last follow-up, he had been accepted to the residential program that had previously rejected him.

In subsequent case studies in our laboratory this social apperception exercise has continued to be helpful, especially with partially recompensated paranoid schizophrenia patients whose social rehabilitation progress has stalled. An experimental study of the effects of the exercise (Schlank, 1987) suggests that it may also have more generalized benefits. The subjects were eight chronic schizophrenic patients in an intensive inpatient psychiatric rehabilitation program. Along with other rehabilitation activities, they underwent problem-solving training in a group, similar to that described by Spivack, Platt, and Shure (1976). After every problem-solving training session, each patient was given a rating on an operationalized scale of progress by the group leader. Concomitant with the problem-solving training, each patient was seen individually by a cognitive therapist. For the first 4 weeks, the cognitive therapy was restricted to discussions of the problem-solving group and its application to living situations. In the second 4 weeks, half the patients began doing the apperception exercise in their individual sessions. After 4 more weeks the second half of the patients began the apperception exercise. The problem-solving group leader was blind to which patients had started the exercise.

Figure 2.3 shows the problem-solving process ratings for the two patient subgroups over the three 4-week epochs of the study. Introduction of the apperception exercise produced a significant change in the progress rate, and by the end of the study the patients who had had 8 weeks of the exercise were doing better in problem-solving than the patients who had had only 4 weeks. The results of this study suggest that even when deficits in relatively molecular functions such as concept modulation are not specifically identified, therapeutic strengthening of such functions can benefit more molar rehabilitation-oriented activities such as problem-solving training.

Laboratory brain imaging techniques such as Positron Emission Tomography (PET) may prove helpful in guiding cognitive interventions. Recent research (Berman, Illowsky, & Weinberger, 1988) suggests that some of the cognitive operations of interest to psychopathologists are associated with identifiable patterns of metabolic activity in the brain. It is interesting that metabolic activation of the frontal lobes is associated with performance of conceptual tasks such as the Wisconsin Card Sorting Test, and patients who have difficulty with such tasks also tend to show abnormal patterns of brain activation. PET images may help predict which patients will benefit from cognitive interventions or help select among different treatment options.

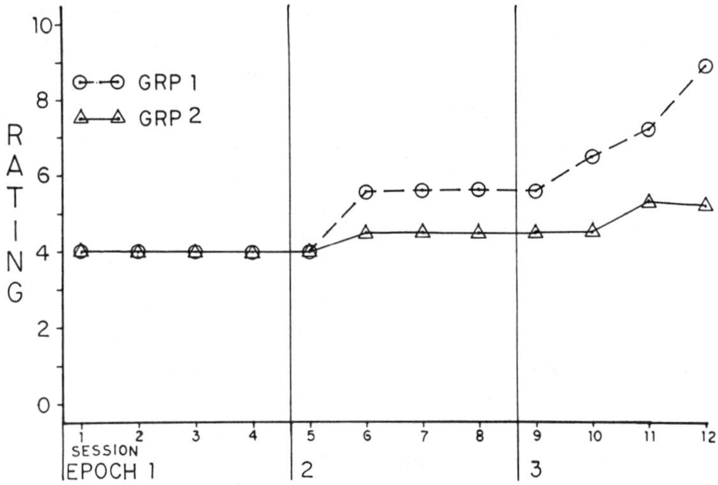

Figure 2.3. Performance of patients in a cognitive problem-solving training group, as measured by therapist's rating. After a baseline period (epoch 1), an apperception exercise was introduced in epoch 2 for Group (GRP) 1, and epoch 3 for Group 2. A repeated measures analysis of variance test yielded a significant interaction for groups by sessions within epochs, indicating that the effect of the exercise was detectable within four sessions.

INTEGRATION STRATEGIES

For optimal impact, assessment and treatment of basic psychological processes should be integrated with a patient's overall rehabilitation program. Moreover, these psychological considerations should be combined with specific skill-training interventions. Three general strategies have evolved for this: the *incorporation strategy*, the *targeted group treatment strategy*, and the *individualized treatment strategy*.

Incorporation Strategy

Certain principles that emerge from the cross-fertilization of rehabilitation with experimental psychopathology can be incorporated into conventional skill-training methods. This makes the methods and the skill trainers more sensitive and responsive to patients' deficient basic psychological processes. This strategy has been pursued most successfully by Robert Liberman and his colleagues at the UCLA Clinical Research Center for Schizophrenia and Psychiatric Rehabilitation. Their guidelines (Liberman, Nuechterlein, & Wallace, 1982) for optimizing the skill-training setting are as follows:

- keep the training setting uncluttered and devoid of distracting stimuli
- use postgraphic charts for clear and simple visual cueing for cognitive strategies
- use mild censure contingent on inappropriate responding as well as praise for appropriate responding
- conduct task analysis and break down tasks into simple steps
- decrease novelty by many repetitions before moving to new material or scenes

Also, even casual observation of skill trainers trained in the UCLA model reveals that in the course of conducting training, care is always taken to anticipate and compensate for possible difficulties in attention and cognition.

The main advantage of the incorporation strategy is that it makes use of existent skill-training technology. It is limited, however, because of the heterogeneity of patients' deficits. Even the most experienced and highly trained skill trainer cannot be expected to assess and respond to every patient's unique constellation of deficits in the course of group sessions. The incorporation strategy should be part of every therapist's repertoire, but it cannot be expected to solve completely the problem of basic psychological deficits.

Targeted Group Treatment Strategy

Another strategy is to develop skill-training modalities that target molecular psychological deficits the same way more molar skill deficits are targeted. The development of the UCLA Interpersonal Problem Solving Module (Donahoe, n.d. a, n.d. b; Eckman, Donahoe, Liberman, & Marder, 1989), which integrates cognitive problem solving with social-skill training, is an example. However, questions remain about whether the more molecular processes prerequisite to social functioning can be efficiently addressed by the interpersonal problem-solving approach (Bellak, Morrison, & Mueser, 1989). A group-training modality that systematically addresses even more molecular psychological deficits has been developed by Brenner and his colleagues at the University of Bern (Brenner, 1987). A variety of attentional and cognitive processes are addressed and quickly integrated with more molar social-interactional skills. Outcome research on the Bern modality indicates that it enhances the effectiveness of social-skill training; however, there is still much to be learned about its specific effects on more molecular functioning and the generalization of its effects to rehabilitation progress. It is now in use in Europe and will probably generate considerable interest in the United States.

Individualized Treatment Strategy

Direct rehearsal of specific processes targeted by laboratory tests is the most individualized approach to treating basic psychological deficits. This approach has the greatest potential for addressing the heterogeneity of patients' problems, but it also would be the most expensive. Also, although outcome studies do suggest that molecular deficits can be modified this way, it is still questionable whether such changes generalize to more molar abilities. Nevertheless, this strategy may be the last resort for patients who do not respond to less individualized approaches. A case treated in our laboratory provides an illustration:

The patient was a 30-year-old male who had spent 7 of his last 10 years in inpatient settings. He had had a relatively normal childhood and adolescence. Shortly after his high school graduation his father died, and this was followed by a rapid loss of the patient's personal and social functioning. He lost his job and refused to seek new employment. His behavior became bizarre and occasionally assaultive. He was repeatedly hospitalized and was diagnosed as having schizophrenia or bipolar disorder at different times. Over the years his social functioning continued to deteriorate and he was institutionalized.

When first seen in our laboratory, his case had just been reviewed with the conclusion that he was unlikely to respond to further treatment and should be transferred to long-term custodial care. Some of the primary symptoms of schizophrenia that had been described during earlier hospitalizations were still in evidence. In interview he showed a distinct tendency to give rambling, tangential, and sometimes incoherent answers to questions. He reported being troubled often by "voices" saying violent things, although he now recognized that these were hallucinations. He expressed a desire to leave the hospital, but could not describe how his behavioral functioning would have to change to make that possible. He attributed most of his problems to the insensitivity or hostility of others. For the past year he had been stably medicated to suppress his hallucinations, thought disorder, and behavioral explosiveness.

The first problem to be addressed was the patient's belligerent noncompliance. He refused to participate in rehabilitation activities or diagnostic testing. If pushed, he quickly became threatening. He was the "ward bully," intimidating other patients for money, cigarettes, and favors. A token economy program was started which selectively reinforced participation in recreational and skill-training activities and punished belligerence and inappropriate social behavior. A "time out from reinforcement" program was instituted for threatening or assaultive behavior. Over a 12-month period his compliance and attendance in groups gradually increased and his problem behaviors decreased. However, he was clearly making no progress in skill acquisition, as reflected in very poor progress ratings from his group therapists. Also, his social behavior was still punctuated by occasional tantrums.

A neuropsychological evaluation indicated cognitive dysfunctions somewhat localized to frontal and right parietotemporal brain areas. A neurological examination noted an asymmetrical gait and a positive Babinski reflex in the left foot, but no other signs of CNS neuropathy. An EEG study and a brain CT scan were negative.

It was hypothesized that the patient's functioning was constrained by a cluster of psychological deficits in span of apprehension, sequential organization and executive functioning, nonverbal short-term memory, and affect regulation. Over the course of the next year a number of cognitive and attentional exercises were prescribed to target the cognitive and attentional deficits. Most of the exercises made use of special education materials designed for working with people with learning disabilities and attention deficit disorder. The patient gradually improved on the exercise tasks. Concomitantly, his performance in skill training began to improve, and his residual behavior problems finally extinguished.

Relaxation training and self-regulation training, which had previously been ineffective, began to produce improvements in his affective self-regulation. He graduated from a problem-solving group in which he had failed twice before. His self-attributions and aspirations also changed. Whereas he had formerly seen himself as a hopeless case who should not be pushed to gain a more independent level of functioning, he became involved in his discharge plan and anticipated a better life outside the hospital. At 10 months after the start of the cognitive and attentional treatment he was retested. Although he still had areas of significant impairment, all the areas that had been specifically targeted showed at least minimal improvement. Almost 2 years after the start of his rehabilitation program he was accepted into a community residential facility. By 1 year after hospital discharge, he was continuing to consolidate his functional improvement.

CONCLUSIONS

Ultimately the best strategy for treating basic psychological dysfunctions in the context of psychiatric rehabilitation will be one that takes advantage of each approach as needed for specific subpopulations. Not all patients need cognitive treatment to benefit from skill training. Some may benefit from a generic group-format cognitive treatment while others may need a more individualized approach.

The problem thus becomes one of assembling a treatment repertoire with varying levels of individualization and designing an assessment procedure capable of determining the required focus and level for individual patients. Large-scale outcome studies will be required to identify the patient characteristics that predict the best, most reliable differential treatment indications. So far the available data suggest that the best predictions will be made by including measures of psychophysiological, attentional, cognitive, and social-behavioral levels of functioning. Until predictive formulas are available, psychological-level treatment in rehabilitation will have to be a hypothetico-deductive process wherein assessments and treatment prescriptions are treated as operational hypotheses to be tested by treatment outcome data in N-of-1 experiments. Given the promise of the research findings to date, it seems reasonable to proceed with carefully controlled case-by-case interventions, and to pursue larger-scale studies to validate the efficacy of psychological interventions in league with judicious pharmacotherapy and structured psychosocial rehabilitation.

REFERENCES

Adams, H., Brantley, P., Malatesta, V., & Turkat, I. (1981). Modification of cognitive processes: A case study of schizophrenia. *Journal of Consulting and Clinical Psychology, 49*, 460–464.

Adams, H., Doster, J., & Calhoun, K. (1977). A psychologically based system of response classifications. In A. Ciminero, H. Adams, & K. Calhoun (Eds.), *Handbook of behavioral assessment* (pp. 47–78). New York: Wiley.

Alumbaugh, R. (1971). Use of behavior modification techniques towards reduction of hallucinatory behavior: A case study. *Psychological Reports, 21*, 415–417.

Azima, H., & Kramer, F. (1956). Effects of partial isolation in mentally disturbed individuals. *Diseases of the Nervous System, 17*, 117–122.

Beck, A. (1976). *Cognitive therapy and the emotional disorders*. New York: International Universities Press.

Bentall, R., Higson, P., & Lowe, C. (1987). Teaching self-instructions to chronic schizophrenic patients: Efficacy and generalization. *Behavioural Psychotherapy, 15*, 58–76.

Berman, K., Illowsky, B., & Weinberger, D. (1988). Physiological dysfunction of dorsolateral prefrontal cortex in schizophrenia: IV. Further evidence for regional and behavioral specificity. *Archives of General Psychiatry, 45*, 616–622.

Bellak, A., Morrison, R., & Mueser, K. (1989). Social problem solving in schizophrenia. *Schizophrenia Bulletin, 15*, 101–116.

Bellak, L., Hurvich, M., & Gediman, H. (1973). *Ego functions in schizophrenics, neurotics and normals*. New York: Wiley.

Bracy, O. (n.d.). A home-based cognitive rehabilitation program. Unpublished manuscript available from Psychological Soft-ware Services, Indianapolis, Indiana.

Brenner, H. (1987). On the importance of cognitive disorders in treatment and rehabilitation. In J. Strauss, W. Baker, & H. Brenner (Eds.), *Psychosocial treatment of schizophrenia*. Toronto: Hans Haber.

Budzynski, T. (1977). Clinical implications of EMG training. In G. Schwartz, & J. Beatty (Eds.), *Biofeedback: theory and research* (pp. 433–448). New York: Academic Press.

Carpenter, W., McGlashan, T., & Strauss, J. (1977). The treatment of acute schizophrenia without drugs. *American Journal of Psychiatry, 134*, 14–20.

Cockshott, J. (1971). The effects of induced anxiety with chronic hospitalized schizophrenics. *Dissertation Abstracts International, 32*, 3631.

Cromwell, R., & Spaulding, W. (1978). How schizophrenics handle information. In W. Fann, I. Karacan, A. Pokorny, & R. Williams (Eds.), *Phenomenology and treatment of schizophrenia* (pp. 127–162). New York: Spectrum.

Dawson, M., & Nuechterlein, K. (1984). Psychophysiological dysfunctions in the development and course of schizophrenic disorders. *Schizophrenia Bulletin, 10*, 204–232.

Dawson, M., Nuechterlein, K., & Schell, A. (1989). *Electrodermal measures in schizophrenia: Episode or vulnerability indicators?* Paper presented at International Congress on Schizophrenia Research, San Diego, CA.

Dienstbier, R. (1989). Arousal and physiological toughness: Implications for mental and physical health. *Psychological Review, 96*, 84–100.

Donahoe, C. P. (n.d.). *Assessment Instrument for Problem-Solving Skills*. (Unpublished). Available from the author at Audie L. Murphy Memorial Veterans Hospital, Psychology Service (116B), 7400 Merton Minter Blvd., San Antonio, TX 78284.

Donahoe, C. P. (n.d.). *The Social Problem-Solving Skills Module*. (Unpublished). Available from the author at Audie L. Murphy Memorial Veterans Hospital, Psychology Service (116B), 7400 Merton Minter Blvd., San Antonio, TX 78284.

D'Zurilla, T., & Goldfried, M. (1974). Problem solving and behavior modification. *Journal of Abnormal Psychology, 78*, 107–126.

Eckman, T., Donahoe, C. P., Liberman, R., &

Marder, S. (1989). *Training solving skills in schizophrenic outpatients.* Paper presented at the annual meeting of the American Psychiatric Association, San Francisco, May.

Ellingson, R. (1954). The incidence of EEG abnormality among patients with mental disorders of apparently nonorganic origin: A review. *American Journal of Psychiatry, 111,* 263–275.

Friedberg, F. (1969). The effects of induced anxiety under verbal and nonverbal conditions on withdrawal in chronic hospitalized schizophrenics. *Dissertation Abstracts International, 30*(1-B), 379–380.

Fujioka, T., & Chapman, L. (1984). Comparison of the 2–7–8 MMPI profile and the Perceptual Aberration—Magical Ideation Scale in identifying hypothetically psychosis-prone college students. *Journal of Consulting and Clinical Psychology, 52,* 458–467.

Fukuda, M., Niwa, S., Hiramatsu, K., Saitoh, O., Kameyama, T., Nakagone, K., Iwanami, A., & Sasaki, T. (1989). *Psychological intervention can partly alter P-300 amplitude abnormalities in schizophrenics.* Paper presented at the annual meeting of the Japanese Biological Psychiatry Society, March, Tokyo.

Glynn, S., & Mueser, K. (1986). Social learning for chronic mental patients. *Schizophrenia Bulletin, 12*(4), 648–668.

Green, M., Ganzell, S., Satz, P., & Vaclav, J. (1990). Teaching the Wisconsin Card Sort to schizophrenic patients. *Archives of General Psychiatry, 47,* 91–92.

Herz, M. (1986). Prodromal symptoms and prevention of relapse in schizophrenia. *Journal of Clinical Psychiatry, 46*(11), Sect. 2, 22–25.

Hogan, R. (1970). Implosive therapy in the short term treatment of psychotics. *Psychotherapy Theory Research Practice, 3,* 25–32.

Honigfeld, G., Gillis, R., & Klett, J. (1966). NOSIE-30: A treatment-sensitive ward behavior scale. *Psychological Reports, 19,* 180–182.

Johnson, M. (1988). Discriminating the origin of information. In T. Oltmanns, & B. Maher (Eds.), *Delusional beliefs: Interdisciplinary perspectives.* New York: Wiley.

Johnson, M., & Raye, C. (1981). Reality monitoring. *Psychological Review, 88*(1), 67–85.

Johnson, W., Ross, J., & Mastria, M. (1977). Delusional behavior: An attributional analysis of development and modification. *Journal of Abnormal Psychology, 86,* 421–426.

Johnston, M., & Holtzman, P. (1979). *Assessing schizophrenic thinking: A clinical and research instrument for measuring thought disorder.* San Francisco: Jossey-Bass.

Kaplan, R. (1975). *The crossover phenomenon: Three studies of the effect of training and information on process schizophrenic reaction time* (Doctoral dissertation, University of Waterloo, Waterloo, Ontario, Canada).

Karras, A. (1962). The effects of reinforcement and arousal on the psychomotor performance of chronic schizophrenics. *Journal of Abnormal and Social Psychology, 65,* 104–111.

Kielhofner, G., Burke, J., & Igi, C. (1982). A model of human occupation: Part 4. Assessment and intervention. *American Journal of Occupational Therapy, 34,* 777–788.

Lezak, M. (1983). *Neuropsychological assessment* (2nd ed.). New York: Oxford University Press.

Liberman, R., & Anthony, W. (1986). The practice of psychiatric rehabilitation: Historical, conceptual and research base. *Schizophrenia Bulletin, 12*(4), 542–559.

Liberman, R., Nuechterlein, K., & Wallace, C. (1982). Social skills training and the nature of schizophrenia. In J. Curran & P. Monti (Eds.), *Social skills training: A practical handbook for assessment and treatment.* New York: Guilford.

Lukoff, D., Wallace, C., Liberman, R., & Burke, K. (1986). A holistic program for chronic schizophrenic patients. *Schizophrenia Bulletin, 12,* 274–282.

Magaro, P. (1984). Psychosis and schizophrenia. In W. Spaulding & J. Cole (Eds.), *The Nebraska Symposium on Motivation: Vol. 31. Theories of psychosis and schizophrenia.* Lincoln, NE: University of Nebraska Press.

McAllister, L. (1970). Modification of performance on the Rod-and-Frame Test through token reinforcement procedures. *Journal of Abnormal Psychology, 75,* 124–130.

Meehl, P. (1962). Schizotaxia, schizotypy and schizophrenia. *American Psychologist, 17,* 827–838.

Meichenbaum, D., & Cameron, R. (1973). Training schizophrenics to talk to themselves: A means of developing self controls. *Behavior Therapy, 4,* 515–534.

Nuechterlein, K., & Dawson, M. (1984a). A heuristic vulnerability/stress model of schizophrenic episodes. *Schizophrenia Bulletin, 10,* 300–312.

Nuechterlein, K., & Dawson, M. (1984b). Information processing and attentional functioning in the developmental course of schizophrenic disorders. *Schizophrenia Bulletin, 10*, 160–203.

Reitman, E., & Cleveland, S. (1964). Changes in body image following sensory deprivation in schizophrenic and control groups. *Journal of Abnormal and Social Psychology, 68*, 168–176.

Rusch, F., Martin, J., & White, M. (1985). Competitive employment: Teaching mentally retarded employees to maintain their work behavior. *Education & Training of the Mentally Retarded, 20*(3), 182–189.

Salzinger, K. (1984). The immediacy hypothesis in a theory of schizophrenia. In W. Spaulding, & J. Cole. *The Nebraska Symposium on Motivation: Vol. 28. Theories of schizophrenia and psychosis*. Lincoln: University of Nebraska Press.

Scheflin, A. (1981). *Levels of schizophrenia*. New York: Wiley.

Schlank, A. (1987). *Effects of a conceptual processing exercise on progress in interpersonal problem solving training* (Master's thesis, University of Nebraska-Lincoln, Lincoln NE).

Schneider, S., & Pope, A. (1982). Neuroleptic-like electroencephalographic changes in schizophrenics through biofeedback. *Biofeedback and Self-Regulation, 7*(4), 479–490.

Schooler, N., & Spohn, H. (1982). Social dysfunction and treatment failure in schizophrenia. *Schizophrenia Bulletin, 8*(1), 85–98.

Serber, M., & Nelson, P. (1971). The ineffectiveness of desensitization and assertive training in hospitalized schizophrenics. *Journal of Behavior Therapy and Experimental Psychiatry, 2*, 107–109.

Shagass, C., Ornitz, E., Sutton, S., & Tueting, P. (1978). Event-related potentials and psychopathology. In E. Callaway, P. Tueting, & S. Koslow (Eds.), *Event-related brain potentials in man* (pp. 443-496). New York: Academic Press.

Shemburg, K., & Leventhal, D. (1972). Outpatient treatment of schizophrenic students in a university clinic. *Bulletin of the Menninger Clinic, 36*, 617–640.

Shuart, W. (1985). Effects of self-instructional training on performance in a social skills training group (Doctoral dissertation, University of Nebraska-Lincoln, Lincoln NE).

Slade, P. (1972). The effects of systematic desensitization on auditory hallucinations. *Behavior Research and Therapy, 10*, 85–91.

Small, M., Giganti, M., & Steinberg, D. (1978). A comparison of thermal biofeedback and relaxation training within a behavior management program. *American Journal of Clinical Biofeedback, 1*, 68–70.

Spaulding, W. (1978). The relationships of some information processing factors to severely disturbed behaviors. *Journal of Nervous and Mental Disease, 166*, 417–428.

Spaulding, W. (1986). Assessment of adult-onset pervasive behavior disorders. In A. Ciminero, H. Adams, & F. Calhoun (Eds.), *Handbook of behavioral assessment* (2nd ed.). New York: Wiley.

Spaulding, W., Garbin, C., & Dras, S. (1989). Cognitive functioning in chronic psychiatric patients and schizotypal college students. *Journal of Nervous and Mental Disease, 177*(12), 717–728.

Spaulding, W., Wyss, H., Littrell, R., & Sullivan, M. (1988). *Explorations in training self-regulation skills in chronic psychiatric patients*. Paper presented at the World Congress of Behaviour Therapy, Edinburgh, U.K., September.

Spivack, G., Platt, S., & Shure, M. (1976). *The problem solving approach to adjustment*. San Francisco: Jossey-Bass.

Spohn, H., Lacoursiere, R., Thompson, K., & Coyne, L. (1977). Phenothiazine effects on psychological and psychophysiological dysfunction in chronic schizophrenics. *Archives of General Psychiatry, 34*, 633–644.

Storms, L., & Broen, W. (1969). A theory of schizophrenic behavioral disorganization. *Archives of General Psychiatry, 20*, 129–144.

Strauss, J., & Carpenter, W. (1981). *Schizophrenia*. New York: Plenum Press.

Stuve, P. (1988). *Acquisition of attentional skills in chronic psychiatric patients: An exploration of video game therapy* (Master's thesis, University of Nebraska-Lincoln, Lincoln NE).

Summerfield, A., Alphs, L., Wagman, A., Funderburk, E., & Strauss, J. (1989). *Monetary reinforcement reduces perseverative errors in patients with schizophrenia*. Paper presented at International Congress on Schizophrenia Research. San Diego, CA.

Valins, S., & Nisbett, R. (1971). Attributional processes in the development and treatment of emotional disorders. In E. Jones, D. Kanouse,

H. Kelley, R. Nisbett, S. Calins, & B. Weiner (Eds.), *Attribution: Perceiving the causes of behavior* (pp. 137–150). Morristown, NJ: General Learning Press.

Wallace, C. (1982). The social skills training project of the Mental Health Clinical Research Center for the Study of Schizophrenia. In J. Curran & P. Monti (Eds.), *Social skill training: A practical handbook for assessment and treatment* (pp. 57–89). New York: Guilford.

Wallace, C., & Liberman, R. (1985). Social skills training for patients with schizophrenia: A controlled clinical trial. *Psychiatric Research, 15*, 239–247.

Wishner, J., & Wahl, O. (1974). Dichotic listening in schizophrenia. *Journal of Consulting and Clinical Psychology, 42*, 460–464.

Wong, S., Massel, H., Mosk, M., & Liberman, R. (1986). Behavioral approaches to the treatment of schizophrenia. In G. Burrows, T. Norman, & G. Rubenstein (Eds.), *Handbook of studies on schizophrenia*, part 2. New York: Elsevier.

Zeisset, R. (1968). Desensitization and relaxation in the modification of psychiatric patients' interview behavior. *Journal of Abnormal Psychology, 73*, 18–24.

Zubin, J., & Spring, B. (1977). Vulnerability: A new view of schizophrenia. *Journal of Abnormal Psychology, 86*, 103–126.

CHAPTER 3

INTEGRATING SYMPTOM ASSESSMENT INTO PSYCHIATRIC REHABILITATION

David Lukoff
Joseph Ventura
Keith Nuechterlein
Robert Paul Liberman

The careful and reliable elicitation, rating, and monitoring of psychopathology are essential to rehabilitation efforts with psychotically disordered patients. The initial assessment of symptomatology, at time of intake or first contact, establishes a baseline understanding of the patient and allows the rehabilitation team to make informed treatment decisions that take into account the patient's clinical condition. For example, patients can be screened for high levels of symptomatology that might preclude assignment to rehabilitation programs with high levels of functional demands or social stimulation. After a baseline has been established, ongoing monitoring of psychopathology may permit identification of prodromal symptoms that may enable patients and their treatment teams to prevent florid relapses and sustain a rehabilitative trajectory. Thus, as a screening tool, an aid to clinical decision making, and for the prevention of relapses, the regular assessment of symptomatology can improve the effectiveness of rehabilitation interventions.

The process by which psychopathology develops in an individual is not well understood, but it is thought to be the outcome of a complex interaction among genetic, vulnerability, stressor, protective, and potentiator factors that operate within an individual as well as in the individual's environment. Stressful life changes in any of these areas, such as the death of a patient's friend or an overstimulating work environment, will affect the occurrence and severity of symptoms. On the other hand, participation in a work-training program that increases the patient's coping skills can operate as a protective factor in the prevention of exacerbations of symptomatology. Symptoms interact with social and occupational functioning in a reciprocal way; that is, psychopathology can affect and be affected by events in the social and work spheres. Symptoms, when severe, may also become stressors, in that their emergence can frighten relatives, coworkers, and often the patients themselves. The interaction of stress, vulnerability, coping, and competence factors is a dynamic process, and therefore the symptom picture of patients varies over time (Liberman, 1986).

Accurate diagnosis of patients is based on the reliable assessment of psychopathology and can be a prerequisite to the choice of an appropriate rehabilitation program. For example, remediation of social withdrawal would be different for a patient with major depression than for a patient with schizophrenia. Cognitive therapy and antidepressant medication aimed at reducing the patient's negative thinking style and irrational beliefs could be helpful in reducing withdrawal if it were secondary to depression, but would not be effective if the withdrawal were the result of delusions of persecution. This chapter focuses on specific techniques for assessing psychopathology that have been developed for use with patients with diagnoses of *Diagnostic and Statistical Manual of Mental Disorders*, 3rd ed., revised (DSM-III-R) psychotic disorders—the majority of the chronically ill (Lukoff & Ventura, 1988). Assessment of psychopathology is a prelude to diagnosis but requires, in addition, a knowledge of the diagnostic criteria and procedures outlined in the DSM-III-R.

In the lexicon of the rehabilitation practitioner, the array of characteristic symptoms of psychiatric disorder and the syndromal diagnosis represent the *impairments* of the patient. Interview-based rating instruments have been developed that are reliable for detecting and monitoring the symptoms of psychiatric patients undergoing rehabilitation. Three such instruments, which can be used by rehabilitation professionals, are reviewed in this chapter: the Brief Psychiatric Rating Scale (BPRS) (Overall & Gorham, 1962), which was designed to assess a wide range of psychopathology including the *positive symptoms* of psychotic disorders (e.g., hallucinations, delusions, and conceptual disorganization); the Schedule for the Assessment of Negative Symptoms (Andreasen, 1982), which was created to assess *negative symptoms* (e.g., affective blunting, amotivation); and Target Symptom Scale (May, 1980).

SYMPTOM MONITORING AS AN AID TO CLINICAL DECISION MAKING

Routine clinical decision making can be aided by the regular assessment of psychopathology as described in vignettes that are based on cases from the University of California at Los Angeles (UCLA) Aftercare Clinic where schizophrenic patients are routinely assessed with the BPRS every 2 weeks. These scores are graphed and regularly consulted in making clinical decisions.

High levels of psychotic symptomatology can interfere with a patient's productive involvement and progress in rehabilitation (Liberman & Foy, 1983; Wing, 1978). Thus, the intensive rehabilitation of highly symptomatic patients is best deferred until their symptoms are more stabilized or in remission; alternatively, a less intense program should be developed for them. However, the mere presence of psychotic symptoms does not preclude treatment. For patients with psychotic disorders, screening criteria for rehabilitation programs must allow for the persisting psychotic symptoms that many patients have even in their best clinical state. Studies have shown that patients with serious mental illnesses such as schizophrenia often have persisting symptoms when they are discharged from the hospital (Brown, Birley, & Wing, 1972; Vaughn, Snyder, Jones, Freeman, & Falloon, 1984). Longitudinal studies have demonstrated that perhaps 50% of schizophrenic patients do not attain a stable clinical remission (Ciompi, 1980). Thus, patients must be assessed not only for the *presence* of symptoms, but also the *intensity* and *stability* of symptoms. When patients with moderately high levels of psychopathology are being rehabilitated, the training sessions should be shorter and the treatment more structured, behavioral, and focused on short-term goals.

Case Examples

Case 1: Symptom Severity and Readiness for Rehabilitation

Two patients were referred to the horticulture program at a time when there was only one opening. The staff noted that Jill had a better work history but was concerned that she had been discharged from the hospital only 1 week earlier. John was younger, had no significant work history, and had been living at home for the previous 2 years following the onset of schizophrenia. The staff arranged interviews with both Jill and John to assess motivation and psychopathology using the BPRS. At the next team meeting, the interviewer reported that both seemed highly motivated, but that Jill was still hearing intrusive voices throughout the day. John also had hallucinations but they occurred only once or twice a week. The staff decided that Jill would be very unlikely to meet the demands for the sustained cognitive and attentional functioning and task involvement required by the program. Therefore, they selected John for the opening and opted to conduct a follow-up interview with Jill to determine if her clinical condition had improved to the point where she, too, could participate in the horticulture program.

Case 2: Negative Symptoms

When symptom reduction is a goal of the rehabilitation intervention, monitoring the targeted symptoms permits evaluation of the effectiveness of the patient's program. When a patient presents with high levels of positive or negative symptoms, vocational rehabilitation must involve interventions to reduce them. For example, the negative symptom of amotivation can adversely affect a patient's ability and energy for participation in training. Psychosocial treatments for negative symptoms, such as token economy (Glynn & Mueser, 1986), have been developed and validated. Sometimes when patients are being taught new vocational or social skills, increases in anxiety occur. In addition to interfering with the training process, anxiety can trigger hallucinations and even full relapses in schizophrenic patients. Relaxation training can be provided in the rehabilitation milieu to reduce anxiety as in the second example below.

John was in a Job Finding Club and was motivated to obtain a job as a telephone receptionist. For the previous 9 months, his training had consisted of answering phones at the Mental Health Center that housed the Job Club. Despite his experience and written recommendations, he had not been offered a job following 6 job interviews. The rehabilitation counselor running the Job Club brought in a video camera and recorder to tape a role-played job interview with John. The video made both John and the counselor aware that while John gave good verbal answers to the usual employment interview questions, he showed almost no expressive hand and facial gestures. These are negative symptoms called "unchanging facial expression" and "paucity of expressive gestures" on the Schedule for the Assessment of Negative Symptoms (SANS).

Employers generally expect some enthusiasm from a prospective employee, but John was showing none. The counselor arranged for John to participate in a social-skills training group available at the Mental Health Center where he could work on improving his expressiveness. In addition, the counselor arranged to monitor John's progress on reducing his negative symptoms by rating the two SANS items—"unchanging facial expression" and "paucity of expressive gestures"—in weekly role-played job interviews at the Job Club. These two symptoms became the target symptoms for regular assessment. The counselor rated John a 1 on the 1–5 scale for the first video interview. John agreed to remain in the social-skills training group until he could achieve a rating of 4 on the scale 2 weeks in a row or until he landed a job. John continued going to interviews and sharing his self-evaluations of his interviewing skills, particularly his expressiveness, with the members of the Job Club. Five weeks later he was offered a job. Although John had received a rating of only 3 in the role-played interview at that point, he told the rehabilitation counselor that the training in expressiveness had already helped him both in job interviews and in other social situations.

Case 3: Social Anxiety

While attending a sheltered workshop as part of his first phase of vocational rehabilitation, Bill was observed to be highly anxious. While at the workshop his hands trembled to the degree that it interfered with his ability to complete the task demands for many of the workshop jobs. Yet, outside the workshop setting, his hands did not tremble. As Bill became increasingly frustrated over his difficulties in completing the job tasks, he was observed to become more tense and agitated. Rather than refer Bill for new medications, his counselor decided to train him to use relaxation techniques. The rehabilitation counselor set up a monitoring procedure to determine whether the relaxation training was helping Bill to reduce his anxiety at the workshop. The counselor asked Bill to monitor his anxiety daily at home each night and again in the morning at the mid-morning break at the sheltered workshop. The counselor also made weekly interview assessments of the target symptom of anxiety. Bill reported that he enjoyed the sessions and was learning to relax both his body and mind. He discovered that his longstanding habit of staying up late watching television and then drinking three cups of coffee in the morning contributed to his feelings of anxiety. As Bill cut down on late hours and coffee and practiced relaxation techniques, his self-ratings of anxiety went down as did the counselor's ratings. The hand trembling at the sheltered workshop diminished as the anxiety rating fell.

Case 4: Medication Change

Medications can be adjusted based upon symptom information collected by a rehabilitation staff member. In the typical outpatient clinic, patient visits may be separated by 2 weeks or a month. Moreover, medication appointments are frequently only 5 to 10 minutes, too brief for a psychiatrist to assess symptoms. Because rehabilitation staff observe patients for longer periods and in more diverse settings, they are in a better position to monitor symptoms and provide valuable information to the prescribing psychiatrist about a patient's medication needs.

Dave, a 27-year-old veteran with schizophrenia in remission, had been participating in an office machine repair training program at the VA hospital for 2 months and was progressing toward graduation. He also took a course on medication self-management which led him and his psychiatrist to decide to switch from daily mellaril tablets to monthly injections of haloperidol decanoate. Two weeks after receiving his first injection, the rehabilitation staff noticed increased apathy and social withdrawal in Dave. Since these negative symptoms had not previously been present, they decided to inform the clinic of their observations and contacted a nurse there. At Dave's next appointment, the prescribing psychiatrist told Dave that he would be given a lower dose to cut down on the side effects of lowered energy and motivation that he was experiencing. The staff at the office machine repair training program and the psychiatrist followed the change in negative symptoms by administering the SANS. Following this lower dose, Dave's vocational progress was no longer impaired by apathy and social withdrawal, reflected both in his SANS ratings and his participation in the vocational rehabilitation program.

SYMPTOM MONITORING AS A TOOL TO PREVENT RELAPSE

Whenever it is possible to intervene to prevent an imminent relapse, rehabilitation personnel should do so. Many patients show a deterioration of cognitive status following a relapse and others do not return to their previous level of functioning after each episode of illness (Herz, Syzmanski, & Simon, 1982). In addition, relapses cause disruptions, both for the individual whose progress is impeded and for the staff who must devote valuable resources to arranging appropriate treatment that frequently requires costly hospitalization. The disruptive effects of a florid relapse on family members and other clients in the rehabilitation program also need to be considered.

Definitions of relapse, for use in rehabilitation program evaluation, need to be based on the level of psychopathology rather than social disturbance or rehospitalization. The latter are not reliable indicators of relapse since they are affected by a wide variety of social factors that are not related to the core illness process. For example, the likelihood that a given patient will be hospitalized is affected by socioeconomic status, race, and sex since behavioral disturbances are differentially tolerated by families of different ethnic backgrounds (Wing, 1978). To avoid this confounding, researchers have developed definitions of relapse that are keyed exclusively to the presence of psychotic symptoms (Lukoff, Liberman, & Nuechterlein, 1986). Table 3.1 shows examples of operational definitions for relapse.

When the focus is on early intervention, detecting a full-blown relapse is too late in the cycle of clinical deterioration. Several definitions of symptomatic exacerbation have been developed that are designed to catch a relapse in the prodromal phase when intervention often can prevent the continued downward course. Relapse in schizophrenia is usually preceded by a prodromal period that the patient, relatives, and the therapist can learn to identify. When Herz and Melville (1980) retrospectively interviewed schizophrenic patients and their relatives about the period preceding a relapse, most were able to report a distinct prodromal period. They found that 87% of patients experienced mood changes and neurotic symptoms prior to the onset of psychotic symptoms. The symptom configuration reported by the patients and relatives showed a high degree of intraindividual specificity and stability across incidents of relapse. As listed in Table 3.2, the symptoms were mostly of a nonspecific dysphoric type (Herz & Melville, 1980). Only a small percentage of patients reported that the period between onset of prodromal symptoms and relapse was less than 1 day. In more than two-thirds of the cases, the duration of such symptoms was more than 1 week, after which the florid psychotic symptoms developed.

Patients can be taught to monitor their own symptoms, to recognize warning signs of relapse, and thereby to become empowered to participate actively in their own treatment decisions. Mendel (1976) developed a program in which schizophrenic patients in the community were trained to recognize their own warning signs. Each patient carried a list of his or her own idiosyncratic symptoms, ranging from "thinking a lot about past hospitalizations" to "trouble sleeping," along with a phone number to call if these warning signs developed.

To teach patients with schizophrenia and other chronic psychotic disorders to manage their illness and treatment, skills-training modules have been designed, field tested, and validated in the areas of symptom self-management and medication self-management (Eckman, et al., 1990; Wirshing, Eckman, & Liberman, 1990). The Symptom Management Module (1986) comprises four skill areas: Identifying Warning Signs of Relapse; Seeking Early Intervention for Warn-

Table 3.1. Brief Psychiatric Rating Scale and Behavioral Anchors Used to Define Types of Relapse in the UCLA Aftercare Clinic

SCALE ITEM	PSYCHOTIC RELAPSE: RATING	PSYCHOTIC RELAPSE: DEFINITION	RELIABILITY COEFFICIENT
Unusual thought content	6 Severe	Full delusion(s) present with much preoccupation *or* many areas of functioning are disrupted by delusional thinking	.93
	7 Extremely severe	Full delusion(s) present with almost total preoccupation *or* most areas of functioning are disrupted by delusional thinking	
Hallucinations	6 Severe	Hallucinations experienced several times a day *or* many areas of functioning are disrupted by hallucinations	
	7 Extremely severe	Hallucinations are persistent throughout the day *or* most areas of functioning are disrupted by hallucinations	.97
Conceptual disorganization	6 Severe	Speech incomprehensible due to severe impairments most of the time	.73
	7 Extremely severe	Speech incomprehensible throughout interview	

SCALE ITEM	OTHER TYPES OF RELAPSES: RATING	OTHER TYPES OF RELAPSES: DEFINITION	RELIABILITY COEFFICIENT
Depression	6 Severe	Deeply depressed most of the time *or* many areas of functioning are disrupted by depression	.90
	7 Extremely severe	Patient deeply depressed constantly *or* most areas of functioning are disrupted by depressive thinking	
Suicidality	6 Severe	Patient wants to kill self. Searches for appropriate means and time *or* suicide attempt that is potentially serious threat to life with patient knowledge of possible rescue	.97
	7 Extremely severe	Patient has specific suicidal plan and intent (e.g., "As soon as ______, I will kill myself by doing X") *or* suicide attempt characterized by plan that the patient thought was lethal or an attempt in secluded environment	
Self-neglect	6 Severe	Patient's hygiene and eating potentially life-threatening (e.g., eats and/or bathes only when prompted)	.78
	7 Extremely severe	Patient's hygiene and eating life-threatening (e.g., does not eat or engage in hygiene)	
Bizarre behavior	6 Severe	Patient has committed unusual petty crimes (e.g., directing traffic, public nudity, contacting authorities about imaginary crimes)	.84
	7 Extremely severe	Patient has committed unusual serious crimes (e.g., setting fires, asocial theft, kidnapping committed in bizarre fashion or for bizarre reasons)	
Hostility	6 Severe	Patient has assaulted others but with no harm likely (e.g., slapped or pushed others *or* destroyed property, knocked over furniture, broken windows)	.89
	7 Extremely severe	Patient has attacked others with definite possibility of harming them or with actual harm (e.g., assault with hammer or weapon)	

Table 3.2. Frequency of Patients Reporting Prodromal Symptoms

PRODROMAL SYMPTOM	FREQUENCY
Nervous and tense	> 70%
Impaired concentration Sleep disturbance Restlessness Depression Reduced enjoyment Preoccupation with one or two things	> 60%
Loss of interest Ideas of reference	> 50%

Note: Adopted from Herz and Melville (1980, p. 804).

ing Signs; Coping with Persistent Psychotic Symptoms, and Avoiding Alcohol and Street Drugs. The skills are taught in a series of eight learning activities that include motivational exercises, videotaped demonstrations, role plays, problem-solving sequences, and in vivo homework assignments.

Figure 3.1 shows the structure of the Symptom Management Module. During the final skill area on avoiding alcohol and street drugs, patients are given models, role-play practice, and coaching to use appropriate communication skills, such as are depicted in Figure 3.2.

Exacerbations in response to rehabilitation should be detected at an early phase when preventive action can be taken. The rehabilitation team is frequently faced with patients who become increasingly symptomatic in ways that interfere with the rehabilitation processes while they are participating in a program. Symptomatic increases may be triggered by stressors in the patient's family or home environment or by outside events. Preventive intervention can include adjustments in the dose or type of medications, crisis services, increased frequency of counseling, or even suspension of the rehabilitation program. When assessments of prodromal symptoms are performed on a regular basis—for example, every 2 weeks—the results can be used to adjust a patient's program to prevent further clinical deterioration.

Case Examples

Case 1: Preventing Exacerbation Associated with Rehabilitation

When Linda, a patient with bipolar disorder, was discharged from a psychiatric hospital following a manic psychotic episode, she went to live at home. Two of her previous hospitalizations, including her recent one, had occurred within 2 months of beginning a new job. But she had been able to work 3 continuous years at a job involving food preparation at a nursing home and thought that she would like to try working again. Linda's parents also preferred that Linda work and be able to afford her own apartment. Linda's parents contacted a halfway house that ran a catering service as part of their vocational training program. The director of the catering program and Linda worked out a plan that would allow Linda to attempt a job again. First, they agreed to start slowly with no more than two catering events per week, about 10 hours of work. Second, Linda was able to talk to her parents to gain their support in concrete ways such as being flexible about mealtimes since

Module: Symptom Self-Management

Skill Area: Avoiding alcohol and street drugs

Behavioral skills learned

- Understand harmful effects of alcohol and street drugs
- Identify benefits of avoiding alcohol and street drugs
- Refuse alcohol and street drugs when invited to use
- Employ alternatives to alcohol and street drugs when feeling dysphoric
- Level with doctor and therapists about use of alcohol and street drugs

Figure 3.1. The structure of a skills-training module includes general skill areas that cover the main content of the functional domains within which are nested specific behavioral competencies required for social and independent living. The skill area, avoiding alcohol and street drugs, from the Symptom Management Module is shown with its constituent behavioral or educational objectives.

Linda might have to work at those times. Third, her psychiatrist was contacted to arrange weekly monitoring during the first 2 months to allay both Linda's and her parents' fears that working might lead to yet another relapse. Fourth, both Linda and her parents were enrolled in the Symptom Self-Management Module, an educational program that teaches how to recognize prodromal signs of relapse.

As shown in Figure 3.3, Linda's psychiatrist used the BPRS to make the weekly assessments and found increases on the Anxiety and on Unusual Thought Content scale items after Linda's first week of work. Her excessive concerns about the "cleanliness" of the food she was preparing, even though not delusional, reminded the psychiatrist of Linda's delusion of being fed poisoned food. Her medication was increased but she was encouraged to continue with the catering. By the sixth week, Linda had acclimated to the demands of working and reported that she felt much less anxious and worried about the food. Her BPRS scores returned to their baseline level. She gradually took on more catering jobs, and her medication dose was lowered. Monitoring of symptomatology with the BPRS was maintained by her psychiatrist as was her own self-monitoring of her warning signs.

Case 2: Preventing Exacerbation Associated with Life Events

Exacerbations in response to major life events can be prevented if prodromal symptoms are noted and early intervention is provided. Rehabilitation usually involves ongoing case management through which surveillance of the patient's entire life situation, including events occurring in social and vocational rehabilitation, is provided. Life changes associated with rehabilitation can themselves produce stress-induced exacerbations that may impede a patient's further progress.

Bill had been participating for 2 months in a Job Finding Club at a community mental

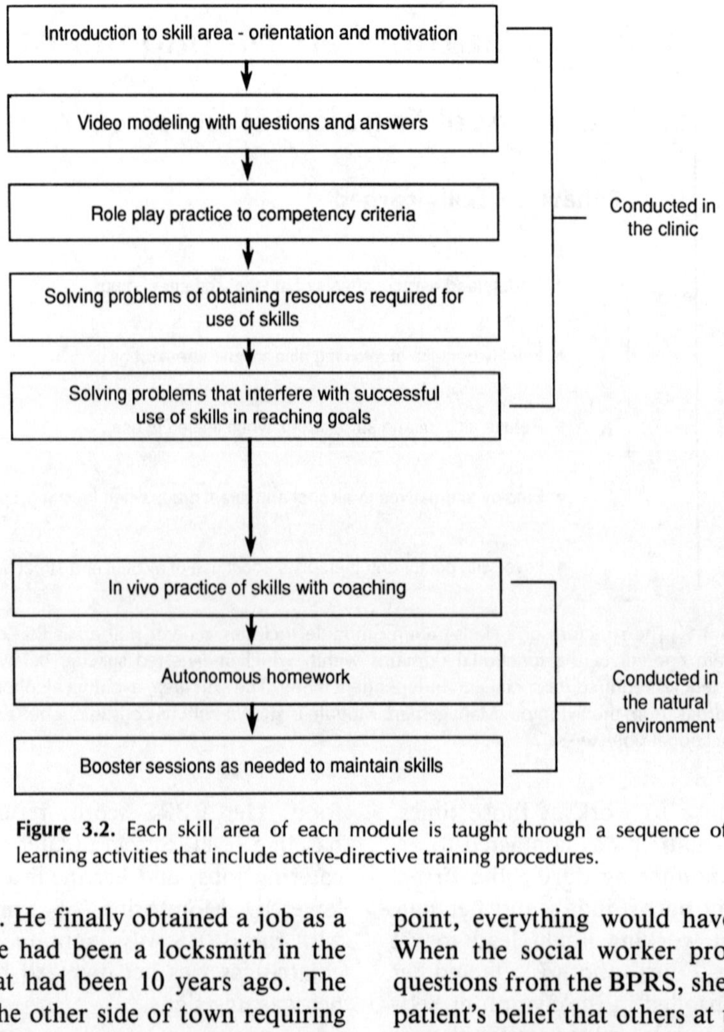

Figure 3.2. Each skill area of each module is taught through a sequence of learning activities that include active-directive training procedures.

health center. He finally obtained a job as a locksmith; he had been a locksmith in the army but that had been 10 years ago. The job was on the other side of town requiring a one-and-a-half hour bus ride and he was concerned that the long commute might make him late for work. Therefore, Bill decided to move to a board-and-care home that was closer to his new job even though it meant leaving the neighborhood where his parents lived.

The social worker connected with the job club helped him find a place to live that was within walking distance of where he would be working. One month after the move, the social worker had a session with Bill and asked him how he was doing. He replied that he enjoyed his job and was pleased that he had retained his locksmithing skills. If the social worker had stopped the interview at this point, everything would have seemed fine. When the social worker proceeded to ask questions from the BPRS, she uncovered the patient's belief that others at the board-and-care were staring at him and talking about him. She noticed the pressure of mild conceptual disorganization for the first time, as shown in Figure 3.4. These prodromal symptoms were of concern to the social worker because she knew that they frequently precede a relapse and they had not been present prior to Bill's beginning his job and moving. Further inquiry revealed that Bill was feeling socially overwhelmed at his new residential facility, which was much larger than his previous one. Bill had not been able to make even a casual friendship in the month he had been there. In addition, he missed having dinner with his parents, something he had done several times a week before the move.

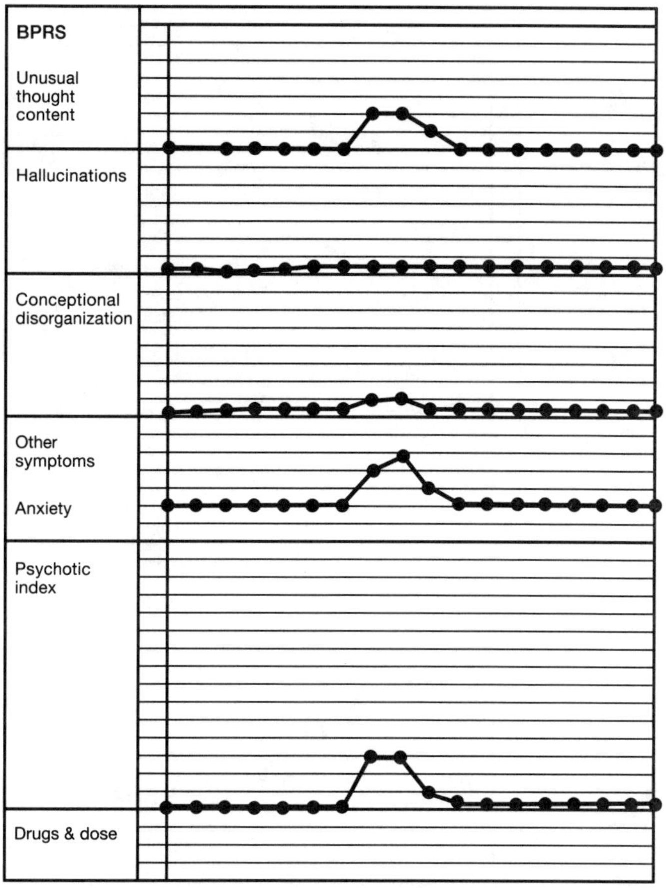

Figure 3.3. Graph of Psychotic Index for Linda. The Brief Psychiatric Rating Scale (BPRS) is used regularly to monitor a patient's psychopathology, adjust medication dose, and guide treatment decisions. In this case, detection of Linda's increase in anxiety and delusions prompted timely and effective clinical intervention.

The social worker immediately scheduled an appointment that afternoon with Bill's psychiatrist to determine whether an increase in medication was warranted. With Bill's consent, she notified the board-and-care manager to suggest that he pay special attention to Bill and assist him in getting acquainted with other residents. Bill's contacts with the social worker were increased to twice a week. Three weeks later Bill's symptoms returned to their previous subclinical level. By carefully monitoring the patient's symptomatology and altering the stressful situation, the social worker was able to avert a potential relapse and enable the patient to sustain his vocational momentum.

Antipsychotic Medication Intervention

With appropriate patients, early intervention with intermittently administered antipsychotic medication strategies can be utilized instead of continuous medication. Recognition of the actual and potential risks associated with maintenance on continuous antipsychotic drugs has grown. These include the risk of temporary and permanent

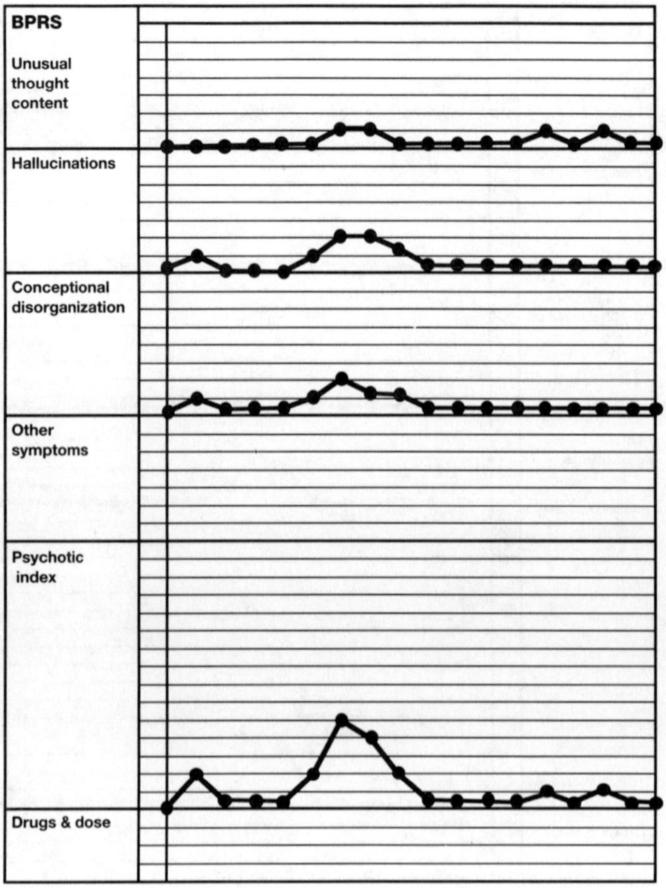

Figure 3.4. Graph of Psychotic Index for Bill. The Brief Psychiatric Rating Scale (BPRS) is used titrate medication and the frequency of psychosocial interventions to protect the patient from stress-induced relapses.

tardive dyskinesia, estimated to occur in upwards of 25% of long-term patients, and distressing extrapyramidal side effects. In addition, there is the possibility that antipsychotic medication may exacerbate the negative symptoms of schizophrenia (Falloon, Watt, & Shepherd, 1978). Diminished social functioning and motivation, two of the most significant negative symptoms, could have a particularly deleterious impact on rehabilitation efforts.

While it has been clearly established that antipsychotic medication offers prophylactic benefits in forestalling relapse, investigators have found that medication can indefinitely prevent relapse for only 22% of patients. In 13% of patients, medications do not seem to be necessary or helpful in preventing relapses, and in 65% relapses are only postponed (Hirsch, Jolley, & Manchanda, 1983). These findings along with the concerns identified above have led to attempts to develop *targeted, intermittent* (Herz, Syzmanski, & Simon, 1982), or *early intervention medication* (Hirsch, Jolley, & Manchanda, 1983) strategies. These approaches are designed to allow patients to remain drug-free with regular monitoring of their clinical state to identify the earliest signs of relapse. If such prodromal signs are detected, a patient is immediately returned to an antipsychotic medication regimen for a time-limited period. This strategy has been shown to reduce the total exposure to antipsychotic medication for many patients.

To be good candidates for intermittent, targeted medication regimens, patients need to be able to tolerate at least several months of no medication without a relapse, and to have the knowledge and skill to self-monitor prodromal symptoms and collaborate actively with caregivers in obtaining early intervention when needed. Cooperative and knowledgeable family members or roommates also need to be involved in the treatment relationship and planning process. When relapses occur in this type of medication strategy, they can be limited in time and severity.

INSTRUMENTS FOR ASSESSING PSYCHOPATHOLOGY

Accurate assessment of symptoms involves two distinct processes to address separately their presence and intensity. Symptoms must first be elicited from the patient through interviewing and observation. Then, they need to be categorized and rated for intensity. Structured interview schedules guide the interviewer in systematically covering all the most clinically significant symptom areas. Both the BPRS for assessing positive symptoms and the SANS for negative symptoms have accompanying structured interview schedules with questions to elicit specific types of psychopathology. In addition, both the BPRS and SANS have manuals that define each symptom in the scale and give clinical examples of the anchor point ratings for the intensity of each symptom. The use of a structured interview and operational rating criteria has been found to increase the level of agreement among raters. Scales with good interrater reliability more accurately measure changes occurring in an individual over time.

Brief Psychiatric Rating Scale

The original BPRS (Overall & Gorham, 1962) was designed for use by clinical observers of inpatient psychiatric populations in psychopharmacological outcome studies. It originally contained 16 symptom categories. The instrument was later expanded to 18 items (Guy, 1976) and then to 24 by the addition of subscales that cover the psychopathology found with outpatients with serious mental disorders (Lukoff, Liberman, & Nuechterlein, 1986). Included are the positive symptoms of greatest importance for assessing the clinical condition of patients with psychotic disorders; hallucinations, delusions, and thought disorder. Appendix 3.1 shows the form or recording ratings for the 24 symptoms covered by the BPRS. The items are rated on a 1 to 7 point scale of increasing severity. A manual containing a semistructured interview and operational definitions for the anchor points has been published (Lukoff, Liberman, & Nuechterlein, 1986). The sections of the manual that cover psychotic symptoms are illustrated in Appendix 3.2. Administration of the interview and rating of symptoms takes 10 to 30 minutes depending upon the interviewer's familiarity with the patient, the number of symptoms present, and the patient's capacity to describe symptoms. The level of symptoms can be readily graphed so that changes in baseline levels of one or more symptoms can be quickly detected and intervention begun.

The BPRS assesses many nonpsychotic prodromal symptoms that have been found to increase before a full-blown relapse, such as anxiety, distractibility, tension, depression, and emotional withdrawal. It has also been used in studies involving prodromal symptoms in the prediction of relapse (Marder, Van Putten, & Mintz, 1984; Subotnik & Nuechterlein, 1988). Therefore, the BPRS is an appropriate instrument to use in a monitoring program to prevent relapses. Because scale items tap affective blunting and motor retardation, the BPRS also can be used to measure negative symptoms.

While other instruments can be used to monitor psychopathology, the BPRS was highlighted here because it is the workhorse of assessment, frequently used in clinical studies, with established reliability and validity. In addition, a manual for its use is available from the UCLA Clinical Research Center for Schizophrenia and Psychiatric Rehabilitation (Box 6022, Camarillo, CA 93011) and the scaling and rating criteria are readily learned.

Schedule for Assessment of Negative Symptoms

Negative symptoms are defined by the absence of or pathologically low levels of affect, motivation, verbal behavior, attentional capacity, social behavior, and motor behavior. The Schedule for the Assessment of Negative Symptoms (SANS) (Andreasen, 1982) was designed to measure the negative symptoms of psychotic disorders. Some consider the negative symptoms to constitute the true core symptoms of schizophrenia and their importance in affecting the functioning and rehabilitation of patients is being increasingly recognized. Brain imaging studies have documented anomalies in brain structure that appear to be related to high levels of negative symptoms. While negative symptoms and depression have been confounded in the past, the SANS allows researchers and clinicians to distinguish between them.

The SANS consists of 30 items covering five major areas: Affective Flattening or Blunting, Alogia, Avolition-Apathy, Anhedonia-Asociality, and Attention. A manual for using the SANS includes a glossary, anchor points, and interview schedule. Each item is assessed by two to seven individual items, a subjective rating and a global rating, all on a 1 to 5 point scale of increasing severity. Administration of the interview takes 20 to 30 minutes depending on the interviewer's familiarity with the patient, the patient's verbal coherence, and the number of symptoms present. Appendix 3.3 shows the form for recording ratings for the 30 symptoms covered by the SANS.

The withdrawal-retardation subscale of the BPRS (which consists of the motor retardation, emotional withdrawal, and blunted affect items) correlates highly with the SANS composite score. If one is interested only in the global level of negative symptoms rather than information about specific symptoms, the BPRS can be used alone. However, the SANS covers symptoms that affect areas of vocational functioning that are of particular interest to rehabilitation staff, such as avolition/apathy, impersistence at work or school, physical anergia, and poor grooming and hygiene. One assessment strategy for negative symptoms is to administer the SANS at intake to obtain a "snapshot" of the patient's deficiencies. Then the specific negative symptoms that were elicited and seem to have a bearing on rehabilitation can be monitored as target symptoms, an assessment technique that is described below.

Target Symptom Ratings

The rating of target symptoms (May, 1980) makes use of the finding that patients tend to have exacerbations of the same symptoms across different episodes of relapse (Herz, Syzmanski, & Simon, 1982; Leff & Wing, 1981). Therefore, it is possible to monitor efficiently the specific symptoms that most sensitively reflect a given patient's clinical condition. Target symptom scales can be used readily by clinicians of all disciplines.

One example of the use of target symptoms was a study by Falloon, Boyd, and McGill (1984) to monitor the psychopathology of patients who were participating in a 2-year study of family, individual, and drug therapy for chronic, relapsing schizophrenia. For each patient in the study, the researchers selected two symptoms that had recurred during previous exacerbations. Care was taken to specify each symptom exactly as it was manifested in that patient. These target symptoms were monitored monthly and rated on a 1 to 7 point scale of increasing severity similar to the procedure in the BPRS. The investigators found that the target symptom scale was sensitive to episodes of relapse and distinguished the treatment conditions better than did the BPRS. It is likely that target symptom scales, because they highlight symptoms that are specific for each patient, reflect individual differences and are more sensitive to changes in clinical state than multidimensional, more comprehensive instruments.

Target symptoms are probably an underutilized method for monitoring both positive and negative symptoms. By focusing on just two or three symptoms that have a bearing on a patient's rehabilitation, staff can save time on assessment yet still be on top of the significant changes occurring in a patient's clinical condition as they affect his or her rehabilitation. These symptoms can be drawn from the BPRS or SANS, although they can be customized to fit the patient's pattern of symptomatology.

CONCLUSION

The reliable assessment of psychiatric symptoms serves a vital function in the rehabilitation of seriously mentally ill patients. Monitoring symptoms aids clinical decision making, such as evaluation of readiness for rehabilitation, and can warn rehabilitation professionals of the appearance of prodromal symptoms suggestive of an imminent relapse. The BPRS is an instrument that has demonstrated reliability and validity in assessing the positive and negative symptoms of psychotic disorders as well as a wide range of other clinically significant symptoms and behaviors. The SANS provides a wide range of negative symptoms relevant to rehabilitation efforts. Finally, rating target symptoms allows for a focused and efficient assessment of key symptoms. These three scales are all brief and relatively easy to learn to administer, which makes them highly useful in the rehabilitation milieu.

REFERENCES

Andreasen, N. (1982). Negative symptoms in schizophrenia: Definition and reliability. *Archives of General Psychiatry, 39*, 784–788.

Brown, G., Birley, J., & Wing, J. (1972). Influence of family life on the course of schizophrenic disorders: A replication. *British Journal of Psychiatry, 121*, 241–258.

Ciompi, L. (1980). Catamnestic long-term study on the course of life and aging of schizophrenics. *Schizophrenia Bulletin, 6*, 606–618.

Eckman, T., Liberman, R. P., Blair, K., & Phipps, C. C. (1990). Teaching medication management skills to schizophrenics. *Journal of Clinical Psychopharmacology, 10*, 33–38.

Falloon, I., Boyd, J., & McGill, C. (1984). *Family care of schizophrenia: A problem-solving approach to the treatment of mental illness.* New York: Guilford Press.

Falloon, I., Watt, D. C., & Shepherd, M. (1978). The social outcome of patients in a trial of long-term continuation therapy in schizophrenia: Pimozide versus Fluphenazine. *Psychological Medicine, 8*, 265–274.

Glynn, S., & Mueser, K. T. (1986). Social learning for chronic mental inpatients. *Schizophrenia Bulletin, 12*, 648–668.

Guy, W. (1976). *ECDEU Assessment Manual.* (DHEW Pub. No. 76-338). Rockville, MD: National Institute of Mental Health.

Herz, M., & Melville, C. (1980). Relapse in schizophrenia. *Archives of General Psychiatry, 137*, 801–805.

Herz, M. I., Syzmanski, H. V., & Simon, J. (1982). Intermittent medication for stable schizophrenic outpatients: An alternative to maintenance medication. *American Journal of Psychiatry, 139*, 918–922.

Hirsch, S. R., Jolley, A. G., & Manchanda, R. (1983). Early intervention medication as an alternative to continuous depot treatment in schizophrenia: Preliminary report. In J. Strauss, W. Boker, & H. Brenner (Eds.), *Psychosocial treatment of schizophrenia.* Toronto: Hans Huber Publishers.

Leff, J., & Wing, J. (1971). Trial of maintenance therapy in schizophrenia. *British Medical Journal, 3*, 599–604.

Liberman, R. P. (1986). Coping and competence as protective factors in the vulnerability-stress model of schizophrenia. In M. J. Goldstein, I. Hand, & K. Hahlweg (Eds.), *Treatment of schizophrenia.* Berlin: Springer-Verlag.

Liberman, R. P., & Foy, D. W. (1983). Psychiatric rehabilitation for chronic mental patients. *Psychiatric Annals, 13*, 539–545.

Lukoff, D., Liberman, R. P., & Nuechterlein,

K. H. (1986). Symptom monitoring in the rehabilitation of schizophrenic patients. *Schizophrenia Bulletin, 12*, 578–602.

Lukoff, D., & Ventura, J. (1988). Psychiatric diagnosis. In R. P. Liberman (Ed.), *Psychiatric rehabilitation of chronic mental patients*. Washington, DC: American Psychiatric Association Press.

Marder, S. R., Van Putten, T., & Mintz, J. (1984). Maintenance therapy in schizophrenia: New findings. In J. M. Kand (Ed.), *Drug maintenance strategies in schizophrenia*. Washington, DC: American Psychiatric Press.

May, P. R. (1980). Strategies for applied researchers in chronic schizophrenia: Choosing the right treatment and measuring outcome. In C. Baxter & T. Melnechuck (Eds.), *Perspectives in schizophrenia research*. New York: Raven Press.

Mendel, W. (1976). *Schizophrenia: the experience and its treatment*. San Francisco: Jossey-Bass.

Overall, J., & Gorham, D. (1962). The Brief Psychiatric Rating Scale. *Psychological Reports, 10*, 799–812.

Subotnik, K., & Nuechterlein, K. H. (1988). Prodromal signs and symptoms of schizophrenic relapse. *Journal of Abnormal Psychology, 97*, 405–412.

Symptom Management Module. (1986). Available from the Camarillo-UCLA Research Center, Box A, Camarillo, CA 93011 (ATTN: Dissemination Coordinator).

Vaughn, C., Snyder, K., Jones, S., Freeman, W., & Falloon, I. (1984). Family factors in schizophrenic relapse: A California replication of the British research on expressed emotion. *Archives of General Psychiatry, 41*, 1169–1177.

Wing, J. (1978). Social influences on the course of schizophrenia. In L. Wynne, R. Cromwell, & S. Matthysse (Eds.), *The nature of schizophrenia: New approaches to research and treatment*. New York: John Wiley.

Wirshing, W., Eckman, T., & Liberman, R. P. (1990). Management of risk of relapse in schizophrenia. In C. Tamminga & S. C. Schulz (Eds.), *Schizophrenia research*. New York: Raven Press.

APPENDIX 3.1. BRIEF PSYCHIATRIC RATING SCALE (BPRS)

This form consists of 24 symptom constructs, each to be rated on a 7-point scale of severity ranging from "Not present" to "Extremely severe" (see below). If a specific symptom is not rated, mark NA = Not assessed. Circle the number headed by the term that best describes the patient's present condition.

NA	1	2	3	4	5	6	7
Not assessed	Not present	Very mild	Mild	Moderate	Moderately severe	Severe	Extremely severe

Rate items 1–10 on the basis of patient's self-report

1. Somatic concern	NA	1	2	3	4	5	6	7
2. Anxiety	NA	1	2	3	4	5	6	7
3. Depression	NA	1	2	3	4	5	6	7
4. Guilt	NA	1	2	3	4	5	6	7
5. Hostility	NA	1	2	3	4	5	6	7
6. Suspiciousness	NA	1	2	3	4	5	6	7
7. Unusual thought content	NA	1	2	3	4	5	6	7
8. Grandiosity	NA	1	2	3	4	5	6	7
9. Hallucinations	NA	1	2	3	4	5	6	7
10. Disorientation	NA	1	2	3	4	5	6	7

Rate items 11–25 on the basis of observed behavior and speech

11. Conceptual disorganization	NA	1	2	3	4	5	6	7
12. Excitement	NA	1	2	3	4	5	6	7
13. Motor retardation	NA	1	2	3	4	5	6	7
14. Blunted affect	NA	1	2	3	4	5	6	7
15. Tension	NA	1	2	3	4	5	6	7
16. Mannerisms and posturing	NA	1	2	3	4	5	6	7
17. Uncooperativeness	NA	1	2	3	4	5	6	7
18. Emotional withdrawal	NA	1	2	3	4	5	6	7

NA	1	2	3	4	5	6	7
Not assessed	Not present	Very mild	Mild	Moderate	Moderately severe	Severe	Extremely severe

19. Suicidality	NA	1	2	3	4	5	6	7
20. Self-neglect	NA	1	2	3	4	5	6	7
21. Bizarre behavior	NA	1	2	3	4	5	6	7
22. Elated mood	NA	1	2	3	4	5	6	7
23. Motor hyperactivity	NA	1	2	3	4	5	6	7
24. Distractibility	NA	1	2	3	4	5	6	7

APPENDIX 3.2. BPRS PSYCHOTIC SYMPTOM DESCRIPTIONS

Descriptions of psychotic symptoms from the Brief Psychiatric Rating Scale with their anchor points for clinicians ratings. The standard interview questions following each set of anchor points are used to elicit reliable symptom information from the patient.

Unusual Thought Content: Unusual, odd, strange, or bizarre thought content. Rate the degree of unusualness, not the degree of disorganization of speech. Delusions are patently absurd, clearly false, or bizarre ideas verbally expressed. Include thought insertion, withdrawal, and broadcast. Include grandiose, somatic, and persecutory delusions even if rated elsewhere.

2	Very mild	Ideas of reference (people stare/laugh at her or him). Ideas of persecution (people mistreat her or him). Unusual beliefs in psychic powers, spirits, unidentified flying objects. Not strongly held. Some doubt.
3	Mild	Same as 2, with full conviction—but not delusional.
4	Moderate	Delusions present but not strongly held, functioning not disrupted *or* encapsulated delusion with full conviction, functioning not disrupted.
5	Moderately severe	Full delusion(s) present with some preoccupation *or* some areas of functioning disrupted by delusional thinking.
6	Severe	Full delusion(s) present with much preoccupation *or* many areas of functioning are disrupted by delusional thinking.
7	Extremely severe	Full delusion(s) present with almost total preoccupation *or* most areas of functioning are disrupted by delusional thinking.

Have things or events had special meanings for you?____________________

Did you see any references to yourself on TV or in the newspapers?____________________

Do you have a special relationship with God?____________________

How do you explain the things that have been happening (specify)?____________________

Have you felt that you were under the control of another person or force?____________________

Grandiosity: Exaggerated self-opinion, self-enhancing conviction of special abilities or powers or identity as someone rich or famous. Rate only patient's statements about him- or herself, not his demeanor.

2	Very mild	Feels great and denies obvious problems.
3	Mild	Exaggerated self-opinion beyond abilities and training.
4	Moderate	Inappropriate boastfulness, claims to be "brilliant," understands how everything works.

5	Moderately severe	Claims to be great musician who will soon make recordings or will soon make patentable inventions—but not delusional.
6	Severe	Delusional—claims to have special powers like ESP (extra-sensory perception), to have millions of dollars, made movies, invented new machines, worked at jobs when it is known that he was never employed in these capacities.
7	Extremely severe	Delusional—claims to have been appointed by God to run the world, controls the future of the world, is Jesus Christ, or President of the United States.

Is there a special purpose or mission to your life?____________________

Do you have any special powers or abilities?____________________

Have you thought that you might be somebody rich or famous?____________________

Hallucinations: Reports of perceptual experiences in the absence of external stimuli. When rating degree to which functioning is disrupted by hallucinations, do not include preoccupation with the content of the hallucinations. Consider only disruption due to the hallucinatory experience. Include thoughts aloud—"gedankenlautwerden."

2	Very mild	While resting or going to sleep, sees visions, hears voices, sounds, or whispers in absence of external stimulation, but no impairments in functioning.
3	Mild	While in a clear state of consciousness, hears nonverbal auditory hallucinations (e.g., sounds or whispers) or sees illusions (e.g., faces in shadows) on no more than two occasions and with no impairment in functioning.
4	Moderate	Occasional verbal, visual, olfactory, tactile, or gustatory hallucinations (1–3 times) but no impairment in functioning *or* frequent nonverbal hallucinations/visual illusions.
5	Moderately severe	Daily *or* some areas of functioning are disrupted by hallucinations.
6	Severe	Several times a day *or* many areas of functioning are disrupted by hallucinations.
7	Extremely severe	Persistent throughout the day *or* most areas of functioning are disrupted by hallucinations.

Have you heard any sounds or people talking to you or about you when there has been nobody around?____________________

Have you seen any visions or smelled any smells others do not seem to notice?____________________

Have these experiences interfered with your ability to perform your usual activities/work?____________________

Suspiciousness: Expressed or apparent belief that other persons have acted maliciously or with discriminatory intent. Include persecution by supernatural or other nonhuman agencies (e.g., the devil).

2–3	Mild	Seems on guard. Unresponsive to "personal" questions. Describes incidents where other persons have harmed or wanted to harm him that sound plausible. Patient feels as if others are laughing or criticizing him/her in public.
4–5	Moderate	Says other persons are talking about him maliciously *or* says others intend to harm him. Beyond likelihood of plausibility—but not delusional.
6–7	Severe	Delusional. Speaks of Mafia plots, the FBI, or others poisoning his food.

Do you ever feel uncomfortable in public, as if people are watching you?________________________

____

Is anyone trying to harm or interfere with you in any way?________________________

____

Are you concerned about anybody's intentions toward you?________________________

____

Have you felt that any people are out to get you?________________________

____

Conceptual Disorganization: Degree to which speech is confused, disconnected, or disorganized. Rate tangentiality, circumstantiality, sudden topic shifts, incoherence, derailment, blocking, neologisms, and other speech disorders. Do not rate *content* of speech. Consider the first 15 minutes of the interview.

2	Very mild	Peculiar use of words, rambling but speech is comprehensible.
3	Mild	Speech a bit hard to understand or make sense of due to tangentiality, circumstantiality, or sudden topic shifts.
4	Moderate	Speech difficult to understand due to tangentiality, circumstantiality or topic shifts on many occasions *or* 1–2 instances of severe impairment, e.g., incoherence, derailment, neologisms, blocking.
5	Moderately severe	Speech difficult to understand due to circumstantiality, tangentiality, or topic shifts most of the time *or* 3–5 instances of severe impairment.
6	Severe	Speech is incomprehensible due to severe impairments most of the time.
7	Extremely severe	Speech is incomprehensible throughout interview.

APPENDIX 3.3. SCALE FOR THE ASSESSMENT OF NEGATIVE SYMPTOMS

For each item that is an observable behavior, multiple sources of information including direct observation by the investigator, family members, and self-report by the patient should be used. The subjective items (8, 14, 19, 25, 29) should be based exclusively on the patient's self-report. It need not bear any resemblance to the behavioral or global ratings. Global ratings should be an overall rating and not a mean score for the component behaviors.

		Questionable	Minimal	Moderate	Marked	Severe
Affective Flattening or Blunting						
1. Unchanging facial expression	0	1	2	3	4	5
2. Decreased spontaneous movements	0	1	2	3	4	5
3. Paucity of expressive gestures	0	1	2	3	4	5
4. Poor eye contact	0	1	2	3	4	5
5. Affective nonresponsivity	0	1	2	3	4	5
6. Inappropriate affect	0	1	2	3	4	5
7. Lack of vocal inflections	0	1	2	3	4	5
8. Subjective complaints of loss of feeling	0	1	2	3	4	5
9. Global rating of affective flattening	0	1	2	3	4	5
Alogia						
10. Poverty of speech	0	1	2	3	4	5
11. Poverty of content of speech	0	1	2	3	4	5
12. Blocking	0	1	2	3	4	5
13. Increased latency of response	0	1	2	3	4	5
14. Subjective rating of alogia	0	1	2	3	4	5
15. Global rating of alogia	0	1	2	3	4	5
Avolition-Apathy						
16. Grooming and hygiene	0	1	2	3	4	5

17. Impersistence at work or school	0	1	2	3	4	5
18. Physical anergia	0	1	2	3	4	5
19. Subjective complaints of avolition and apathy	0	1	2	3	4	5
20. Global rating of avolition-apathy	0	1	2	3	4	5

Anhedonia-Asociality

21. Recreational interests and activities	0	1	2	3	4	5
22. Sexual interest and activity	0	1	2	3	4	5
23. Ability to feel intimacy and closeness	0	1	2	3	4	5
24. Relationships with friends and peers	0	1	2	3	4	5
25. Subjective awareness of anhedonia/asociality	0	1	2	3	4	5
26. Global rating of anhedonia-asociality	0	1	2	3	4	5

Attention

27. Social inattentiveness	0	1	2	3	4	5
28. Inattentiveness during mental status testing	0	1	2	3	4	5
29. Subjective complaints of inattentiveness	0	1	2	3	4	5
30. Global rating of inattentiveness	0	1	2	3	4	5

CHAPTER 4

FUNCTIONAL ASSESSMENT

Jerome V. Vaccaro
Deborah B. Pitts
Charles J. Wallace

Psychiatric rehabilitation has been defined as the recovery of social, occupational, and instrumental role functioning to the fullest extent possible through learning procedures and environmental supports (Liberman, 1988). When restoration of functioning is limited by continuing symptomatic impairments and disabilities, rehabilitation efforts aim to (a) help the individual acquire the maximum feasible competencies needed to enact desired social, occupational, and instrumental roles, and (b) build social and task environments that support role functioning.

Psychiatric assessment of a person with a major mental disorder is a necessary first step in treatment and rehabilitation planning. The clinical diagnostic process, with its focus on the occurrence and intensity of symptoms and other impairments, is supplemented by information gathered in a comprehensive functional assessment. Functional assessment provides information about an individual's ability to perform everyday activities independently, to satisfy personal needs, and to meet reasonable environmental expectations. It is a planned and ongoing process of collecting, integrating, and interpreting information regarding an individual's past and current adaptation, and formulating recommendations to maximize future adaptation. In conducting a functional assessment clinicians pinpoint and review an individual's strengths, weak-

Parts of this chapter were reproduced from C. J. Wallace, 1986, Functional Assessment in Rehabilitation, in *Schizophrenia Bulletin, 12* 604–630. *Schizophrenia Bulletin*, a publication of the National Institute of Mental Health, is in the public domain and thus reproduction of excerpts from it is permitted.

nesses, and goals, as well as survey factors in the environment that can facilitate or impede adaptation.

While many concur with the value of functional assessment in the comprehensive care of individuals with chronic mental illness, implementation of functional assessment in routine clinical practice has been slow. Three obstacles to the widespread use of functional assessment are (a) inadequate time and personnel resources, (b) lack of training in the use of assessment principles and instruments, and (c) lack of guidelines for the selection of the most appropriate assessment instruments for particular patients and settings. For example, clinical staff who are trained and experienced in performing diagnostic assessments are often ill equipped to use the procedures that are integral to functional assessment. This underscores the need for research and development in the area and for dissemination and training of staff to perform functional assessments. We will provide an overview of the current state of functional assessment and a description of requisite training and resource deployment for using currently available techniques. We will review considerations in selection or design of assessments that meet individual patient and program needs, and will endorse two assessment protocols that meet these needs.

FRAMEWORK FOR FUNCTIONAL ASSESSMENT

The concept of functional assessment in rehabilitation derives from the expansion of assessment beyond the medical diagnosis of disease and residual functioning of damaged body parts to a broader assessment of performance in an environmental context. Functional assessment in psychiatric rehabilitation can be more specifically defined as the process of collecting, integrating, and interpreting information for the purpose of planning rehabilitation interventions in the following domains:

- the specific social, occupational, and instrumental roles in which the individual desires to engage
- the specific coping skills and competencies needed by the individual to engage in desired roles
- the specific psychiatric, cognitive, and/or volitional impairments that may impede acquisition or use of coping skills and competencies needed to engage in desired roles and that will require medical intervention or prosthetic supports in the environment
- the specific environmental demands and supports that will impede or enhance the individual's ability to engage in desired roles

The authors' ordering of this framework in a hierarchy is intentional and informed by the model of human occupation that identifies an individual's valued roles as the starting point for data collection and analysis in functional assessment (Smith, 1990).

Roles

The process of functional assessment begins with the identification of goals that are congruent with the patient's desired life roles. This first step of role definition serves to guide future assessment and interventions. It provides the patient with a road map, allowing him to understand the connection between his individual goals and rehabilitation interventions. Without this, there is a risk that patients will not see the benefit of addressing their skill deficits, possibly leading to poor compliance with interventions.

Peter is a 27-year-old man who has been diagnosed as having schizophrenia and being cocaine dependent. Attempts had been made to engage him in treatment on many occasions, all to no avail. He was seen by rehabilitation counselors, who identified a series of deficits in social and independent living skills. For example, he had poor self-care and grooming skills and was not able to carry on meaningful and productive conversations. Staff suggested he enroll in social skills-training classes targeted to these deficits, but he declined. Finally, he was enrolled in a skills-training group where he outlined a number of roles that he saw as being desirable for himself. These included his being an independent homemaker, improving his standing within his family, and securing steady employment. He and his counselors then developed a plan that clearly linked the skills-training programs to his desired roles. He now attends classes to improve his self-care and grooming habits and his conversation skills, and sees these as important in establishing himself independently in the community and relating successfully to family members and potential employers.

Roles define one's place in social interaction, appropriate attitudes one assumes, and requisite tasks one performs. Roles thus serve as a source of identity. We all see ourselves in relation to others in terms of the roles we occupy. There are a variety of roles we each assume, grouped into social, occupational, psychosexual, and personal self-care spheres. It is often necessary to invest considerable time and effort in helping mentally ill individuals to articulate realistic and feasible roles and goals.

Coping Skills and Competencies

In the next phase of functional assessment, an analysis of coping skills and competencies requires clinicians, in league with their patients, to take an inventory of the skills and abilities needed to enact specific social, occupational, and instrumental roles. For example, physical, social, emotional, and intellectual skills are needed for engagement in living, learning, and working environments (Anthony & Cohen, 1984). In addition, perceptual-motor processes, problem-solving, planning, and communication skills are directly related to successful engagement in roles with an occupational dimension (Kielhofner, 1985).

Social skills are generically necessary for satisfactory performance in roles such as friend, family member, worker, and consumer (Liberman, 1982). Components of social skills include affective, cognitive, and motoric domains of functioning. Social skills include *receiving skills*, so that one is aware of what is being communicated along affective and cognitive dimensions; *processing skills*, so that one is able to translate cognitively what is received into a set of options for action and choose appropriate courses of action; and *sending skills*, so that one communicates the chosen alternative in an effective manner.

Skills essential for adaptive functioning have also been described in terms of major life domains, such as daily living skills, vocational skills, and recreational skills. For individuals with mental disorders, independent living requires skills in such areas as medication self-management, symptom self-management, self-care and grooming, meal preparation, money management, and use of public transportation (Anthony & Liberman, 1986). Vocational skills include the abilities and competencies to select an appropriate job, to execute job-specific tasks, to persist in a job-search, and to sustain a job despite challenges and frustrations.

Impairments

The third step in functional assessment involves elicitation and rating of the positive and negative symptoms that characterize each individual's mental disorder. The nature and severity of these symptoms may change over time and as a result of treatment. For example, schizophrenic patients' hallucinations and delusions often have episodic courses, remitting and exacerbating in response to changes in medication and socioenvironmental stress. As noted by Lukoff and coauthors in Chapter 3, symptoms of psychiatric illness also intrude upon affect and cognition. In addition, cardinal features of schizophrenic and affective disorders are the cognitive distortions and defects in motivation that are presumably a result of neurotransmitter system abnormalities. By regularly monitoring target symptoms, rehabilitation staff can improve the effectiveness of their interventions.

Environmental Demands and Supports

The fourth step in functional assessment requires evaluation of the physical and psychosocial aspects of the environment in which the patient will live or work and which must support the patient's chosen roles and acquired skills. Instruments available for evaluating the environment have tended to focus on institutional conditions and depend upon self-report inventories or direct observation.

The Multiphasic Environmental Assessment Procedure, developed by Moos and Lemke (1979), was designed to assess the social and physical environments of nursing homes, residential care settings, and other group living settings. It consists of five components, covering areas such as physical and architectural resources, policy and program resources, resident and staff resources, and the sheltered care environment. The Ward Atmosphere Scale (Moos, 1974) is a 100-item or 40-item true/false questionnaire for use with staff and patients of a psychiatric unit. Ten components cover areas such as involvement, support, spontaneity, management of anger and aggression, and program clarity.

While questionnaire instruments, such as those developed by Moos and his colleagues, can tap qualitative aspects of the environment indirectly through the perceptions of individuals participating in the environment, more reliable and valid methods for assessing the environment have recently become available through the use of direct behavioral observation, in which ratings are made of actual interactions over time.

Developed and validated by Paul (1987), the Observational Assessment Instrumentation for Service and Research includes the Time Sample Behavioral Checklist, the Staff-Resident Interaction Chronograph, and the Computerized Planned Access Observational Information System. The Staff-Resident Interaction Chronograph provides a continuous time- and situation-specific data base on psychosocial activities of clinical staff—the nature, amount, content, and distribution of verbal and nonverbal interactions that staff provide to patients in hospital or community settings. The Chronograph is employed by technician-level observers who summarize the data by computer for clinicians to make decisions regarding staff training, development, and utilization.

INSTRUMENTS AND METHODS FOR FUNCTIONAL ASSESSMENT

It should first be stated that no single, definitive instrument, interview process, or data source is available for comprehensive functional assessment in psychiatric rehabilitation. Functional assessment in psychiatric rehabilitation must be flexible enough for measurement of the variability in the functional course and outcome of mental disorders, both between individuals and in any particular individual over time. Practitioners of psychiatric rehabilitation are encouraged to develop functional assessment protocols or packages from currently available instruments for evaluating role functioning; coping skills and competencies; psychiatric, cognitive, and volitional impairments; and environmental demands and supports. Examples of two instruments—the Independent Living Skills Survey (ILSS) and the Occupational Case Analysis and Rating Scale (OCAIRS)—that facilitate data collection for individually and environmentally relevant and meaningful rehabilitation recommendations are given in the case example for Sam, pp. 88–91.

The mental health and rehabilitation literature abounds with instruments that can be used in functional assessment, and many reviews are available. Assessment instruments measure vocational functioning (Anthony, Cohen, & Danley, 1988; Boston, 1988), social skills (Liberman, 1982), behaviors that contribute to functional performance (Kuehnel & Liberman, 1988), target symptoms and impairments (Lukoff, Liberman, & Nuechterlein, 1986), social functioning (Beattie & Stevenson, 1984), broad ranges of client characteristics (Anthony & Farkas, 1982), and social adjustment (Weissman, 1975, Weissman & Sholomskas, 1982). Overviews have been published of available instruments used to assess functional living skills (Halpern & Fuhrer, 1984; Wallace, 1986) and instruments used by occupational therapists and others (Asher, 1989; Newman, 1980; Ciarlo, Edwards, Kiresuk, Newman, & Brown, 1981). A summary of a broad array of functional assessment instruments is reproduced in Table 4.1.

It is not within the scope of this chapter to review all available instruments, but rather to provide the clinician with a framework for selecting instruments for data collection. We encourage clinicians to review and consider building a full complement of instruments from which they may select one or more, depending on the specific individual with whom they are working and the social and task environments in which the individual will enact valued roles.

Before they administer assessment instruments such as questionnaires, interviews, or direct observation, practitioners working in rehabilitation must grasp several general principles that are discussed in the following sections of this chapter. These principles are the (a) engagement of the patient in an active process of goal setting; (b) selection of sources of data for functional assessment; (c) responsibility and competencies required by mental health or rehabilitation professionals for functional assessment; (d) monitoring of functional changes; and (e) integration and interpretation of data into a longitudinal pattern as rehabilitation proceeds.

Engagement of Patient in Goal Setting

As its starting point, assessment must be able to engage and assist the patient in articulating a set of goals for social, occupational, and instrumental role functioning. Therefore, careful attention should be paid to the therapeutic relationship and rapport that succeed in generating an active dialogue between assessor and patient resulting in the establishment of meaningful goals. Once this is accomplished, formal evaluation of skills and deficits leading to rehabilitation planning may begin.

In working with their patients, clinicians often fear that unreasonable goals and expectations will be identified by individuals with chronic mental disorders. As a result, clinicians often move to establish treatment and rehabilitation plans based on their assessment of patients' deficits, without regard for coupling these with patients' goals. When patronized in this manner, patients often feel their own needs are not being considered, leading to poor compliance with recommended interventions. We recommend an approach in which patients are actively encouraged to elaborate their goals and then target interventions so that these goals are realized.

Keith is a 26-year-old man who was recently diagnosed as having paranoid schizophrenia. When psychotic symptoms were controlled with antipsychotic medications, he engaged in a rehabilitation planning effort with an occupational therapist who was a member of a community mental health center treatment team. When first asked to identify his goals, he said he wanted to enter college and complete his bachelor's degree. He hadn't been in school for 6 years, and said he wanted to matriculate as a full-time student in a prestigious school in engineering. The clinician felt this was unrealistic. On further exploration, it was learned that Keith had felt happiest when he was in school, and he now thought this would be the best way to realize his goal of being "happy and independent." Once this goal of becoming independent and more pleased with himself was identified, he was helped by his therapist to set as a long-term goal resumption of his schooling at a local trade school. He then began to work with his ther-

Table 4.1. Major Characteristics of Instruments Measuring Functional Living Skills of the Chronically Mentally Ill

INSTRUMENT	AREAS ASSESSED	TIME FRAME OF ASSESSMENT	DATA COLLECTION METHOD
Katz Adjustment Scale (KAS)—Katz & Lyerly (1963)	Symptoms, expected activities, recreation/leisure activities	Past "few" weeks	Form R; 205-item questionnaire completed by significant other Form S; 138-item questionnaire completed by patient
Personal Adjustment & Role Skills Scale (PARS)—Ellsworth et al. (1968)	Symptoms, substance abuse, general community functioning	Past month	5 versions of PARS, all questionnaires of 29 to 79 items completed by significant other
Social Behaviour & Adjustment Scale (SBAS)—Platt et al. (1980)	Symptoms, role performance, objective burden, household distress	Past month	Semistructured interview conducted with significant other that covers 329 items
Psychiatric Status Schedule (PSS)—Spitzer et al. (1970)	Symptoms, instrumental role performance	Past week (symptoms) Past month (role performance)	Patient version: 321 items rated during structured interview; informant version: items rated during structured interview
Psychiatric Evaluation Form (PEF)—Endicott & Spitzer (1972b)	Symptoms, instrumental role performance	Past week (symptoms) Past month (role performance)	28 items completed by experienced clinician using all sources of information
Current & Past Psychopathology Scale (CAPPS)—Endicott & Spitzer (1972a)	PEF + past adjustment, symptoms, & personality	PEF + from age 12 to 1 month before evaluation	PEF + 13 items of current symptoms + 130 items of Psychiatric History Scale completed by experienced rater
Social Adjustment Scale (SAS)—Weissman et al. (1971)	General and interpersonal performance & satisfaction in 6 instrumental roles	Past 2 months (SAS, SAS-II) Past 2 weeks (SAS-SR)	SAS: 42 items rated during interview with patient; SAS-SR: 42-item questionnaire completed by patient; SAS-II: 52 items for chronic patients rated in interview
Social Stress & Functioning Inventory (SSFIPD)—Serban (1978)	Performance and stress in 21 areas of community living	Not reported	174 performance items and 130 stress items rated during interview with patient
Denver Community Mental Health Questionnaire (DCMHQ)—Ciarlo & Riehman (1977)	Distress, isolation, drug and alcohol abuse, productivity, use agencies, satisfaction with service	Past 24 hours to past month	61 items rated during interview with patient
Community Adaptation Schedule (CAS)—Burnes & Roen (1967)	Behavior, affect, desire for change in 34 areas of functioning	Current	212-item questionnaire completed by patient
Rehabilitation Evaluation (REHAB)—Baker & Hall (1983)	"Deviant" behavior and "general" behaviors (speech, interaction, etc.)	Past week	7 deviant behavior items and 15 general behavior items completed by trained institutional staff

Note: Reprinted from Wallace (1986, pp. 606–607), with permission.

apist to target skills and deficits in the areas of grooming and conversational abilities. He saw these as essential to accomplish his goal of entering school. Three months later, he entered a mechanics school.

Sources of Data for Functional Assessment

Sources of data for functional assessment can include a review of a patient's past and current treatment and rehabilitation records; the observation of actual performance, preferably in natural environments (Paul, 1987); interview of the individual and key members of his or her support system; and the administration of questionnaires and tests.

Procedures may include standardized tests, questionnaires, performance checklists, activities, and tasks designed to evaluate specific abilities. The use of standardized test and interview procedures must be accompanied by an understanding of their scientific properties, including their validity, reliability, sensitivity, and specificity. Psychiatric rehabilitation interventions based on data having low validity and reliability can yield an inaccurate and distorted clinical image of an individual's functional performance. For example, if the sensitivity of an instrument is low, clinicians risk underidentifying the existence of conditions or true problems, and individuals may not receive needed interventions. Conversely, when the specificity of an instrument is low, clinicians risk identifying problems that do not exist and individuals may receive interventions that are not needed.

In addition, the design of a functional assessment in psychiatric rehabilitation will be influenced by the mission of an agency. For example, crisis stabilization units need to stress rapid assessment of patients' abilities to live independently and manage their symptoms, while long-term community adjustment programs may stress detailed assessment of leisure and basic conversation skills, and abilities to manage persistent symptoms. Moreover, the fiscal and staff resources of a rehabilitation setting delimit the scope of practice, the target population served, and thus the form and extensiveness of the assessment procedures. Data sources selected for use must yield information consistent with the mission and philosophy of the setting so that rehabilitation goals are congruent with agency resources and priorities. For instance, agencies with no in-house vocational rehabilitation capability are best served by using functional assessment instruments that yield basic information regarding vocational skills and then referring patients to appropriate agencies for more extensive assessment and training.

Functional Assessment: Responsibility and Competencies

Functional assessment as a process does not belong to any one disciplinary or professional group. The most efficient and progressive systems of care recognize the importance of a truly interdisciplinary clinical effort. This involves careful assignment of specific assessment tasks to appropriate members of the team, coupled with adequate communication among these members to integrate the functional assessment. Table 4.2 outlines the areas of functional assessment addressed by each of a number of disciplines in state hospital or community mental health settings. With an interdisciplinary team structure in place, and with proper supervision from senior clinicians, data collection may be managed so that it is both efficient and comprehensive.

Raymond is a 24-year-old man who was referred to the assessment team at a community mental health center for a comprehensive diagnostic and functional assessment. The team consisted of a psychiatrist, psychologist, occupational therapist, and case manager. The psychiatrist performed a clinical interview and administered two standardized instruments for diagnostic and symptom monitoring purposes, the Present State

Table 4.2. Discipline of Clinician and Functions Assessed in a Comprehensive Functional Assessment

DISCIPLINE OF CLINICIAN	FUNCTIONS ASSESSED
Nursing Assistant	Self-care and grooming
Nurse	Physical health, substance abuse, motor behavior
Psychiatrist	Psychiatric symptoms, role functioning
Psychologist	Attitude and motivation, attention and memory, communication skills
Social Worker	Family interactions, social interactions
Occupational Therapist	Role functioning, vocational and cognitive functioning

Examination and the Brief Psychiatric Rating Scale. The psychiatrist also engaged Raymond in a goal-setting process, in which he was helped to identify future goals.

Initially, Raymond could not identify any goals, but then said that he wanted to become a productive member of his family. He said he would also like to make some friends and socialize more. In addressing these concerns, the psychiatrist found that Raymond suffered from a number of psychiatric symptomatic impairments. These included incessant auditory hallucinations, persecutory delusions, blunted affect, tangential thinking, and severe distractibility. His attention and concentration were severely impaired, and he imagined he could write words on his hand with his fingers. He said he did this to "preserve" his thoughts. These symptomatic impairments greatly impaired his role functioning, in that he could not engage with family members in productive dialogue, performed poorly in his vocational skills program, and had no social contacts.

The psychologist worked with the family to identify their areas of concern and to target skills they might need in order to communicate effectively with Raymond and support his treatment and rehabilitation. She found that the family directly provided for many of Raymond's day-to-day needs, often at their emotional and financial expense. For example, due to his poor grooming and self-care skills they would sometimes shave him and would generally plan his days due to his skills deficits in the area of social problem solving.

The occupational therapist performed an assessment utilizing the Occupational Case Analysis and Rating Scale and the Independent Living Skills Survey. Raymond identified his primary role as a family member, and could not identify any desired future or past work roles. He was able to describe his daily routine, which was quite impoverished. Raymond evidenced poor attention and concentration, and was unable to perform several simple, concrete tasks assigned to him. He was highly distractible, and had poor problem-solving abilities. He and his family identified skills deficits in the areas of grooming and self-care, cooking, and money management.

The case manager performed an assessment using knowledge tests from several skills-training modules. She learned that Raymond had little information about the medications he was taking and could not identify community resources for leisure activities or public transportation. She also learned that his problem-solving skills were poor.

The team assembled its findings and made comprehensive recommendations to the family, outlining a rehabilitation plan that was comprehensive in scope and continuously

provided by members of a community mental health team. This included addressing his psychiatric impairments with medication, enrolling him in skills-training modules to improve his medication management and leisure skills, and seeing that his basic needs such as housing and food were addressed.

Monitoring of Functional Changes

While functional assessment is used for initial screening and diagnostic purposes, it must also be used for monitoring changes over time in an individual's adaptive functioning. Repeated measurement of role functioning; coping skills and competencies; psychiatric, cognitive and volitional impairments; and environmental demands and supports permit clinicians to evaluate the efficacy of rehabilitation interventions that have been provided. It is also important since there is variability within any one person's course of schizophrenia or other chronic mental disorder.

Periods of relapse and incapacity may alternate with periods of remission, with improved social, occupational, and instrumental role functioning. It is essential to keep track of a person's functional level so that appropriate rehabilitation goals and interventions can be keyed to the individual's capacity for learning and need for support. In addition, persons with chronic mental disorders may not persist in their engagement with rehabilitation activities or use of psychotropic medications, resulting in regression. Periodic functional assessments are then essential to determine the level of environmental supports that an individual will need at any given time as a result of these ups and downs in clinical course. The following vignette illustrates the importance of ongoing assessment.

Sarah is a 23-year-old woman with a diagnosis of Recurrent Major Depressive Disorder. She became increasingly dysfunctional over a period of 2 years. As her depression worsened she became isolated from others and had no social contacts for over 6 months, lost interest in recreational pursuits, and spent most of her time alone. Once she developed a relationship with her psychiatrist and took medication to control her depression, a functional assessment was performed. Her poor grooming skills and conversational abilities were targeted for intervention. Repeat assessment at 6 months revealed that she now groomed herself properly without prompting, and that her conversational abilities had greatly improved. She was now attending a community socialization group for young single individuals, and interventions were adjusted to target her deficient vocational skills.

Integration and Interpretation of Data

The integration and interpretation of the data collected during a functional assessment leads the clinician to formulate a *functional diagnosis*, identify *functional changes*, and determine a *functional prognosis* (Smith, 1990). Functional diagnosis highlights the functional deficits, functional assets, and most important, the relationship among roles, competencies, impairments, and environmental demands and supports. Functional changes can be observed by comparing patients' status over time, or by comparing behaviors to normative data sets across populations. Functional prognosis can include the likelihood of spontaneous return without rehabilitation and long-term projections in performance; and it can also highlight milestones in therapy.

APPLICATION OF THE FUNCTIONAL ASSESSMENT FRAMEWORK

In the following section we will apply the four-level framework for functional assessment presented earlier in this chapter through the use of a clinical vignette in which two instruments are utilized. These instruments, the Occupational Case Analysis and Rating Scale (OCAIRS), and the Independent Living Skills Survey (ILSS), are presented as tools for functional assessment that clinicians may consider for use in their own practice.

Occupational Case Analysis and Rating Scale

The OCAIRS, developed by Kielhofner and Kaplan (1989), is based on the model of human occupation and has been used by occupational therapists to guide collection, integration, and interpretation of data for functional assessment in psychiatric rehabilitation. The practice and profession of occupational therapy arose out of the belief of early 20th century mental health practitioners that the functional capacities of their psychiatric patients could be improved through orchestrating social and task environments. In this model the term *occupation* comprises an individual's roles and how the individual enacts these roles.

The OCAIRS is composed of a semistructured interview, a rating scale, and a summary form. The interview consists of a predetermined sequence of questions from which the interviewer can elaborate, eliciting information in 11 domains, including personal causation, values and goals, interests, roles, habits, skills, output, physical environment, social environment, feedback, and historical data. In addition to evaluating each of these domains, the rater makes global judgments about the individual's functioning. The completed ratings are organized to provide a profile of the individual's strengths and weaknesses.

Because the instrument is largely based on the respondent's self-perception, observation of actual performance is necessary to evaluate the relationship between the individual's perception and his or her actual level of functioning. Additional assessment instruments, based on the model of human occupation, can be used in conjunction with the OCAIRS and incorporated into the narrative report. These include the Role Checklist (Oakley, 1981), in which information is collected about an individual's past, present, and future roles; the Occupational Questionnaire (Riopel, Kielhofner, & Watts, 1986), in which information is collected about an individual's daily routine and degree of interest, value, and personal causation in daily activities; and the Interest Checklist (Matsutuyu, 1967), designed to gather data on an individual's interest patterns.

The OCAIRS was originally designed for use with psychiatric patients having depression and schizophrenia; however, the interview appears relevant to most psychiatric patients with the possible exception of very low functioning, institutionalized populations who are unable to cooperate in an interview and whose verbal responses are unlikely to be reliable. Interrater reliability, as assessed using intraclass correlation coefficients, is reasonably good for the majority of individual component ratings (Casales, 1984; Kaplan, 1984). The OCAIRS has adequate content validity (Weinstein, 1984) and concurrent validity with the Global Assessment Scale (Brollier, Watts, Bauer, & Schmidt, 1988).

Independent Living Skills Survey

The ILSS (Wallace, 1986) was developed to provide a detailed assessment of the community living skills of chronically mentally ill patients residing with significant others or in residential care facilities such as family-care and board-and-care homes. Nine domains are assessed, including eating habits, grooming skills, domestic activities, food preparation skills, health maintenance skills, economic skills, use of public transportation, leisure activities, and job-seeking skills. The nine domains were selected based on a review of 15 previously validated measures of the functioning of chronically mentally ill patients and developmentally disabled patients supplemented by interviews with community social workers and operators of residential care facilities.

This instrument can be used to gather information on the community living skills of individuals through a questionnaire administered to the patient or to caregivers. Direct observation of the component skills can also supplement the information gained from self-report.

Each skill is elicited by specific questions designed to assess the frequency with which an individual is able to perform certain tasks autonomously and appropriately. A 5-point scale is used with anchors referring to the frequency and degree of problem with each skill, ranging from "never" to "always." Finally, the evaluator is asked to make a global assessment of the individual's level of functioning on an 11-point scale.

The ILSS was designed for use with patients residing in the community as well as with hospitalized patients, to gauge their readiness for independent living. It may be used with individuals across a wide spectrum of functioning, from those at relatively high levels to those who are more chronically disabled and dysfunctional. One special advantage of the ILSS lies in its providing specific information on deficits in community living skills that can become targets or goals for rehabilitation. Studies have indicated that the ILSS is reliable and valid (Wallace, 1986), including being predictive of long-term vocational outcomes (Liberman, Massel, Mintz, Arruda, & Nugent, 1990).

Case Example

Sam, a 23-year-old man, experienced the insidious onset of a schizophrenic disorder at the age of 16 when he showed social withdrawal and poor school performance. He had been a good student, and was an accomplished musician, having begun performing publicly at the age of 8. Sam progressively developed auditory hallucinations, persecutory delusions, and a formal thought disorder. His social network became constricted so that he had no friends or social contacts aside from his mother and stepfather at the time of assessment.

A functional assessment was conducted by Sam's case manager, a member of the interdisciplinary team at a community mental health center. The case manager involved Sam, his mother, and stepfather in the assessment through interviews, and also directly observed Sam's behavior in a variety of settings. The following are the results of the OCAIRS and the ILSS. The findings are organized according to the four level model presented in this chapter: the *roles* in which an individual desires to engage, the *coping skills* and competencies needed to engage in those roles, the psychiatric, cognitive and volitional *impairments* that may impede acquisition or use of skills, and the *environmental demands and supports* that will impede or enhance efforts to engage in desired roles.

Role Functioning

Current. Sam stated that his primary role was being a family member, but he was unable to describe the activities or obligations of such a role. His engagement in playful and productive activity was severely restricted and he found it difficult to perform meaningful daily activities routinely and adequately. He described a minimally organized daily schedule of activities, slept late, and did very little in a day. He indicated that on weekends he had "more energy," but did not elaborate a schedule of activities.

Sam said he valued "communicating with his mother," "keeping a realistic view," and "getting things to work." He imagined the long-term future would be "a nightmare" and expected to be "kind of footloose."

Future. He identified roles of living independently, having a job on a part-time basis, and playing his musical instrument again. On prompting, he said he would also like to have some social acquaintances.

Past. Sam remembered a significant role as student, saying his best time was when he was in the fourth grade. He remembered being a "terror," "growing quickly," and "being obnoxious and provocative with (his) classmates, but not the teacher." He stated that his worst time was in "high school, when (he) should have been pulling better grades." He indicated that he did not graduate and had no diploma. In addition, he reported never having been employed.

Skills

Social and problem-solving skills. Communication, planning, and problem-solving skills were present but impaired by psychotic intrusions. Sam stated that he had social difficulties, in that he was "not practical" in his decision making and problem solving.

Eating. Sam was able to eat neatly without prompting. He chewed his food properly and at a reasonable pace. He required prompting to eat a balanced diet, as he preferred to eat junk foods without regard to their nutritional content.

Grooming. Sam bathed each day without being told to do so. He shampooed his hair several times a week, and had no noticeable body odor. His hair was neatly brushed and cropped, and he brushed his teeth and shaved daily, all without prompting. He dressed normally and changed his clothing appropriately, also without prompting.

Domestic activities. Sam kept his room neat and clean, and made his bed daily with some prompting by his mother. He required prompting to change his bed linen on a regular basis, but did so when asked. Sam needed some prompting to wash his clothes. He was able to cook a limited number of simple meals for himself and did so without prompting at appropriate times. He regularly washed his dishes promptly after using them.

Health. Sam cared for his own health appropriately, and had no medical problems. He took prescribed medications faithfully and followed suggestions of health care professionals.

Money management. Sam did not manage his money independently and received public support. His mother cashed his check for him and directed much of his spending. He was taken by the family to stores and they paid his bills through their own checking account. He did not participate in budgeting his money. His use of the telephone was not excessive, thus causing no financial problems in this area.

Transportation. Sam did not have a driver's license, nor did he use public transportation, which was available. He was driven to appointments and to stores by his family.

Leisure. Sam could not identify any hobbies in which he was involved. He did say that he wanted to resume his former hobby of building model cars. He never socialized, did not use community recreational facilities, and was reluctant to go for walks or to movies. He went out to a restaurant with his family on one occasion in the month preceding evaluation.

Job-seeking or job-related skills. Sam never held a job and was not seeking one. He had no concrete job aspirations but said he would like to develop such direction.

Impairments

Volition. Sam expressed little confidence in his abilities and rarely anticipated successful outcomes of action. He proudly described his present attempt "to try and recover his life," but was unable to outline any steps he would take to build his skills in areas where he lacked confidence. He described himself as "lazy" and "not being like most people."

There was a major reduction in his belief about his effectiveness and in his scope of interests.

Cognitive. Sam evidenced poor attention and concentration, and was unable to focus his attention on assigned tasks for longer than several minutes at a time. He was also highly distractible and had poor problem-solving abilities.

Psychiatric. Sam evidenced severe persecutory delusions and auditory hallucinations which intruded on his functional activities. The hallucinations were deprecatory in nature, consisting of multiple voices. He also evidenced a moderately severe formal thought disorder. His affect was severely blunted.

Environmental Analysis

The physical and psychosocial environments were both rich with resources for encouraging and reinforcing adaptive behavior, yet, as noted previously, his engagement in activities was severely limited.

Physical environment. The physical environment supported the performance of valued activities to some extent. Finances were not a problem, nor was transportation. Observation of the home environment noted a rich set of leisure opportunities and access to other resources. He lived with his mother and stepfather in a spacious home where he had the privacy of his own room. His mother provided him with financial support without apparent conflict.

Psychosocial environment. The values and attitudes of his significant others definitely supported successful role performance. His comments reflected their active support of his goals and active collaboration in his daily life. His mother was eager to see him function at a higher level and was prepared to participate in and finance his rehabilitation.

Functional Diagnosis

Sam saw himself as engaging in only one primary role, that of "family member." Past roles included that of student and musician, but not worker. Future desired roles included being a worker and achieving independence. Sam's engagement in recreational and productive activity was severely restricted and he found it difficult to perform meaningful daily activities routinely and adequately. He essentially had no productive activity to anticipate, engage in, or use to structure his day.

Skill competencies were primarily in the domains of self-care and home-care management. Skill deficits were in the domain of affiliative social skills, money management, transportation, leisure, and vocational functioning. Sam was not taking any psychotropic medications at the time of the initial psychiatric assessment and expressed dissatisfaction with previous medications he had taken. Psychotic symptoms clearly continued to impair his skill utilization and acquisition, and his cognitive deficits impaired his ability to receive and process information. Finally, there was a major reduction in his belief about his personal effectiveness, in his scope of interests, and in his personal values.

Functional Changes

Sam had had limited psychiatric treatment and rehabilitation and as a result had become progressively more restricted in the scope of his daily activities. He perceived little of his past functioning as adaptive. Despite the previous but limited psychiatric rehabilitation, personal maturation, and a supportive social and physical environment, he remained disabled.

Functional Prognosis

Sam could certainly benefit from focused and prioritized rehabilitation interventions, and was likely to be able to work and live independently in the future. Several factors contributed to a good prognosis for him: he was motivated to engage in a rehabilitation effort, had supportive social and physical environments, had not had an adequate trial on psychiatric medications, had excellent self-care and home-care management skills, and had a history of engaging in a regular occupational activity (as a student and musician) with success. Risk factors included his lack of employment history, progressive social isolation, failure of psychotic symptoms to remit despite limited psychiatric interventions, and significant reduction in perceived self-efficacy.

Rehabilitation efforts would best be directed toward helping Sam build a daily routine that incorporates areas of interest and pleasure, and that is congruent with his stated desire to "recover" his life. Daily activities could include preparation for completing his high school diploma, musical practice, and daily monitoring of his symptom status. Social-skills training focusing on medication and symptom self-management would also be helpful.

Given his youth, his limited exposure to occupational opportunities, and his continuing psychiatric problems, vocational testing and counseling were not recommended at the time of initial functional assessment. Sam had not developed sufficient personal knowledge regarding his interests, abilities, and values to make a meaningful occupational choice. When his stamina and psychiatric condition have improved, *and* he began to express a specific desire for employment, vocational counseling and supportive employment options could be introduced.

Sam would benefit from a gradual introduction into the work force. Early efforts could focus on building his stamina for work and gaining knowledge about his skills and values. Given his level of self-care skills and his ability to complete home-management activities when directed, it was recommended that semisupervised apartment living be explored. This should be coupled with a structured social program to prevent him from remaining socially isolated.

CONCLUSIONS

Functional assessment is an ongoing, carefully planned process of collecting, integrating, and interpreting information regarding an individual's past and current adaptation. The result of this process is the rehabilitation plan for maximizing future adaptation. Functional assessment should be organized so that a summary is provided of the patient's desired roles, coping skills and competencies, impairments, and environmental demands and supports.

If the purpose of functional assessment is to determine broad areas of living skills for which rehabilitation may be desirable, then one or another of the more comprehensive and inclusive instruments outlined in Table 4.1 may be appropriate, such as the Social Adjustment Scale (Weissman, 1971). An advantage of these instruments is that they are useful for evaluating entire rehabilitation programs and describing the characteristics of patients who participate in them. Furthermore, they often include assessments of psychopathology and antisocial behaviors that, even at very low frequencies of occurrence, may impede successful adaptation to community life among patients who are skilled enough to prepare their own food, seek a job, or care for their personal possessions. If significant others are available, then instruments that use information from both patients and informants may be particularly appropriate.

If, however, the purpose of the assessment is to pinpoint behaviors that will be a focus of the rehabilitation plan, then one of the more specific instruments may be appropriate, such as the Independent Living Skills Survey. Unfortunately, the psychometric adequacy of these instruments is not generally as well documented as that of the more comprehensive instruments; furthermore, the more specific the instruments, the more limited is the range of patients to whom they can be successfully administered. Furthermore, assessment useful for developing and monitoring rehabilitation procedures should be guided by procedures that can be feasibly implemented.

Indeed, the most appropriate assessment procedures for planning rehabilitation may involve administration of the very instruments that are part and parcel of the specific rehabilitation procedures to be used. For example, an assessment in use at the University of California at Los Angeles Center for Schizophrenia and Psychiatric Rehabilitation consists of role-play exercises and information inventories extracted from social and independent living skills-training modules developed at that center.

For most settings, the most desirable functional assessment package would include a set of instruments, ranging from those that are global through those that engage patients in the actual tasks they will perform in their rehabilitation. Such a packet should be tailored to the individual patient and program so that it accurately addresses identified needs and goals, which then fit into existing or planned interventions.

REFERENCES

Anthony, W. A., & Cohen, B. F. (1984). Functional assessment in psychiatric rehabilitation. In A. Halpern & M. Fuhrer (Eds.), *Functional assessment in rehabilitation* (pp. 79–100). Baltimore, MD: Brookes.

Anthony, W. A., Cohen, M. R., & Nemec, P. B. (1986). Assessment in psychiatric rehabilitation. In B. Bolton (Ed.), *Handbook of measurement and evaluation in rehabilitation* (pp. 299–312). Baltimore, MD: Brookes.

Anthony, W. A., Cohen, M. R., & Danley, K. S. (1988). The psychiatric rehabilitation model as applied to vocational rehabilitation. In J. A. Ciardiello & M. B. Bell (Eds.), *Vocational rehabilitation of persons with prolonged psychiatric disorders* (pp. 59–80). Baltimore, MD: Johns Hopkins University Press.

Anthony, W. A., & Farkas, M. A. (1982). A Client-outcome planning model for assessing psychiatric rehabilitation interventions. *Schizophrenia Bulletin, 8*, 13–38.

Anthony, W. A., & Liberman, R. P. (1986). The practice of psychiatric rehabilitation: Historical, conceptual, and research base. *Schizophrenia Bulletin, 12*(4), 542–559.

Asher, I. E. (1989). *An annotated index of occupational therapy evaluation tools.* Rockville, MD: American Occupational Therapy Association.

Baker, R., & Hall, J. N. (1983). *Rehabilitation evaluation of Hall and Baker (REHAB).* Aberdeen, Scotland: Vine Publishing.

Barris, R. (1982). Environmental interactions as extension of the model of occupation. *American Journal of Occupational Therapy, 36*, 637–644.

Beattie, M., & Stevenson, J. (1984). Measures of social functioning in psychiatric outcome research. *Evaluation Review, 8*, 631–644.

Bigelow, D. A., Brodsky, G., Steward, L., & Olson, M. (1982). The concept and measurement of quality of life as a dependent variable in evaluation of mental health services. In G. J. Stahler & W. R. Tash (Eds.), *Innovative approaches to mental health evaluation.* New York: Academic Press.

Boston, B. (1988). Vocational assessment of persons with psychiatric disorders. In J. A. Ciardiello & M. D. Bell (Eds.), *Vocational rehabilitation of persons with prolonged psychiatric disorders* (pp. 177–195). Baltimore, MD: Johns Hopkins University Press.

Boston, B., & Cook, D. W. (Eds.). (1980). *Rehabilitation client assessment.* Baltimore, MD: University Park Press.

Brollier, C., Watts, J. H., Bauer, D., & Schmidt, W. (1988). A concurrent validity study of two occupational therapy evaluation instruments. *Occupational Therapy in Mental Health, 8*, 4.

Brollier, C., Watts, J., Bauer, D., & Schmidt, W. (1988). A content validity study of the assessment of occupational functioning. *Occupational Therapy in Mental Health, 8*, 4.

Brown, M., Gordon, W. A., & Diller, L. (1983). Functional assessment and outcome measurement: An integrative review. In E. L. Pan, T. E. Backer, & C. L. Vash (Eds.), *Annual review of rehabilitation.* New York: Springer-Verlag.

Burnes, A. J., & Roen, S. R. (1967). Social roles and adaptation to the community. *Community Mental Health Journal, 3*, 153–158.

Casales, A. (1984). Unpublished research project, Baltimore, MD: Towson State University.

Christiansen, C. H. (in press). Occupational performance assessment. In C. H. Christiansen,

& C. Baum (Eds.), *Human performance deficits*. Thorofare, NJ: Slack.

Ciarlo, J. A., Edwards, D. W., Kiresuk, T. J., Newman, F. L., & Brown, T. R. (1981). *Final report: The assessment of client/patient outcome techniques for use in mental health programs*. Washington, DC: Department of Health and Human Services.

Ciarlo, J. A., & Riehman, J. (1977). The Denver Community Mental Health Questionnaire: Development of a multidimensional program evaluation. In R. D. Coursey, G. A. Specter, S. A. Murrel, & B. Hunt (Eds.), *Program evaluation for mental health: Methods, strategies, and participants*. New York: Grune & Stratton.

Coulton, C. (1979). Developing an instrument to measure person-environment fit. *Journal of Social Service Research, 3*, 159–173.

Cone, J. D. (1985). *The Pyramid Scales*. Available from Pro-Ed, 5341 Industrial Oaks Blvd, Austin, TX 78735.

Cubie, S., & Kaplan, K. (1982). A case analysis method for the model of human occupation. *American Journal of Occupational Therapy, 36*, 645–656.

Ellsworth, R. B., Foster, I., Childers, B., Arthur, G., & Kroeker, D. (1968). Hospital and community adjustment as perceived by psychiatric patients, their families and staff. *Journal of Consulting and Clinical Psychology, 32*, 1–41.

Endicott, J., & Spitzer, R. L. (1972a). Current and Past Psychopathology Scales (CAPPS): Rationale, reliability, and validity. *Archives of General Psychiatry, 27*, 678–687.

Endicott, J., & Spitzer, R. L. (1972b). What! Another rating scale? The Psychiatric Evaluation Form. *Journal of Nervous and Mental Disease, 154*, 88–104.

Frey, W. D. (1984). Functional assessment in the 1980's: A conceptual stigma and a technical challenge. In A. S. Halpern & M. J. Fuhrer (Eds.), *Functional assessment in rehabilitation*. Baltimore, MD: Brookes.

Fuhrer, M. J. (1987). *Rehabilitation outcomes: Analysis and measurement*. Baltimore, MD: Brookes.

Glynn, S., & Mueser, K. T. (1986). Social learning for chronic mental inpatients. *Schizophrenia Bulletin, 12*, 648–668.

Habeck, R., Frey, W., Sheppard, C., Galvin, D., & Allen, L. (1986). Functional assessment reflects trends in rehabilitation practice, technology. *The Interconnector*. East Lansing, MI: University Center for International Rehabilitation, Michigan State University.

Halpern, A. S., & Fuhrer, M. J. (Eds.). (1984). *Functional assessment in rehabilitation*. Baltimore, MD: Brookes.

Harding, C. M., & Strauss, J. S. (1985). The course of schizophrenia: An evolving concept. In M. Alpert (Ed.), *Controversies in schizophrenia*, (pp. 339–350). New York: Guilford Press.

Kaplan, K. (1984). Short-term assessment: The need and a response. *Occupational Therapy in Mental Health, 4*, 29–45.

Kaplan, K., & Kielhofner, G. (1989). *Occupational Case Analysis Interview and Rating Scale*. Thorofare, NJ: Slack.

Katz, M. M., & Lyerly, S. B. (1963). Methods for measuring adjustment and social behavior in the community: I. Rationale, description, discriminative validity and scale development. *Psychological Reports, 13*, 502–535.

Kaufert, J. M. (1983). Functional ability indices: Measurement problems in assessing their validity. *Archives of Physical Medicine and Rehabilitation, 64*, 260–267.

Kielhofner, G. (Ed.). (1985). *A model of human occupation: Theory and application*. Baltimore, MD: Williams and Wilkins.

Kiernat, J. M. (1982). Environment: The hidden modality. *Journal of Physical and Occupational Therapy in Geriatrics, 21*, 3–12.

Kuehnel, T., & Liberman, R. P. (1988). Functional assessment. In R. P. Liberman (Ed.), *Psychiatric rehabilitation of chronic mental patients*. Washington, DC: American Psychiatric Press.

Liberman, R. P. (1982). Assessment of social skills. *Schizophrenia Bulletin, 8*, 62–83.

Liberman, R. P., Massel, H. K., Mintz, J., Arruda, M. J., & Nugent, S. (1990). *Psychiatric symptoms and the functional capacity for work*. Paper presented at the Annual Meeting of the American Psychiatric Association, May, New York.

Lifchez, R. (1979). The environment as a social support system for independent living. *Archives of Physical Medicine and Rehabilitation, 60*, 467–476.

Lukoff, D., Liberman, R. P., & Nuechterlein, K. H. (1986). Symptom monitoring in the rehabilitation of schizophrenic patients. *Schizophrenia Bulletin, 12*(4), 578–593.

Matsutuyu, J. (1967). The interest checklist.

American Journal of Occupational Therapy, 32, 628–630.

McDowell, I., & Newell, C. (1987). *Measuring health: A guide to rating scales and questionnaires*. New York: Oxford University Press.

Moos, R. H. (1974). *Evaluating treatment environments: A social ecological approach*. New York: Wiley.

Moos, R. H., & Lemke, S. (1979). *Multiphasic environmental assessment procedure*. Palo Alto, CA: Stanford University Press.

Nagi, S. Z. (1977). The disabled and rehabilitation services: A national overview. *American Rehabilitation, 2*, 26–33.

Neville, A., & Kielhofner, G. (1983). *Modified Interest Checklist*. Unpublished workbook. Chicago: National Institutes of Health.

Newman, F. L. (1980). Global scales: Strengths, uses and problems of global scales as an evaluation instrument. *Evaluation and Program Planning, 3*, 257–268.

Oakley, F. The model of Human Occupation in Psychiatry (unpublished master's research project, Virginia Commonwealth University, 1982).

Paul, G. L. (Ed.). (1987). *Observational assessment instrumentation for service and research*. Champaign, IL: Research Press.

Platt, S., Weyman, A., Hirsch, S., & Hewett, S. (1980). The Social Behavior Assessment Schedule (SBAS): Rationale, contents, scoring, and reliability of a new interview schedule. *Social Psychiatry, 15*, 43–55.

Riopel, N., Kielhofner, G., & Watts, J. (1986). The relationships between volition, activity pattern, and life satisfaction in the elderly. *American Journal of Occupational Therapy, 40*, 278–283.

Rogers, J., Weinstein, J., & Figone, J. (1978). The interest checklist: An empirical assessment. *American Journal of Occupational Therapy, 32*, 628–630.

Serban, G. (1978). Social Stress and Functioning Inventory for Psychotic Disorders (SSFIPD): Measurement and prediction of schizophrenics' community adjustment. *Comprehensive Psychiatry, 19*, 337–347.

Smith, R. O. (1990). Synthesizing and interpreting functional assessment data for meaningful recommendations. In C. B. Royeen (Ed.), *Assessing function*. AOTA Self Study Series. Rockville, MD: American Occupational Therapy Association.

Spitzer, R. L., Endicott, J., Fleiss, J. L., & Cohen, J. (1970). The Psychiatric Status Schedule: A technique for evaluating psychopathology and impairment in role functioning. *Archives of General Psychiatry, 23*, 41–55.

Taylor, C. B., Liberman, R. P., & Agras, W. S. (1982). Treatment and evaluation in behavior therapy. In J. M. Lewis, & G. Usdin (Eds.), *Treatment planning in psychiatry*. Washington, DC: American Psychiatric Press.

Wallace, C. (1986). Functional assessment in rehabilitation. *Schizophrenia Bulletin, 12*, 604–630.

Watts, J. H., Brollier, C., Bauer, D., & Schmidt, W. (1988). A comparison of two evaluation instruments used with psychiatric patients in occupational therapy. *Occupational Therapy in Mental Health, 8*, 4.

Watts, J., Kielhofner, G., Bauer, M., Gregory, M., & Valentine, D. (1986). The assessment of occupational functioning: A screening tool or use in long-term care. *American Journal of Occupational Therapy, 40*, 231–240.

Weinstein, B. (1984). Unpublished research project. Baltimore, MD: Towson State University.

Weissman, M. M. (1975). The assessment of social adjustment. *Archives of General Psychiatry, 32*, 357–365.

Weissman, M. M., Paykel, E. S., Siegal, R., & Klerman, G. L. (1971). The social role performance of depressed women: Comparisons with a normal group. *American Journal of Orthopsychiatry, 41*, 390–405.

Weissman, M. M., & Sholomskas, D. (1982). The assessment of social adjustment by the clinician, the patient, and the family. In E. I. Burdock, A. Sudilovsklу, & S. Gershon (Eds.), *The behavior of psychiatric patients: Quantitative techniques for evaluation*. New York: Marcel Dekker.

Wood, P. H. N. (1980). Appreciating the consequences of disease: The classification of impairments, disabilities, and handicaps. *The WHO Chronicle, 34*, 376–380.

World Health Organization (WHO). (1980). *International classification of impairments, disabilities, and handicaps: A manual of classification relating the consequences of disease*. Geneva: Author.

CHAPTER 5

SOCIAL SKILLS TRAINING

Patrick W. Corrigan
Mark L. Schade
Robert Paul Liberman

Social skills training has become an essential component of current psychiatric rehabilitation strategies (Anthony & Nemec, 1984; Liberman et al., 1986). Mentally disabled patients have serious deficits in interpersonal behavior and social functioning (Zigler & Phillips, 1961, 1962). Patients may be alienated from their friends and families, unable to communicate appropriately with others, and unable to find and maintain work. In addition, many patients have difficulty coping with the requirements of daily living, which include planning and carrying out important instrumental tasks, such as dealing with social agencies, negotiating treatment with caregivers, or cashing a check. These deficits, in conjunction with psychiatric symptoms, severely limit the disabled individual's capacity for functioning effectively outside of the supervised or custodial settings.

Antipsychotic medications may alleviate severe psychiatric symptoms, such as hallucinations, delusions, mood swings, and neurovegetative symptoms. However, medications have been less effective in controlling the negative symptoms associated with psychiatric disorders, including deficits in social functioning, and they do not provide patients with the skills needed to survive in the community. Social skills training is a psychosocial intervention specifically designed to meet the needs of socially dysfunctional patients. Social skills training represents a structured application of behavioral learning techniques aimed at helping patients build a repertoire of skills that improve their ability to function adequately in the community.

Behavioral assessment of the individual's deficits provides information which guides the focus of training. Information may be drawn from observations of the patient's performance in role play or simulated interactions, as well as from direct observation of behavior in natural settings. Patients' self-reported perceptions of their social environments, their reactions to problem situations, and data obtained from family members and significant others in the patients' environment may all yield information relevant to the training effort. Repeated assessments throughout the course of training allow evaluation of patients' progress in acquiring the targeted skills.

Key elements of social skills training programs include didactic presentation of relevant information, modeling, repeated rehearsal of the skills via role-play exercises, contingent use of material and social reinforcers, corrective feedback to shape the targeted behaviors, and homework assignments designed to promote the use of newly acquired skills in real-life situations.

EFFICACY OF SOCIAL SKILLS TRAINING

In evaluating the effectiveness and usefulness of social skills training programs, a number of important issues must be addressed. First, it is essential to determine whether such programs result in the acquisition of the desired skills. It must be shown that patients do in fact learn or relearn skills as a consequence of the training procedures. Second, for patients to receive the maximum benefit from skills training, they must be able to use their newly acquired skills in a variety of actual situations outside the treatment setting. In other words, newly acquired behaviors should transfer to novel situations and settings outside the training environment if training is to be considered successful. Third, it must be demonstrated that the acquisition of social skills improves the patients' capacity to adjust to the community. If patients actually do use their skills in the community, they should stay out of the hospital longer and experience fewer and less severe relapses of psychiatric symptoms. Finally, successful training may affect other areas of patients' lives. The effects of social skills training on patients' satisfaction with and general quality of life needs to be demonstrated.

Acquisition of Social Skills

Three primary classes of behavior are often targeted for modification using skills-training techniques (Fecteau & Duffy, 1986; Morrison & Bellack, 1984; Wallace et al., 1980; Wallace, Boone, Donahoe, & Foy, 1985). *Response topography* includes specific nonverbal and paralinguistic behaviors such as voice volume and fluency, eye contact, and hand gestures. *Content-related behaviors* constitute a more molar class of behaviors, such as expressing appreciation, making a positive statement, and requesting additional information. *Cognitive problem-solving skills* include perceptual, attentional, information processing, and generative skills that facilitate an individual's ability to utilize topographic skills effectively. Accurately perceiving social situations, identifying emotions, self-monitoring, generating and evaluating response alternatives, and determining the appropriateness of one's behavior for a particular situation are examples of cognitive–social skills.

Results of research suggest that many specific verbal and nonverbal behaviors are successfully acquired by patients in skills-training programs (Morrison & Bellack, 1984; Wallace et al., 1980). For example, training in social and conversational skills in fourteen 90-minute training sessions for seven long-stay, mixed-diagnosis female residents of a token economy ward resulted in increased eye contact, better posture, less psychotic talk, and improved general conversational ability (Fecteau & Duffy, 1986). In another study, 28 male chronic schizophrenic patients were randomly assigned to either a life skills-training program or to a control condition (Brown & Munford, 1983). Patients in both groups received 20 hours of programmed treatment activities per week for 3 months. The skills-training program focused on topographic and content-related behaviors in the areas of interpersonal skills, nutrition, health, personal finances, time management, and community networking skills. Change scores on self-report measures and role-play assessments indicated that individuals in the training program successfully learned skills in these areas.

In a Veterans Affairs (VA) day hospital program, social skills training and stress management training was provided to 34 male outpatients (Frisch, Elliott, Atsaides, Salva, & Denney, 1982). The patients' performances on taped role-play situations and a simulated interaction task revealed that individuals assigned to social skills training alone, or in conjunction with stress management training, demonstrated greater acquisition of the targeted skills than patients assigned to a minimal treatment control condition.

Some skills-training programs focus on the acquisition of cognitive social skills in addition to overt behaviors. For example, training curricula have been designed to target social perception and cognitive self-management skills (Becker, Heimberg, & Bellack, 1987; Van Dam-Baggen & Kraaimaat, 1986), problem solving (Hansen, St. Lawrence, & Christoff, 1985) and information processing skills (Wallace, 1982). Wallace and Liberman (1985) reported the results of a controlled trial of social skills training for 28 male schizophrenic patients. The patients were randomly assigned to either an intensive social skills-training program or to an equally intensive holistic health therapy program. Skills training focused on *receiving* and *processing* components of interpersonal problem-solving skills, as well as *sending* appropriate responses. In addition, patients assigned to this program received behavioral family therapy that emphasized training in communication and problem-solving skills. Holistic health therapy focused on coping with life stressors through the use of yoga, meditation, walking, and jogging. Patients in this treatment group received supportive, insight-oriented family therapy. Patients in both programs received 6 hours of scheduled treatment daily for 9 weeks. Only individuals in the skills-training program were judged to have successfully acquired receiving and processing skills, based on their improved performance on questions designed to assess their ability to attend to and accurately perceive problem situations, to interpret interpersonal cues, and to generate, evaluate, and select reasonable response alternatives.

A multiple-baseline design was utilized to examine the effectiveness of interpersonal problem-solving training for six schizophrenic patients and one depressed patient in a partial hospitalization program (Hansen et al., 1985). Discussions of problem situations were audiotaped and rated for the presence of each skill component and for the overall effectiveness of the solutions generated by the patients. Performance on all skill components improved with training. Moreover, the investigators compared ratings of the patient's responses to those of a normal, nonpsychiatric sample and found that the psychiatric patients initially generated less effective solutions than normal individuals. However, the solutions of the psychiatric patients were as effective as those of normal individuals by the end of training.

Nezu (1986) evaluated the use of social problem-solving skills training with 32 individuals who met Research Diagnostic Criteria (RDC) for unipolar depression. Patients were randomly assigned to problem-solving therapy, problem-focused therapy, or a waiting-list control group. Problem-solving training focused on teaching subjects to define problems and formulate a range of possible solutions while problem-focused treatment was essentially a group psychotherapy program in which individuals were encouraged to discuss their problems with other group members. Both treatment programs consisted of eight weekly sessions ranging in length from 90 to 120 minutes. An analysis of group members' responses to a self-report inventory of problem-solving skills indicated that individuals who received skills training developed more effective problem-solving skills than their counterparts who received the other therapies.

Despite the fact that recent evidence indicates that both topographic and cognitive processing skills can be successfully acquired by psychiatric patients, a number of methodological problems remain. The quality of dependent measures assessing the acquisition of skills is questionable. Despite the fact that indices taken from role plays have excellent reliability, the validity of the measures is uncertain. Little association between role-play behavior and observation of behaviors in natural environments has been found (Bellack, Hersen, & Lamparski, 1979; Bellack, Hersen, & Turner, 1978). Therefore, it is unclear exactly what successful role playing is measuring. Similarly, measures of problem solving are dubious as well. The Means-End Problem Solving Test (MEPS) is the standard in this area but has failed to show adequate psychometric properties (Butler & Meichenbaum, 1981). New technologies for assessing the social functioning of residential patients in real-life settings are now available but have yet to be widely used (Paul, 1986, 1987a,b; in press a,b).

Evaluation of skills acquisition by psychiatric patients continues to be limited by the lack of data on competent social behavior in normal individuals (Morrison & Bellack, 1987). Little information is available regarding specific components of skilled social functioning, and few investigators make an effort to include nonpsychiatric validation samples in their research designs. Consequently, it is difficult to identify those skill components that are likely to be most relevant to normal functioning. Moreover, skills trainers are left with no objective criterion against which to measure deficits and improvements in social functioning.

Possible interactions between skills-training procedures and patient characteristics have not been adequately investigated. While effective training programs have been described for both depressed and schizophrenic individuals (Liberman, Massel, Mosk, & Wong, 1985), many studies suffer from a lack of reliable diagnostic assessment. Virtually no information is available on the learning of skills by patients having different types of cognitive and attentional deficits. Such deficits need to be assessed to clarify the relationships between cognitive-attentional processes and acquisition of socially skilled behavior.

Generalization of Skills-Training Effects

For patients to obtain maximum benefit from skills training, they must be able to use their newly acquired skills in a variety of real-life settings outside the training situation; however, the evidence suggesting generalization of these skills is mixed. Generalization of skills can be divided into *stimulus generalization*, in which patients perform targeted skills in social environments that differ from the training situation; *response generalization*, in which the repertoire of trained responses is flexible, leading to the performance of similar, but functionally different skills; and *durability*, in which acquired skills are maintained long after training is complete (Brown, 1982).

Numerous authors have been able to demonstrate that trained skills will transfer to different situations (Falloon, Lindley, McDonald, & Marks, 1977; Goldsmith & McFall, 1975; Hersen, Eisler, & Miller, 1974; Kazdin, 1974; Liberman, Mueser, & Wallace, 1986; McFall & Lillesand, 1971; Wallace & Liberman, 1985). However, other studies have not been as successful, finding that acquired behaviors do not transfer to other settings (Cole, Klarreich, & Fryatt, 1982; Frederiksen, Jenkins, & Foy, 1976; Hersen et al., 1974). Response generalization has been difficult to test as well, with both normative data and specific criteria by which to judge change in this construct lacking. Typically, assessment on response generalization has focused on whether functioning within independent domains such as work or recreation have improved. Early findings in this area have been largely negative (Bellack, Hersen, & Turner, 1976; Brown & Munford, 1983; Hersen, Eisler, & Miller, 1973; McFall & Lillesand, 1971; McFall & Twentyman, 1971). However, results from a recent study suggest that improved identification of problem components and increased generation of relevant solutions may generalize to related interpersonal behaviors (Hansen et al., 1985). These investigators found that 7 chronically disabled individuals were able to enlarge their repertoire of responses to problem situations.

The use of cognitively oriented skills-training techniques has yielded better generalization of the skills to related behaviors. For example, a cohort of schizophrenics at high risk for relapse received 30 hours per week of social skills training that focused on teaching patients actively to "solve" their problems. Results showed improvement not only on targeted skills but also in social functioning skills that were not trained (Wallace & Liberman, 1985). Similarly, in a study of skills training within the family context, Falloon and his coworkers (1977) found that first weekly, then biweekly, and finally monthly training sessions resulted in generalized improvements in employment, friendships, and functioning within the home.

Evidence regarding the durability of social skills has largely been positive when training has been sufficiently intensive, long term, and comprehensive. Several studies have shown that acquired skills are still performed at adequate levels 1 to 3 months later (Brown, 1982; Frisch et al., 1982; Jaffe & Carlson, 1976; Wallace et al., 1985). Other studies have shown that skills can be maintained over much longer periods of time (Holmes, Hansen, & St. Lawrence, 1984; Liberman et al., 1986; Monti, Curran, Corriveau, Delancey, & Hagerman, 1980), with two studies demonstrating that skills were reported at significant levels 2 years after training (Kindness & Newton, 1984; Longin & Rooney, 1975). However, contradictory evidence from two other studies shows that skills were not maintained after 2 to 3 months had passed (Spencer, Gillespie, & Ekisa, 1983; Van Dam-Baggen & Kraaimaat, 1986). Future research needs to account for the divergence in findings over generalization and maintenance variables. Relationships between specific variables and outcome need to be discerned. The discrepant findings may be attributed to differences in the diagnosis of the samples, aspects of the training procedures, or means of assessment.

Strategies for Promoting Generalization

Generalization may be advanced by using transfer strategies to guide skills training (Trower, 1986). Skills trainers need to make deliberate plans to include generalization promoting procedures into the treatment approach. Several of these strategies are summarized in Table 5.1.

Maintenance and generalization of skills are likely enhanced by overlearning, such that the greater the exposure to skills training, the longer the skills will be performed after training has ended. Skills-training programs of a few sessions' duration underestimate the vigor with which maladaptive behaviors are retained and the recalcitrance with which new skills are regularly performed. Criterion-based programs have been suggested as well in which training is repeated until the patient can perform the behavior at target levels. Liberman and his

Table 5.1. Generalization Strategies

Overlearning
Multiple training modules
Homework assignments
Use of natural reinforcers and caregivers
Problem-solving strategy
In vivo practice
Fading of training structure and supervision
Intermittent reinforcement
Teaching patients to use self-management

colleagues (1982) have suggested that several years of ongoing education with repeated booster sessions are necessary for adequate generalization and maintenance of skills in schizophrenics and those with cognitive dysfunctions that create learning disabilities. It is becoming increasingly clear that interdiction of the severely disabled person's maladaptive patterns will require lengthy and comprehensive intervention strategies to improve generalization and maintenance of skills.

Skills need to be trained in a range of different situations to foster stimulus generalization. Thus, conversational skills need to be trained for interpersonal situations, work skills for vocational settings, leisure skills for recreational settings, and medication management skills for responsible and compliant pharmacotherapy. By training skills in different situations, responses will be specific to a wide range of discriminative stimuli. Corrigan, Davies-Farmer, and Lome (1988) have outlined a comprehensive curriculum for severely disabled mental patients, based on Lazarus's (1981) multimodal system, including problem solving, health maintenance, sex and dating, relapse prevention, and cognitive remediation skills. Results of a 3-year study have shown that this comprehensive approach was able to decrease relapse rates significantly in 18 chronic schizophrenics.

In addition to a broad curriculum, several other strategies have been recommended to improve generalization skills. Trower (1986) suggested homework as an important transfer strategy. Hospital staff have been shown to be helpful in aiding patients to carry out homework. In a recent study with severely regressed, schizophrenic inpatients, generalization of basic conversation skills occurred when the therapists relayed the homework assignments to on-ward nursing staff as well as to patients (Martinez-Diaz et al., 1983). Nursing staff provided occasional prompts and reinforcement for patients engaging in their assignments.

Stokes and Baer (1977) have recommended that training occur in vivo. Skills that are carried out in the community enhance generalization and maintenance of the target behaviors. In this way, the contingencies and expectations specific to the trained milieu and the community can be blurred and the control over the stimuli and responses involved in training can be loosened. Different situational responses can be trained concurrently as well, thereby enhancing response generalization. Kazdin (1975) proposed that training programs use reinforcers that occur in natural situations, and that these reinforcers be given on intermittent schedules with family members managing the contingencies.

Symptom Remission and Relapse

A major goal of social skills training is to improve the patient's ability to function effectively in real-life settings. Beyond improvement in role functioning, successful training should also be associated with reductions in the frequency and severity of psychiatric symptoms, thereby helping to reduce relapse and rehospitalization. Presumably, skills acquired through training will protect an individual against relapse by strengthening his or her ability to cope with stressors and challenges from the natural environment.

Comprehensive social skills training can reduce clinical symptoms in psychiatric patients. Among schizophrenic inpatients and outpatients who are stabilized on medication, intensive social skills training significantly lowered symptoms (Falloon et al., 1982; Liberman, Falloon, & Wallace, 1984; Wallace & Liberman, 1985). Similarly, schizophrenics who participated in a day hospital program and concurrently received social skills training showed symptom reductions that were more durable over a 6-month follow-up period than did patients who were in the day hospital program but did not receive skills training (Bellack, Turner, Hersen, & Luber, 1984). Social skills training also alleviated depression for unmedicated depressed outpatients (McKnight, Nelson, Hayes, & Jarrett, 1984; Nezu, 1986) and for medicated depressed inpatients (Miller, Norman, & Keitner, 1989). It had clinical effects equivalent to antidepressant medication (Bellack, Hersen, & Himmelhoch, 1983) and was associated with a lower rate of dropout from treatment than medication or cognitive therapy (Bellack et al., 1983; Miller et al., 1989).

Hogarty et al. (1986) determined the effects of psychosocial treatments on preventing or postponing exacerbation of psychiatric symptoms by following 90 schizophrenic and schizoaffective patients at high risk for relapse. Patients were assigned to four treatment groups; some of the patients were on neuroleptic medications alone, while others received behavioral family therapy, social skills training, or a combination of both, in addition to medication. Relapse was defined as a change from "nonpsychotic" status at discharge to "psychotic" status, or was indicated by a team consensus that a severe clinical exacerbation of psychotic symptoms had occurred. Examination of relapse rates in the total sample 12 months after treatment indicated that both behavioral family therapy and social skills training were associated with lower relapse rates. While 41% of the patients in the drug control group relapsed during the follow-up period, about 20% of those patients assigned to either family therapy or to skills training experienced relapse, and none of the patients who received both family therapy and skills training relapsed. Moreover, data from a subsample of verifiably drug compliant individuals revealed a similar pattern of results.

Information on relapse over longer periods of time is available as well. Relapse and rehospitalization data have been reported for a controlled clinical trial comparing social skills training with holistic health therapy (Wallace & Liberman, 1985). Clinical relapse was defined as a substantial increase in psychiatrist ratings of symptomatology (Wallace, 1982). Nine months after treatment, 21% of the patients who received social skills training had relapsed, compared to 50% of the patients in holistic health therapy. A standard state hospital treatment control group from a concurrent study (Vaughn et al., 1982) yielded a 56% rate of relapse during the same 9-month period. By the end of the full 24-month follow-up period, 50% of the skills-training group members, and 79% of the holistic health therapy patients had experienced clinical relapse. Patients in the social skills group spent an average of 54 days in the hospital during these 2 years, and were rehospitalized a total of 16 times. By comparison, the holistic health group accumulated a total of 30 rehospitalizations, with group members spending an average of 87 days in institutional care. This study is notable for the inclusion of a lengthy follow-up and the use of multiple measures of psychiatric relapse. A longer follow-up period was used for 19 patients in a 3-month social skills-training program in a transitional halfway house setting (Friedlob, Janis, & Deets-Aron, 1986). Five years after treatment, 63% of the patients had successfully avoided rehospitalization and remained in the community. Although no control group was included in this study, the rehospitalization rate of approximately 37% compares favorably to rates reported elsewhere (Hogarty, Anderson, & Reiss, 1987; Wallace & Liberman, 1985).

The recent data on social skills training and psychiatric symptom relapse are encouraging, and indicate that skills-training programs place patients at lowered risk for relapse. However, relapse rates differ from study to study, and may fluctuate depending on a number of factors including lack of comparable definitions of relapse. The length of the follow-up period is critical. Skills-training programs demonstrate greater relapse-prevention effects within a year after treatment. Relapse rates increase with longer follow-up, suggesting that social skills training-programs effectively delay, rather than prevent, major exacerbations of psychiatric symptoms (Hogarty et al., 1987; Hogarty et al., 1986). The intensity and duration of the skills-training program is also important. Studies that include comprehensive, frequent training sessions over a year's time, followed by intermittent "booster" sessions, would be expected to demonstrate better relapse prevention than studies that use brief, limited skills-training programs (Bellack et al., 1984; Wallace & Liberman, 1985).

Since medication compliance affects relapse rates, could social skills training exert its antirelapse effects simply by facilitating adherence to medication regimens? Several investigators examined the interaction between social skills training and the administration of neuroleptic drugs (Falloon et al., 1982; Hogarty et al., 1986; Hogarty et al., 1987; Wallace & Liberman, 1985). Though significant interactions were not found, trends suggested that medication compliance is improved by social skills training; however, compliance did not fully account for the relapse protection afforded by social skills training.

The use of skills training to improve the coping capacities of patients and relatives appears to yield even greater protection against relapse. In a study of 36 schizophrenics considered at high risk for relapse because they lived with a high "expressed emotion" relative, subjects were randomly assigned to either a family skills-training or supportive therapy condition (Falloon et al., 1982). Family skills training focused on communication and problem-solving skills within the family unit and was carried out in the family home once a week for 3 months and then once every 2 weeks for 6 months. Family training ended with monthly booster sessions for the next 15 months. Patients in the supportive therapy condition met with an individual therapist for the same period of time. Results revealed that patients who received family therapy experienced relapse rates of 6% in 9 months and 11% in 2 years, while for the control group, relapse rates of 44% and 78%, respectively, were experienced. It is of note that, in this study, in vivo training and the involvement of the patient's natural support network may have produced greater generalization than in other studies where training was based in a hospital or clinic and relied on simulations of the patient's real-life relationships.

Quality of Life

Although research suggests that social skills training can improve social competence and decrease psychotic symptoms, little attention has been paid to whether this technology can improve the satisfaction patients feel in their day-to-day lives. Quality of life is a broad construct, so vast that it defies any singular definition. Quality of life can be measured by patients' self-ratings of their subjective satisfaction with their existence, by ratings made by significant others of patients' level of social functioning, and by objective indicators of material or social attainments (Lehman, Ward, & Linn, 1982). Malm and his associates (1981) described eight domains that make up a satisfying existence: sufficient medical and psychiatric care, a range of human relationships, the material goods necessary for life, communication and transportation services, fruitful working conditions, safety from crime and natural disasters, access to leisure and recreation activities, and inner spiritual life. Given the limited and dysfunctional life-style of most severely disabled psychiatric patients, the ability of social skills training to affect any of these domains may be the ultimate measure of the worth of this technology.

Quality of life can be measured by having the patient rate his or her level of participation in everyday life. While instruments have been developed to tap patients' subjective experience of "quality of life" (Carpenter, Heinrichs, & Hanlon, 1986; Klerman, 1977; Lehman, Ward, & Linn, 1982; Malm, May, & Dencker, 1981), only a few studies have assessed quality of life of persons with severe psychiatric disabilities. Liberman et al. (1986) measured this construct vis-à-vis Strauss and Carpenter's (1972, 1974, 1977) four levels of functioning before and after social skills training. Results showed that patients' everyday lives improved in two areas: positive symptoms significantly diminished while employment activity improved. In the same study, families rated their schizophrenic young adult offspring on several domains using the Katz Adjustment Scales, Revised (KAS-R). In contrast with the control group, the relatives of patients who received social skills training reported that they were more satisfied with the activities of their children who were now busy with church, friends, family, and leisure activities. However, the skills-training program was confounded by concurrent behavioral family therapy such that improved ratings on the KAS-R may have represented more benevolent attitudes regarding the severely disabled family member as a result of increased knowledge about the disease.

Liberman and several colleagues (1984) used completed homework assignments as an indicator of the impact of social skills training on social adjustment. They reasoned that if this form of training was able to improve the rate of completion of individually meaningful homework tasks, then the interventions had some utility in affecting the patient's daily life. Results from a multiple-baseline, single-subject experimental design found that social skills training improved the subjects' completion of homework tasks in hospital, family, and community settings. In another study, Marzillier and Winter (1978) searched for reasons 4 subjects who had demonstrated clear improvement in social functioning on single-subject designs after social skills training did not improve overall. They concluded that extratherapeutic change requires skills training to be one component of an overall treatment approach. They subsequently provided relaxation and cognitive interventions for these individuals, finding that overall functioning was enhanced.

From a community perspective, social skills training indirectly increases patients' quality of life to the extent that relapse decreases, thereby diminishing patients' stay in the hospital (Hogarty et al., 1986), and enabling them to return to a community in which they can enjoy the privileges society has to offer. Unfortunately, the potential of social skills training in particular, and community mental health in general, have failed to be realized (Bellack & Mueser, 1986). A majority of the chronic, mentally ill residing in urban environments and receiving outpatient care have marginal lives at best (Klerman, 1977; Lehman, Ward, & Linn, 1982). Given the plight of the severely disabled outpatient, improvement of community applications of skills training is clearly indicated. In reviewing the literature on community support programs, Test (1984) found that community treatment generally surpasses inpatient care for most outcome variables. Future research on the effect of skills training on quality of life must include evaluations of the system in which training occurs and in which the patient will be placed (Shepherd, 1986).

MODELS OF SOCIAL SKILLS TRAINING

Social skills training is no longer in its first generation having demonstrated its validity as a behavior change technology. Now approaching its third decade, social skills training is meeting the challenge to formulate models that address the limitations of its efficacy as well as guide future research endeavors. Until recently, skills training was without clear conceptual definition. Curran (1979) warned, "Unless we reach consensus about constructs we are addressing, we are likely to be building a Tower of Babel" (p. 325). Since that time, however, several models have been developed to chart current and future skills-training technology.

Stress-Vulnerability-Coping-Competence Model

The stress-vulnerability model describes the relationship between biological predispositions of psychosis and other major mental disorders, and contemporary environmental stressors that, when superimposed on a vulnerable person, bring about the onset of illness or relapse (Nuechterlein & Dawson, 1984a; Zubin & Spring, 1977). Even everyday, microstressors can accumulate, overcoming mentally ill individuals' ability to cope, and leading to exacerbation of symptoms (Birley & Brown, 1970; Brown & Birley, 1968). Acquisition of skills can protect some individuals against stress-induced relapse by conferring on them the ability to manage stressors through adaptive life skills. Skills can also enable individuals to galvanize more effectively a social support network to aid in stress management. In addition, overlearned skills that result in long periods of reinforcement and improved quality of life may actually promote salutary changes in the brain, thereby reducing psychobiological vulnerability.

Biological vulnerability and social functioning have a reciprocal relationship (see Figure 5.1). Prolonged vulnerabilities, especially during the prodromal years of schizophrenia or in combination with environmental stressors causing the onset of symptoms, interfere with the acquisition of skills typically important during the developmental years of adolescence and young adulthood. The skills repertoire of chronic psychiatric patients is subsequently limited without the social and coping skills necessary to deal with the demands and challenges of independent living in the community. At the same time, patients with few skills find it more difficult to cope with stressors (Wallace, 1984; Zigler & Phillips, 1961, 1962) and are unable to build a supportive network around themselves which could serve as a protective buffer against environmental stressors (Liberman et al., 1984). Moreover, the relapse of symptoms impedes the retrieval of whatever minimal skills may have been learned earlier. In a vicious cycle, the lack of a sufficient social and coping repertoire unmasks further vulnerability to stress with increased likelihood of relapse of symptoms.

Topographic Behavior Model

Social skills-training procedures were developed in the context of operant and social learning conceptions of abnormal behavior. In this view, social dysfunction comprises specific, observable behavioral excesses (e.g., hostile remarks) and deficits (e.g., poor eye contact) that prevent the individual from behaving appropriately in social situations. These problem behaviors are not necessarily global or stable in nature, but are likely to occur at particular times and places with specific individuals (Mischel, 1968, 1973; Ullmann & Krasner, 1975). Social skills deficits result from inadequate learning experiences or from lack of contingent reinforcement in the person's current social environment. Social skills-training techniques are based on the presumption that the capability to respond in situationally appropriate ways can be acquired through structured learning situations (Morrison & Bellack, 1987). Since social behaviors are learned and maintained as a function of the consequences that they elicit from other people, repeated practice with positive social reinforcement is used to shape and strengthen appropriate behavior. The provision of information and feedback, and the use of modeling further promote skills acquisition.

Strong emphasis is placed on ongoing assessment of skills deficits by observing patients in realistic situations. Self-report by patients and reports of significant others may provide important additional information. The parameters of the deficits are identified by specifying the types of deficits that are observed and the relevant characteristics of the situations in which they tend to occur. The skills trainer, thus, must conduct a functional assessment of when, where, and with whom the problem behavior occurs.

Based on the information gathered through a variety of procedures, specific problems are identified and the patient and the trainer together develop positive training

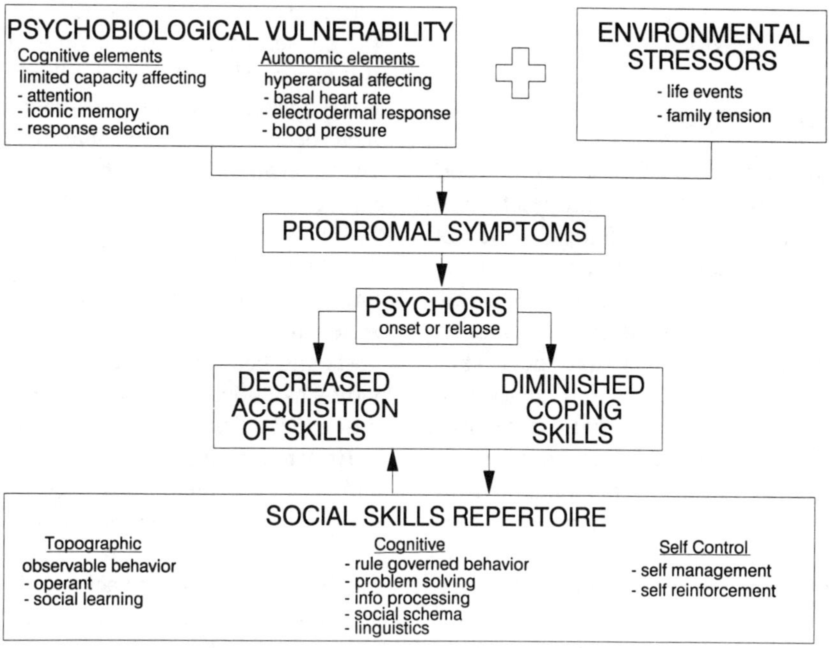

Figure 5.1. The relationship between psychobiological vulnerability and social functioning is mediated by promodal and psychotic symptoms, stressors, and skill development. Stressors, impinging upon vulnerable individuals, can result in early signs of relapse. The experience of florid psychotic symptoms interferes with the performance of existing coping skills and with the acquisition of new skills, resulting in atrophy of the individual's social repertoire and a limited ability to cope with future stressors.

goals that are attainable within the patient's learning capacities (Liberman et al., 1986). Goals are specific, high-frequency behaviors that will provide ample opportunity for practice and feedback. During training, the patient engages in a role play of a problem situation that has occurred recently or is likely to occur again in the near future, often using other group members to participate in relevant roles. For the first role play or "dry run" of each problem situation, the patient is instructed to act as if he or she were in the actual situation. Assets, deficits, and excesses in the patient's performance are noted, and the patient is praised for appropriate behaviors and efforts. Other group members are encouraged to offer positive feedback.

In subsequent role plays, the trainer demonstrates the target behaviors, prompts the patient to perform specific responses, and reinforces successive approximations to the desired goal. Component behaviors are added one by one. As one component skill (e.g., eye contact) is mastered, others (e.g., facial expression, vocal tone, loudness, posture, speech content) are sequentially introduced. After each role-play, appropriate elements of the patient's performances are praised and corrective feedback is given. Generalization of the newly learned behavior to real-life situations is promoted by giving homework assignments to practice the skills in the natural environment and providing positive feedback for successful performance. Transfer of skills may be further facilitated by repeated practice and overlearning, by fading and structure and frequency of training, and by enlisting the help of friends, family members, psychiatric staff, and others to ensure that the natural environment is socially responsive and reinforcing to the patient's performance of appropriate social behavior.

Cognitive Models

Despite the success of topographic models, this viewpoint has been criticized for representing a reflexive view of social functioning in which a limited number of specific skills are developed for responding to a relatively small number of selected situations. An alternative view holds that social skills are dynamically inductive and generative, building social repertoires that are flexible, with behaviors being adapted to meet the changing needs of the interpersonal environment. From this perspective, social competence is derived from rule-driven events (Argyle, 1986; Harre & Secord, 1972) and thus, social skills-training methods should be concordant with the means by which these rules are cognitively processed or represented. Models that have arisen from this perspective have looked beyond behavioral formulations, deriving theoretical foundations from other disciplines including information science, social psychology, and linguistics.

Problem Solving

Problem solving has been identified as a mechanism or mediator of social functioning; in this model, social interactions represent puzzles that need to be deciphered and subsequently acted on. Human beings are viewed as rational agents who choose means (various coping and social skills) that will help them satisfy ends (instrumental or affectional consequences) (Trower, 1982). Means-end analysis led to development of training methods for clinical work with psychiatric populations (D'Zurilla & Goldfried, 1971; Platt, Siegel, & Spivack, 1975; Spivack, Platt, & Shure, 1976). The prototype training method to teach patients problem solving comprises five steps: identifying the elements of problem situations; generating a range of alternative, potential solutions to these elements; selecting one of these alternatives; implementing it; and evaluating the chosen option after a time to determine if it effectively met the individual's needs and goals. More recently, cost-benefit analyses have been applied to problem-solving models to evaluate the efficacy of each alternative (Beach & Mitchell, 1978; D'Zurilla, 1986). Solutions are judged in terms of the feasibility of carrying out the alternatives and their respective reinforcement value. After anticipating the short- and long-term costs and benefits of each solution, the individual can select the solution that affords the best expected utility.

Effective problem-solving skills have been shown to correlate positively with social competence and inversely with severe psychopathology (D'Zurilla, 1986; Phillips, 1978). Platt and Spivack (1972a, 1972b, 1975) studied the abilities of severely disabled patients to conduct means-end analyses and found that schizophrenics were significantly inferior to normals in generating solutions and evaluating their efficacy post hoc. A recent replication of this finding documented that the problem-solving efficacy of 7 chronic psychiatric patients was significantly below the skills of 20 "normals" living in the community (Hansen, St. Lawrence, & Christoff, 1985).

Direct training of social problem solving has been shown to remediate these deficits. Siegel and Spivack (1976a, 1976b) first trained patients on the problem-solving steps. Unfortunately, while they found a wide range of positive results, their method was largely anecdotal making their findings difficult to interpret. In two subsequent studies, Coche and his colleagues used the Means-End Problem Solving Test (MEPS) to measure outcome on problem-solving-training programs with chronic patients. However, results were mixed, finding positive effects on the first study (Coche & Flicke, 1975) but negative results on the second (Coche & Douglas, 1977). Bellack and his colleagues (1990) have criticized the MEPS, maintaining that the measure has yet to be validated.

Social problem-solving training has been shown to raise scores on self-report measures of this construct (Bedell, Archer, & Marlowe, 1980). Edelstein and his colleagues (1980) found that individuals trained on problem-solving skills improved their ability to respond to hypothetical problems they might encounter after leaving the hospital. Hansen et al. (1985) were able to increase the problem-solving skills of a chronic inpatient group to a level comparable to that of a normal criterion group.

Information-Processing Models

More recent models have incorporated the principles of information science, focusing on the different stages mediating social information from input to response. Social perception, an early processing stage, is viewed as jeopardized when the input of interactional stimuli is distorted or compromised by psychobiological abnormalities, resulting in impaired social skill and social competence (Morrison & Bellack, 1981). Application of social skills depends on the ability to read the social environment accurately. Social perception includes listening to the content of messages, interpreting emotions, getting clarification, determining the relevance of one's own behaviors, and correctly timing responses (Bellack & Hersen, 1978; Wallace et al., 1980).

Perceptual deficits affect social functioning on several levels. Severely disabled psychiatric patients are less consistent and certain of the accuracy of their interpersonal judgments (Livesay, 1981). Similarly, Trower, Bryant, and Argyle (1978) have found that schizophrenics are poor perceivers, being susceptible to inaccurate stereotypes, halo effects, and attribution errors. Chronic patients also show a series of facial affect recognition difficulties (Morrison, Bellack, & Mueser, 1988). Morrison and Bellack (1981) have found that impaired perception affects the quality of responses as well—subjects with poor social perception have diminished assertive abilities. Adult psychiatric inpatients who were unable to identify the level of assertion–aggression in six "negative" videos showed poor performance on a role-play test.

Several studies have examined whether perception of social cues can be trained. Finch and Wallace (1977) applied a combination of instruction, modeling, and feedback to chronic psychotics, training patients to attend not only to the relevant interpersonal cues but to discriminate when they were not attending. They found this strategy to be a useful adjunct to more traditional skills-training procedures. Liberman et al. (1986) described an attention-focusing procedure used to enhance conversation skills training in thought-disordered, regressed schizophrenics. This training procedure oriented the patient's attention to relevant training curricula while minimizing demands on information processing capacities. Results of a multiple-baseline, single-subject design revealed improved conversational skills after traditional training interventions had been unsuccessful.

Several models have outlined the cognitive processing of social interactions from social perception to behavioral output. D'Zurilla (1986) described the problem-solving process in terms of problem perception and solution appraisal. McFall (1982) described the information process as the decoding, decision making, and encoding of social information. Wallace (1982; Wallace et al., 1980) produced the most comprehensive and best-tested model, dividing the entire social act into receiving, processing, and sending skills (see Table 5.2). Receiving variables include the processes by which patients identify the content of past and current messages as well as the concomitant emotions and intents communicated by another person. Processing variables define the situational goal toward which the individual may strive and generate options for achieving this end. Sending variables are the observable behaviors the individual expresses. Schizophrenics have been shown to have deficits in receiving, processing, and sending skills that inter-

Table 5.2. Interpersonal Problem-Solving Skills

Receiving Skills
Perceives social cues
Identifies rules and goals specific to situation
Processing Skills
Generates alternatives and their probable consequences
Evaluates feasibility and attainment of goals
Sending Skills
Implements to maximize contingency
Performs verbal and nonverbal components

fere with interpersonal functioning. These deficits are a function in part of the chronicity of the disease and the individual's social deprivation (Wallace, 1984).

Wallace augments his training program with a series of questions designed to facilitate the acquisition of skills at each stage of information processing. For example, questions to elicit and train receiving skills include "What were your short- and long-term goals? At what level of self-disclosure should you be? Is one person doing most of the talking?" This model was tested in a treatment program in which 28 schizophrenic patients were randomly assigned to problem-solving training or to "holistic health therapy" for a 9-week inpatient period (Liberman et al., 1986; Wallace, 1982; Wallace & Liberman, 1985). A comprehensive assessment of outcome found that patients in the skills-training program improved significantly on social skills, symptoms, and adjustment measures with the effects maintained at a 24-month follow-up. These findings suggest that the division of social skills into receiving, processing, and sending skills is useful for developing treatment programs.

A social information-processing model based on information science has described social cognition as a serial search process in which information proceeds through successive stages until the target of the momentary search is achieved (Bellack, Morrison, & Mueser, 1989). An example of this model is summarized in Figure 5.2. The operation begins with the perception of social stimuli, encoded meaningfully vis-à-vis previously acquired information. Social cues are held in short-term storage where the information can be lost if not acted upon or consolidated into long-term memory. Social cues can lead to the individual's searching his or her memory for appropriate responses and generating a hierarchy of these responses, with behaviors at the apex more likely to be reinforced. A response is selected and acted out in terms of a set of motor skills. Research has demonstrated that the psychiatrically impaired and disabled have numerous processing deficits showing either specific limits to cognitive functioning at different stages of the information process or an overall, generalized dysfunction. Identification of the manner in which cognitive dysfunction inhibits the chain of processing stages may direct the application of specific interventions toward that defective mechanism, thereby enhancing social functioning.

Severely depressed individuals have been shown to have information-processing deficits. This group exhibits diminished attention largely focused on self issues (Ingram, Lumry, Cruet, & Sieber, 1987). In addition, depressives tend to interpret incoming information and recall stored data in a dysphoric light (Ingram, 1984). Several stages have been identified as dysfunctional in schizophrenics as well. They perform poorly on tasks measuring selective and sustained attention (Nuechterlein, 1983; Spring et al., 1983), iconic memory (Asarnow, Nuechterlein, & Marder, 1983; Sacuzzo & Braff, 1981), recall memory (Koh, 1978), response selection (Broen, 1968), and executive functioning (Weinberger, Berman, & Illowsky, 1988; Weinberger, Berman, & Zec, 1986). Nuechterlein and Dawson (1984b) have developed a theory accounting for many specific deficits in terms of an overall dysfunction. Drawing upon Kahneman's (1973)

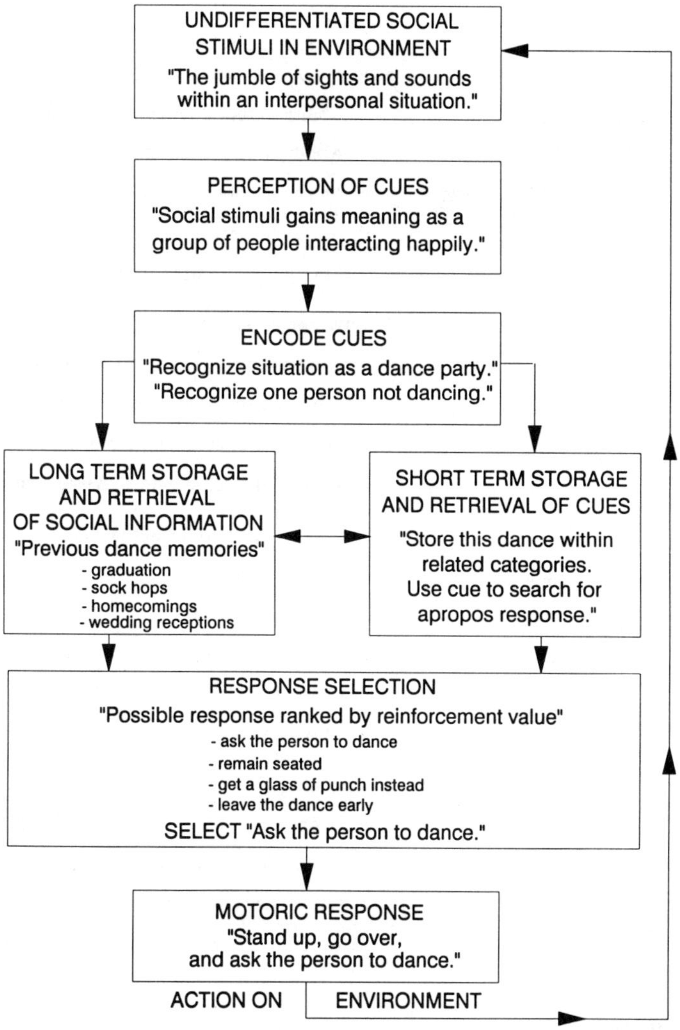

Figure 5.2. An individual attending a dance may perceive and cognitively process the stimuli in the situation, finally selecting a response from among the alternatives in his or her memory storage and using that response effectively in action.

theory of information capacity, they concluded that schizophrenics manifest limited capacity and are thus unable to handle effortful cognitive tasks.

Social Schema

Rather than limiting the focus to the processing of situational information, a more elaborate conceptualization of social skills involves social schemata that represent norms affecting interpersonal skills. Argyle, Furnham, and Graham (1981) listed the situational variables that need to be represented in social schemata; these variables are exemplified in Table 5.3. Given that social behavior is defined vis-à-vis these situational norms, social competence depends on how accurately one's personal schemata mirror these variables.

As a construct, schemata represent the templates through which social information is encoded as well as the blueprints that direct complex social functioning. As tem-

Table 5.3. Situational Variables Represented in Social Schemata: Shopping for Food

1. Goals
   - a. Instrumental: To purchase food for dinner. To stay within budget.
   - b. Affectional: To be friendly with the cashier. "She's always friendly to me"
2. Roles
   - a. Shopper
   - b. Cashier
   - c. Stock person
   - d. Store manager
3. Rules (for shopper)
   - a. Collect food and carry to cashier
   - b. Must have enough money
   - c. No shoplifting
   - d. Be friendly but serious; no horseplay
   - e. Do not open boxes or jars in store
4. Sequence of behavior
   - a. Find a cart
   - b. Find the food
   - c. Bring food to register in cart
   - d. Wait for prices to be totaled
   - e. Pay for food
   - f. Wait for food to be bagged
   - g. Exit
5. Repertoire of skills
   - a. Ability to recall desired food items
   - b. Ability to find food
   - c. Ability to count money
   - d. Ability to steer cart
   - e. Ability to be courteous to cashier
6. Environmental setting
   - a. Long aisles restricting movement of carts
   - b. Narrow aisles easily jam; discourages friendly interactions
   - c. Bright lights, cold temperatures adds to sterility of store
   - d. High-tech machines decrease staff-shopper interaction
7. Language: setting-relevant jarbon
   - a. Bargain aisle
   - b. Blue light specials
   - c. Save your double-value coupons
   - d. Grade A milk
   - e. 50% lean ground chuck
8. Attitudes
   - a. I hope I can remember everything I need
   - b. I don't like it when people block the aisles
   - c. I hope they have Brand X soup on sale
   - d. I want to get my shopping done quickly
9. Emotions
   - a. Impatient
   - b. Businesslike
   - c. Overstimulated
   - d. Happy to get out

plates, schemata affect social perception such that incoming data may be identified in terms of stereotypes (Trower, 1979). The attractiveness stereotype (Dion, Berscheid, & Walster, 1972) would fit this category, with individuals tending to assign labels on the basis that "what is beautiful is good." For example, a stranger whose appearance is bedraggled and whose actions are bizarre is labeled mentally ill. A schema-based stereotype related to physical attractiveness has functional importance because psychiatric patients who are viewed as more physically attractive are greeted with more social support and experience better social adjustment (Farina, Burns, & Austad, 1986; Farina, Fischer, & Sherman, 1977).

These social templates can develop into self-fulfilling prophecies. For example, the initial judgment of an unkempt person directs subsequent responses of most people to avoid such an individual. In turn, the street person who experiences the displeasure and avoidance of others may consequently withdraw from the normalizing potential of social interaction and acquire even more bizarre behaviors. Self-fulfilling prophecies derived from idiosyncratic social schemata may strengthen characteristic psychotic symptoms that can, in turn, inhibit appropriate social functioning. Thus, paranoid individuals with a rigid schema may force all social information into a limited template congruent with persecutory or grandiose views of self or others (Magaro, 1980; Magaro, Johnson, & Boring, 1986). Social data that do not conform to a paranoid schema are modified to fit the template, thereby forming the delusional elaborations characteristic of this disorder. Similarly, severely depressed individuals have been shown to possess schemata that distort incoming information to conform to a highly negative view of self, others, and the future (Beck, 1967; Ingram & Hollon, 1986).

Attribution theorists have written extensively about social schemata, specifically focusing on the attempts ordinary people make to comprehend the causes and implications of events they witness (Ross, 1977). Behavioral attributions lead to inferences regarding the disposition of the actor and to predictions about future occurrences of the act. Individuals use these attributions to guide their responses to social situations.

Attributions are probably governed by logical and empirical rules; in fact, Ross (1977) has outlined two examples: the covariance principle and the discounting principle. Attributions based on the covariance principle conform to rules of inferential logic in which causality is judged from several occurrences of like events. An individual who experiences a coworker as hostile day after day is likely to attribute an angry interaction about coffee money as a recurrence of this pattern. The discounting principle allows attributions to be determined from single occurrences in which causality is evaluated from the individual's previous knowledge of the actor's disposition, goals, and so forth. Hence, the angry coworker might be judged differently if people were aware that he was cranky because of a recent illness.

However, many attributions are not dictated by the laws of inference and deduction; indeed, social judgments are often marked with biases and poor judgment heuristics (Ross, 1977; Tversky & Kahneman, 1974). Several examples of these biases that can skew social perception and social responses are listed in Table 5.4. People typically base judgments about others' actions on the actor's presumed internal dispositions while judgment of one's own actions are attributed to environmental influence (Trower, 1982). For example, persons may be more likely to label the "character" of a hostile coworker as intrinsically flawed while they may attribute their own angry transgressions to momentary hassles from the boss. Attribution theory suggests that the templates guiding social perceptions may be biased and lead to an ego-centered view of the situation.

As blueprints, social schemata influence skills by guiding the specific behavioral elements that make up an interaction. Trower (1979) described the sequencing of skills in which well-learned responses are strung together and automatically performed in serial order without conscious mediation. *Social routines* and *scripts* are examples of these sequences, both of which are limited in terms of the amount of conscious control the individual has when acting out the schema. Social routines (Trower, 1979) represent face-to-face interactions with highly prescribed patterns of behaving that are applicable to multiple settings. Goffman (1972) subdivided routines into supportive interchanges, such as greeting and departing rituals, and remedial interchanges, such as requests, assertive statements, and apologies. The "Western Greeting" has been studied in detail and is defined by two people sighting each other, face-to-face orientation and mutual glance, eyebrow flash, smile, open palm greeting, and gesture with a head toss (Ken-

Table 5.4. Examples of Biases in Social Cognition

Attribution Biases

1. Assign causes to dispositions in others and to environment in self:

   "My spouse is an angry person."

   "I'm irritable because of pressures on the job."

2. Take credit for success and externalize blame for failure:

   "I worked hard for this promotion."

   "The project failed because too many people were involved."

3. Misattribution of arousal:

   "Although I've had six cups of coffee this morning, I'm upset because my daughter didn't kiss me goodbye."

4. Just-world attribution:

   "Everyone gets his or her just desserts—she must have done something to provoke the attack."

Judgment Heuristic Biases

1. Misconception of regression to the mean:

   "Frank was always the best salesman, moving twice as much merchandise as any other worker. Last month, though, Frank sold no more than anyone else. Frank is slipping and is no longer a good salesman."

2. Illusory correlations:

   "Susan noticed that older women at work received more respect than she. Thinking it had to do with their appearance, she dyed her hair grey."

3. Inaccurate judgments based on favorable descriptions:

   "Mary got all A's her first three years of high school. Therefore, she will get an A in Senior Algebra."

4. Inattention to previous probabilities:

   "Even though the last 20 women Harry met were offended by his strong approach, he remains certain that it works."

5. Ignorance of base rates:

   "I've met several homeless people who were mentally ill—it must be true that most chronic psychiatric patients become homeless."

don & Ferber, 1973). Remedial routines keep social interactions from being mired in disagreement by remediating problems that occur. The apology interchange includes an acknowledgement of rule breaking, an account of guilt or embarrassment, and a promise not to repeat the behavior.

Unlike routines, scripts tend to be specific to a social interaction. Schank and Abelson (1977) have identified more than 100 activities within routine situations that are defined by specific scripts including riding a bus, visiting a dentist, and asking for directions. Harre (1977) viewed these examples as standardized routines such that individuals easily share the same social space when acting out the respective parts of the script. Harre also described nonstandardized routines, situations that may be experienced as awkward because the rules are not readily apparent. For example, outsiders who find themselves within a family's private script may struggle for the response that best fits the cadence of the situation.

Severely disabled psychiatric patients, unfamiliar with the routines and scripts prescribed in a social interaction, will find themselves unable to respond rapidly to social cues with appropriate reactions. For example, a chronic patient who has not frequently attended parties may be unaware that an introductory statement made by a guest should be returned with a similar response. In another example, a chronic patient may not understand that receipt of his change after payment of the bill at a restaurant is typically followed by saying thanks for the service and leaving a tip. In both situations, the patient appears rude from lack of knowledge.

Trower (1982) described the means by which social templates and behavioral blueprints interact, borrowing from the feedback loop model of Miller, Galanter and Pribram (1960). Individuals test the social situation vis-à-vis their templates to come to some understanding of the parameters of the interaction. From this understanding, the individual is able to operate on the situation by selecting one of several scripts that will meet his or her goal. This process occurs relatively automatically with little conscious mediation. However, as the person subsequently tests whether this script meets the need of the social situation and finds the goal is not attained, a choice may be made whether to continue searching for appropriate scripts or to exit the situation and withdraw.

As noted earlier, schizophrenics have been shown to lack the necessary perceptual skills to find and appropriately encode situational cues. Therefore, their understanding of situational parameters is hampered and subsequent operations on the interaction are skewed. For example, the paranoid schizophrenic may misconstrue a friendly greeting from a new neighbor as a suspicious intrusion and select a respond-to-the-home-invader script as a basis for reacting. The nonparanoid schizophrenic on the other hand, may not be able to comprehend the friendly introduction at all. No script is selected and the individual withdraws.

Like a character in a play, each person follows a script that permits some latitude for varying responses (Harre & Secord, 1972). Move out of the limits defined in that context, and the role seems inappropriate and the person appears socially maladroit. Roles are so closely defined by the situation in which one finds oneself that individuals may assume a chameleon-like appearance as they move from situation to situation and from role to role (Barker & Wright, 1955; Mischel, 1973).

The mentally ill seem to be distinguished from normals by a constricted number of roles. Research has suggested that severely disabled psychiatric patients interact consistently with others, particularly in unstructured situations in which expected social roles and behavior are not clearly defined (Endler, 1973; Mariotto, 1978; Mariotto & Paul, 1975; Moos, 1969). Thus, patients may respond the same to the nurse on the ward, the minister at church, a friend at the local coffee shop, and their parents at home. Psychiatric patients seem to have a limited number of templates with which to interpret social situations and blueprints with which to respond to these interpretations. The generative quality characteristic of flexible social skills is lacking.

A schematic model of social competence allows researchers to define the components of interpersonal behavior in terms of templates and blueprints and then use these definitions to determine the psychiatric patient's profile of interpersonal strengths and weaknesses. Factor analyses have outlined normative schemata for several social interactions (Argyle et al., 1979). In reviewing these findings, Argyle (1986) determined that some situations included more rules than others (e.g., a tutorial had more rules than a conversation with a friend). By determining the concordance between validated scripts and the social schemata used by patients, their level of social competence can be defined (Trower, 1980, 1982).

The methods used to define adaptive schemata can also be used to define the parameters of abnormal schemata. What situations do the severely mentally disabled find problematic and what aspects of these situations are difficult? In a classic study, Goldsmith and McFall (1975) used the reports of 16 patients to identify a set of common social problems. Typical problem areas included: dating, making friends, having job interviews, relating to authorities, relating to service personnel, and interacting with people they perceived as more intelligent or attractive. Up to this time, the goals of social skills training had been based on the trainer's intuitions. Richardson and Tasto (1976) performed a factor analysis of patients' statements about social fears thereby generating seven groups of interpersonal problems: criticism, assertiveness, confrontation, heterosocial closeness, intimacy, conflict with parents, and interpersonal loss.

Treatment programs have been based on schematic views. Goldsmith and McFall (1975) were able to train patients on a series of adaptive responses to their difficult situations, finding improvements in self-report measures, an interpersonal role-play test, and a naturalistic interpersonal interaction test. More recently, Magaro, Johnson, and Boring (1986) have taught patients minute increments of scripts until an appropriate social role is learned as a unit. Magaro and West (1983) tested this approach with a group of schizophrenics by teaching them the sequential components of conversational skills. As the specific skills of the patients increased, their schizophrenic symptoms diminished.

Linguistic Models

Social interactions consist of instrumental and affectional messages that are largely communicated through paralinguistic and nonverbal expressions. As schemata can divide the morass of social interactions into meaningful structures, so can conversational analyses divide everyday speech into analyzable units. These analyses have provided a model for understanding interpersonal communication (Coulthard, 1984). Conversation has been divided into content and process elements. Content variables are the words and gestures used in communication while process variables include relative speaking time, interruptions, and silences.

Several taxonomies represent aspects of the conversational act. Searle (1975) divided content into five speech acts: *representative acts* in which a belief is conveyed by asserting, agreeing, suggesting, and hinting; *directive acts* that are used to influence the behavior of others by questioning, requesting, commanding, or pleading; *commissives* that commit the individual to some future course of action; *expressives* that declare affective states; and *declaratives* that terminate social relationships via expressions of rejection. Trower et al. (1978) proposed a taxonomy dividing speech into instructions, questions, comments, informal chatter, performance utterances, social routines, expression of emotions, and content messages. Stiles (1978) has discussed the content of communications in terms of a self-other continuum. Individuals who manifest the self extreme of the continuum tend to monopolize conversation with many opinions rather than questioning the attitude of others. These people are considered *ego-centered* and are experienced as aversive by others.

Taxonomies such as these and others have been used to analyze the interplay of conversation. They have described dominant and submissive interactions on the assertive-aggressive continuum (Galassi & Galassi, 1977) and they have been used to analyze the speech patterns of seriously disabled psychiatric patients. Research needs to specify further the interactional speech deficits in severely disabled groups. For example, the speech of schizophrenics may be dominated by directive acts in which patients are either requesting a specific need to be fulfilled or are answering a pointed question asked of them. Moreover, they may use self-statements excessively and be relatively oblivious to the comments or goals of others. As the patients' repertoires increase during social skills training, the amount of informational conversation and inquiries about others may be expected to increase.

Process variables describe the flow of relevant content elements. Chapple (1970) described synchronous and asynchronous patterns in dyads, experienced as the give and take of floor time during conversations. In synchronous dyads, one person is listening while the other is speaking. Asynchronous patterns are marked by both parties speaking at the same time or sharing awkward silences for lengths of time. Good conversationalists share discussion by yielding the floor frequently, asking questions, and incorporating silences into their statements (1977). Similarly, socially attractive speakers are able to use the cues of their partners to discern when it is time for them to begin again to talk (1978). These cues include the pitch of the voice (Brazil, 1975) and the subtle movements of the head, hands, and eyes (Scheflen, 1964). Because their cognitive deficits impair their receiving skills and use of scripts, chronic psychiatric patients have been found lacking on many process variables including turn-taking, looking, smiling, gesturing, and posture (Cappella, 1985; Trower, 1980).

In many ways, applications of conversational analysis mirror the topographic approach to skills training. A module may use the information from these analyses to train specific microskills. An example of a dialogue between a trainer, a patient named Mike, and his friend Sue, using linguistic processes, may sound something like this:

Trainer: Mike, I'd like you and Sue to practice some of the conversation skills you've learned. Sue, why don't you start?

Sue: How are you, Mike?

Mike: Okay.

Sue: It's kind of cold today. Do you like the cold weather?

Mike: Not much.

Sue: What did you do over the holidays?

Mike: Nothing.

The trainer has noticed that Mike is stuck in a directive response set, offering one word answers for the questions asked of him. This form of responding can be improved by asking Mike to elaborate on what he is thinking. First, though, the current level of responding needs to be shaped by reinforcing even the smallest approximation to having a conversation.

Trainer: Mike, I like the way you're paying attention to what Sue is saying. Good job! Can you say a little more about what you're thinking, too? For example, tell us what you did over the holidays.

Mike: Well, I went to my mother's house. I ate dinner. Then I went out on the front porch and had a smoke.

Sue: Did you get any gifts?

Mike: I got some new pants and a nice green shirt. Oh, and I got a new Bible.

Sue: Did you have a big tree?

Mike: Yeah, and I decorated it. I put on all the ornaments, starting on the top. I liked the red ornaments the best.

Mike has greatly increased the quantity of what he is saying. However, his speech is so dominated by "I" statements that Sue may quickly lose interest. The trainer next could diminish the self-dominated talk by asking Mike to question Sue about her holidays.

Self-Control Model

In the self-control model, cognitive–behavioral training is aimed at those cognitive processing tasks that can increase the patient's ability to manage his or her own social behavior flexibly (Kanfer, 1970, 1971, 1975; Kanfer & Karoly, 1972). Self-control is the process by which a person initiates some act that attempts to improve the probability of desired social interactions and outcomes. Self-control is viewed as a feedback loop characterized by self-monitoring, self-evaluation, and self-reinforcement. Self-monitoring refers to the process of observing one's own behavior, the situations in which it occurs, and the consequences that follow it. Observable behaviors, such as "crazy talk," as well as internal events, such as social anxiety, may be monitored. The next step of self-evaluation occurs when a patient's estimate of his or her performance, based on self-monitoring, is compared to internal or external criteria for appropriate behavior. It is important that performance criteria be realistically attainable, and that the initiation of appropriate social behavior be attributed to internal, rather than external, causes (Rehm, 1977, 1984). Self-reinforcement refers to the self-administration of overt or covert rewards or punishments contingent upon the outcome of the self-evaluation process. Self-reinforcement supplements external reinforcement in controlling behavior and serves to maintain appropriate functioning when external reinforcers are delayed or unavailable (Rehm, 1977).

The self-control model has been applied to psychiatrically disabled individuals, primarily depressed patients. Rehm (1977, 1982, 1984) described depression in terms of six primary aberrations in self-control behavior:

1. Selective monitoring of negative events
2. Selective monitoring of immediate as opposed to delayed consequences of behavior
3. Overly stringent self-evaluative criteria
4. Inaccurate attributions of responsibility
5. Insufficient self-reward
6. Excessive self-punishment

According to this formulation, deficits in self-monitoring occur in part because of the tendency for depressed individuals to attend selectively to negative, unpleasant events to the relative exclusion of pleasant events. This negative self-monitoring results in social escape and avoidance behavior that precludes receiving positive reinforcement from the environment. Additionally, self-monitoring deficits may result from attending selectively to immediate rather than delayed outcomes of behavior. For example, the depressed housewife who must make some tough decisions about the unhappy situation in her marriage is likely to focus on and be overwhelmed by the immediate angry repercussions that will meet her efforts and overlook the ultimate, long-term benefits for the family when communication is restored.

Problems of self-evaluation are hypothesized to occur as a result of failure to make accurate internal attributions of causality and a tendency to set overly stringent criteria for success (Rehm, 1977). Inaccurate internal attributions occur when a patient makes excessive external attributions of causality and perceives no relationship between performance and consequences, or makes accurate or excessively internal attributions of causality but perceives himself or herself to be incompetent and ineffective (i.e., unable to obtain positive consequences). Stringent self-evaluative criteria result from unrealistically high standards for success and positive self-evaluation or from low thresholds for negative self-evaluation.

Behavioral interventions aimed at alleviating self-control deficits in depressed individuals have been demonstrated to diminish symptoms of depression and compare favorably to assertiveness skills training (Rehm, 1984; Rehm et al., 1979). The utility of this approach has provided an impetus for self-control skills as an adjunct to skills-training programs for psychiatrically disabled patients (Becker, Heimberg, & Bellack, 1987; Miller et al., 1989; Hersen & Bellack, 1976; Hersen, Bellack, & Himmelhoch, 1982). For example, social skills training, with an emphasis on self-control skills, was delivered to a diagnostically heterogeneous sample of inpatient and outpatient psychiatric patients who reported experiencing social anxiety and/or skill problems in social situations. Skills training consisted of seventeen 90-minute weekly sessions and 3 monthly sessions. Training focused on the acquisition of basic social skills (e.g., observing, listening, giving and receiving feedback, eye contact, speech loudness), specific social responses (e.g., making and refusing requests, giving and receiving compliments, initiating and maintaining conversation, positive and negative assertiveness), and self-management skills (i.e., self-monitoring, setting concrete and realistic goals and subgoals, setting realistic self-standards, and appropriate self-reinforcement). Comparisons between patients who participated in social skills training and those who received conventional psychiatric treatment alone indicated that the social skills group improved more than the control group on self-report measures of social anxiety and assertiveness (Van Dam-Baggen & Kraaimaat, 1986). Self-control procedures for schizophrenics, using instructions, self-talk, and reinforcement, have been demonstrated to reduce inappropriate verbalizations and improve performance on cognitive-intellectual tasks (Meichenbaum, 1969, 1973; Meichenbaum & Cameron, 1973). It may be difficult to gain compliance with self-monitoring, self-evaluation, and self-reinforcement assignments; the complexity of the procedures may have to be reduced and overlearning used to compensate for the cognitive dysfunctions of severely disabled psychiatric patients (Wallace, Robinson, & Webster, 1978).

FUTURE DIRECTIONS FOR SKILLS TRAINING

Traditional behavior therapy approaches, as well as models based on social psychology, linguistics, and information science, have greatly expanded the scope of skills training. The series of modules for training an array of social and community adaptation skills—comprising Trainers' Manuals, Patients' Workbooks, and Demonstration Videos—has incorporated principles from each of the models of social skills articulated in this chapter (UCLA Social & Independent Living Skills Program, 1990). Each module—such as those that teach Basic Conversation Skills, Symptom and Medication Management, and Recreation for Leisure—consists of specific skill areas and educational objectives that are trained through the same seven learning activities (Wallace et al., 1985). Because of their "user friendly" format and portability, these modules represent a major advance in research and clinical practice.

Despite these improvements, however, researchers and clinicians need to be mindful of the limits of these viewpoints and respond to challenges for future developments in technology. For example, the stepwise logical training method implicit in means-end analyses of social problems has been criticized as not accurately reflecting real-life problem solving (Bellack, Morrison, & Mueser, 1989). The combined evidence suggests that social behavior, rather than being a logical stepwise event, may be better portrayed as probabilistic skills based on multiple, interacting elements in the individual and his or her environment. Does this imply that the chronically mentally ill need to be trained on these seemingly infinite combinations of situational variables? Future research needs to investigate the forms of real-life social interactions and the most efficient means by which individuals with severe deficits can be trained to produce effective responses.

On the other hand, while probabilistic problem solving may be a characteristic of normal populations, cognitively dysfunctional patients may yet benefit from rote learning of a logical and linear problem solving process. For example, in one study, schizophrenic patients improved their social skills when taught the logical sequence of problem solving even though normal controls showed worsening of their skills when exposed to the same training (Wallace, Robinson, & Webster, 1978).

In addition to these concerns, there exists a fundamental fallacy in establishing the criteria for patients' social competence as "real life" and "normal" levels of conversation and social interactions. It would be equally erroneous to teach paraplegic individuals to walk with artificial legs using the same kinesis as normals or to teach retarded adolescents to use the same jargon and swagger as nonretarded adolescents when dating or shopping in a store. If the minimal acceptable behaviors requisite for social competence can be defined and set as realistic and attainable goals, this criterion may then yield improvement in mentally impaired persons' social acceptance and quality of life.

SUMMARY

Social skills training with severely disabled psychiatric patients entered its second generation when treatment outcome studies demonstrated that this behavioral change strategy not only expands their social repertoire of skills but also is associated with reduced frequency of symptomatic relapse. For the next generation, challenges and tasks include improving the generalization and durability of outcome as well as the patient's quality of life. Evidence regarding generalization of skills to situations outside the training milieu and to responses other than microbehaviors targeted in most training modules has been equivocal. The view of generalization as a naturally occurring "irradiation" process has changed to a belief that an active strategy needs to be incorporated into skills-training programs. Ultimately, the value of social skills training must also be assessed in terms of its ability to enable patients to improve their quality of life. Whether or not social skills training enhances patients' life satisfaction outside the tightly structured treatment milieu is only now beginning to be evaluated in outcome studies.

A scientific analysis of the mechanisms involved in the acquisition and utilization of social skills can point toward future directions for research and program development. Social skills and social competence are counterweights to the adverse effects of stress and vulnerability on the course and outcome of psychotic disorders. Topographic, cognitive, and self-control models of social competence and social skills training provide blueprints for the design of specific training techniques. The topographic model developed from operant and social learning perspectives. Cognitive models were built on the fields of social psychology, linguistics, and information processing, which added new constructs like information processing stages, social schemata, scripts, and conversational analyses to our understanding of competent social functioning. The self-control model provides a useful conceptualization of social skills deficits observed in psychiatric patients and a technology for training and maintaining socially skilled functioning in the community in the absence of immediate external reinforcers. Future research needs to address the relative potency of each construct as well as its utility in forming effective treatment strategies.

The various models of social functioning combine to form an overall model of social competence, as illustrated in Figure 5.3. This model distinguishes between social skills (i.e., cognitive, verbal, and nonverbal behaviors that must be used to achieve community survival needs and a reasonable quality of life) and social competence (i.e., the impact of these skills on the relevant interpersonal field). Social skills are the target of assessment and training; these skills depend on the individual's being able to carry out the specific topographic behaviors, possess the necessary schemata, processing skills, and linguistic elements, and self-manage the range of behaviors and contingencies. Coping with social challenges and problems require the appropriate use of these social skills. They equip an individual to neutralize stressors, to perceptually control the meaning of experiences so that stress is minimized, to modulate the emotional consequences of stressful events, and to reconstitute social support and assistance in solving problems.

Social competence results from appropriate use of the skills and is measured by the individual's status in social situations and by the reinforcement the individual receives

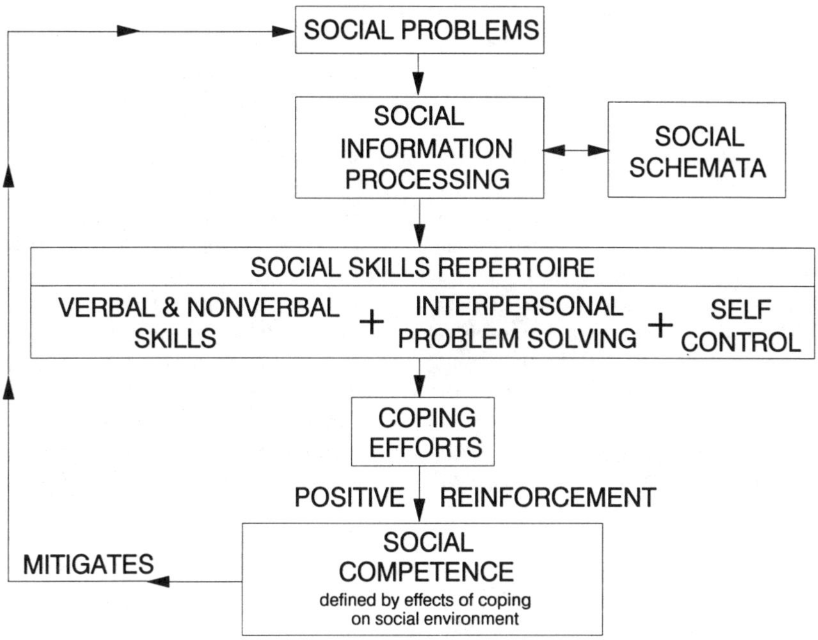

Figure 5.3. Social competence is defined by the positive consequences that accrue to individuals who successfully direct their coping efforts toward challenges and problems in the environment. Success in coping requires mobilization of social schemata, cognitively processing social information, and implementing appropriate problem-solving, verbal, nonverbal, and self-control skills.

in instrumental and affectional relationships. The value of coping and a broad use of social skills in many areas of life is reflected in the unequal distribution of coping and competence in society. Greater social advantages accrue to those who make more use of these adaptive mechanisms, such as the educated, and the affluent (Pearlin & Schooler, 1978).

The cultural issues relevant to social competence bear further investigation as well. Script theory and conversational analysis have yielded constructs that may advance current definitions of "normal and appropriate" social functioning and enhance the ability of social skills trainers to identify relevant, socially valid treatment goals for severely disabled patients. However, few attempts to define these behaviors in terms of a cultural context have been made. Social norms and mores undoubtedly vary between cultures, but the impact of culturally bound expectations for behavior have not been examined under the light of skills-training technology. Whose culture do current conceptualizations of social competence represent? Is it a disservice to train severely disabled patients from various ethnic, socioeconomic, and cultural backgrounds in interpersonal behaviors that may be foreign to their family and friends? In its second generation, research on social skills training needs to examine the manner in which appropriate social functioning is defined in different cultural contexts as well as to generate and validate more effective training techniques.

REFERENCES

Anthony, W. A., & Nemec, P. B. (1984). Psychiatric rehabilitation. In A. S. Bellack (Ed.), *Schizophrenia: Treatment, management, and rehabilitation* (pp. 375–413). Orlando, FL: Grune & Stratton.

Argyle, M. (1986). Social skills and the analysis of situations and conversations. In C. R. Hollin & P. Trower (Eds.), *Handbook of social skills training: Clinical application and new directions* (Vol. 2, pp. 185–216). Elmsford, NY: Pergamon Press.

Argyle, M., Furnham, A., & Graham, J. A. (1981). *Social situations*. Cambridge: Cambridge University Press.

Argyle, M., Graham, J. A., Campbell, A., & White, P. (1979). The rules of different situations. *New Zealand Psychologist, 8*, 13–22.

Asarnow, R. F., Nuechterlein, K. H., & Marder, S. R. (1983). Span of apprehension performance, neuropsychological functioning, and indices of psychosis proneness. *Journal of Nervous and Mental Disorder, 171*, 662–669.

Barker, R. G., & Wright, H. T. (1955). *Midwest and its children: The psychological ecology of an American town*. Evanston, IL: Row Peterson.

Beach, L. R., & Mitchell, T. R. (1978). A contingency model for the selection of decision strategies. *Academy Management Review, 3*, 439–447.

Beck, A. T. (1967). *Depression: Clinical, experimental, and theoretical aspects*. New York: Harper.

Becker, R. E., Heimberg, R. G., & Bellack, A. S. (1987). *Social skills training treatment for depression*. Elmsford, NY: Pergamon Press.

Bedell, J. R., Archer, R. P., & Marlowe, H. A. (1980). A description and validation of a problem solving skills training program. In D. Upper & S. M. Ross (Eds.), *Behavior group therapy, 1980: An annual review* (pp. 185–213). Champaign, IL: Research Press.

Bellack, A. S., & Hersen, M. (1978). Chronic psychiatric patients: Social skills training. In M. Hersen & A. S. Bellack (Eds.), *Behavior therapy in the psychiatric setting* (pp. 169–195). Baltimore, MD: Williams & Wilkins.

Bellack, A. S., Hersen, M., & Himmelhoch, J. M. (1983). A comparison of social skills training, pharmacotherapy, and psychotherapy for depression. *Behavior Research and Therapy, 21*, 101–107.

Bellack, A. S., Hersen, M., & Lamparski, D. (1979). Role-play tests for assessing social skills: Are they valid? Are they useful? *Journal of Consulting and Clinical Psychology, 47*, 335–342.

Bellack, A. S., Hersen, M., & Turner, S. M. (1976). Generalization effects of social skills training with chronic schizophrenics: An experimental analysis. *Behavioral Research and Therapy, 14*, 391–398.

Bellack, A. S., Hersen, M., & Turner, S. M. (1978). Role-play tests for assessing social skills: Are they valid? *Behavior Therapy, 9*, 448–461.

Bellack, A. S., Morrison, R. L., & Mueser, K. T. (1989). Social problem solving in schizophrenia. *Schizophrenia Bulletin, 15*, 101–116.

Bellack, A. S., & Mueser, K. T. (1986). A comprehensive treatment program for schizophrenia and chronic mental illness. *Community Mental Health Journal, 22*, 175–189.

Bellack, A. S., Turner, S. M., Hersen, M., & Luber, R. F. (1984). An examination of the efficacy of social skills training for chronic schizophrenic patients. *Hospital and Community Psychiatry, 35*, 1023–1028.

Birley, J. L. T., & Brown, G. W. (1970). Crisis and life changes preceding the onset or relapse of acute schizophrenia. *British Journal of Psychiatry, 116*, 327–333.

Brazil, D. C. (1975). *Discourse intonation: Discourse analysis monographs 1*. Birmingham: English Language Research.

Broen, W. E. (1968). *Schizophrenia: Research and theory*. New York: Academic Press.

Brown, G. W., & Birley, J. L. T. (1968). Crisis and life changes and the onset of schizophrenia. *Journal of Health and Social Behavior, 9*, 203–214.

Brown, M. (1982). Maintenance and generalization issues in skills training with chronic schizophrenics. In J. P. Curran & P. M. Monti (Eds.), *Social skills training: A practical handbook for assessment and treatment* (pp. 90–116). New York: Guilford Press.

Brown, M. A., & Munford, A. M. (1983). Life skills training for chronic schizophrenics. *Journal of Nervous and Mental Disease, 17*, 1466–1476.

Butler, L., & Meichenbaum, D. (1981). The assessment of interpersonal problem-solving skills. In P. C. Kendall & S. D. Hollon (Eds.), *Assessment strategies for cognitive-behavioral interventions* (pp. 197–221). New York: Academic Press.

Cappella, J. N. (1985). Production principles for turn taking rules in social interaction: Socially anxious vs. socially secure persons. *Journal of Language and Social Psychology, 4*, 193–210.

Carpenter, W. T., Heinrichs, D. W., Hanlon, T. E. (1986). Interpersonal and pharmacologic treatment in schizophrenia: A comparative study of new approaches. *Psychopharmacology Bulletin, 22*, 854-859.

Chapple, E. (1970). Experimental production of transients in human interaction. *Nature, 228*, 630-633.

Coche, E., & Douglas, A. A. (1977). Therapeutic effects of problem-solving training and play-reading groups. *Journal of Clinical Psychology, 33*, 820-827.

Coche, E., & Flick, A. (1975). Problem solving training groups for hospitalized psychiatric patients. *Journal of Psychology, 91*, 19-29.

Cole, J. R., Klarreich, S. H., & Fryatt, M. J. (1982). Teaching interpersonal coping skills to adult psychiatric patients. *Cognitive Therapy and Research, 6*, 105-112.

Corrigan, P. W., Davies-Farmer, R. M., & Lome, H. B. (1988). A curriculum based psychoeducational program for the chronic, mentally ill. *Psychosocial Rehabilitation Journal, 12*, 71-73.

Coulthard, M. (1977). *An introduction to discourse analysis*. London: Longman.

Coulthard, M. (1984). Conversation analysis and social skills training. In P. Trower (Ed.), *Radical approaches to social skills training*. New York: Methuen.

Curran, J. P. (1979). Methodological issues and future directions. In A. S. Bellack & M. Hersen (Eds.), *Research and practice in social skills training*. New York: Plenum Press.

Dion, K., Berscheid, E., & Walster, E. (1972). What is beautiful is good. *Journal of Personality and Social Psychology, 24*, 285-290.

D'Zurilla, T. J., & Goldfried, M. R. (1971). Problem solving and behavior modification. *Journal of Abnormal Psychology, 78*, 107-126.

D'Zurilla, T. J. (1986). *Problem solving therapy: A social competence approach to clinical intervention*. New York: Springer.

Edelstein, B. A., Couture, E., Cray, M., Dickens, P., & Lusebrink, N. (1980). Group training of problem-solving with psychiatric patients. In D. Upper & S. M. Ross (Eds.), *Behavior group therapy, 1980: An annual review*. Champaign, IL: Research Press.

Endler, N. (1973). The person versus the situation—a pseudo issue? A response to Alker. *Journal of Personality, 41*, 287-303.

Falloon, I. R. H., Boyd, J. L., McGill, C. W., Razani, J., Moss, H. B., & Gilderman, A. M. (1982). Family management in the prevention of exacerbations of schizophrenia: A controlled study. *New England Journal of Medicine, 306*, 1437-1440.

Falloon, I. R. H., Lindley, P., McDonald, R., & Marks, I. M. (1977). Social skills training of outpatient groups: A controlled study of rehearsal and homework. *British Journal of Psychiatry, 131*, 599-609.

Farina, A., Burns, G. L., & Austad, C. (1986). The role of physical attractiveness in the readjustment of discharged psychiatric patients. *Journal of Abnormal Psychology, 95*, 139-143.

Farina, A., Fischer, E. H., & Sherman, S. (1977). Physical attractiveness and mental illness. *Journal of Abnormal Psychology, 86*, 510-517.

Fecteau, G. W., & Duffy, M. (1986). Social and conversational skills training with long-term psychiatric inpatients. *Psychological Reports, 59*, 1327-1331.

Finch B. E., & Wallace, C. J. (1977). Successful interpersonal skills training with schizophrenic inpatients. *Journal of Consulting and Clinical Psychology, 45*, 885-890.

Frederiksen, L. W., Jenkins, J. O., & Foy, D. W. (1976). Social skills training to modify abusive verbal outbursts in adults. *Journal of Applied Behavioral Analysis, 9*, 117-127.

Friedlob, S. A., Janis, G. A., & Deets-Aron, C. (1986). A hospital-connected halfway house program for individuals with long-term neuropsychiatric disabilities. *American Journal of Occupational Therapy, 40*, 271-277.

Frisch, M. B., Elliott, C. H., Atsaides, J. P., Salva, D. M., & Denney, D. R. (1982). Social skills and stress management training to enhance patients' interpersonal competencies. *Psychotherapy: Theory, Research, and Practice, 19*, 349-358.

Furnham, A., & Argyle, M. (1981). Responses of four groups to difficult social situations. In Argyle, M., Furnham, A., Graham, J. A. (Eds.), *Social situations*. Cambridge: Cambridge University Press.

Galassi, M. D., & Galassi, J. P. (1977). *Assert yourself! How to be your own person*. New York: Human Sciences Press.

Goffman, E. (1972). *Relations in public: Microstudies of the public order*. Harmondsworth: Penguin.

Goldsmith, J. B., & McFall, R. M. (1975). Development and evaluation of an interpersonal skills training program for psychiatric inpatients. *Journal of Abnormal Psychology, 84*, 57-68.

Hansen, D. J., St. Lawrence, J. S., & Christoff, K. A. (1985). Effects of interpersonal problem-solving training with chronic aftercare patients on problem-solving component skills and effectiveness of solution. *Journal of Consulting and Clinical Psychology, 53*, 167–174.

Harre, R. (1977). The ethogenic approach: Theory and practice. In L. Berkowitz (Ed.), *Advances in experimental social psychology* (Vol. 10). New York: Academic Press.

Harre, R., & Secord, P. F. (1972). *The explanation of social behavior*. Oxford: Blackwell.

Hersen, M., & Bellack, A. S. (1976). Social skills training for chronic psychiatric patients: Rationale, research findings, and future directions. *Comprehensive Psychiatry, 17*, 559–580.

Hersen, M., Bellack, A. S., & Himmelhoch, J. M. (1982). Skills training with unipolar depressed women. In J. P. Curran & P. M. Monti (Eds.), *Social skills training: A practical handbook for assessment and treatment* (pp. 159–184). New York: Guilford Press.

Hersen, M., Eisler, R. M., & Miller, P. M. (1973). Development of assertive responses: Clinical measurement and research considerations. *Behaviour Research and Therapy, 11*, 505–521.

Hersen, M., Eisler, R. M., & Miller, P. (1974). An experimental analysis of generalization in assertive training. *Behaviour Research and Therapy, 12*, 295–310.

Hogarty, G. E., Anderson, C. M., & Reiss, D. J. (1987). Family psychoeducation, social skills training, and medication in schizophrenia: The long and short of it. *Psychopharmacology Bulletin, 23*, 12–13.

Hogarty, G. E., Anderson, C. M., Reiss, D. J., Kornblith, S. J., Greenwald, D. P., Javna, C. D., & Madania, M. J. (1986). Family psychoeducation, social skills training, and maintenance chemotherapy in the aftercare treatment of schizophrenia. *Archives of General Psychiatry, 43*, 633–642.

Holmes, M. R., Hansen, D. J., & St. Lawrence, J. S. (1984). Conversational skills training with aftercare patients in the community: Social validation and generalization. *Behavior Therapy, 64*, 84–100.

Ingram, R. E. (1984). Toward an information processing analysis of depression. *Cognitive Therapy and Research, 8*, 371–385.

Ingram, R. E., & Hollon, S. D. (1986). Cognitive therapy of depression from an information processing perspective, In R. E. Ingram (Ed.), *Information processing approaches to clinical psychology* (pp. 261–284). New York: Academic Press.

Ingram, R. E., Lumry, A. E., Cruet, D., & Sieber, W. (1987). Attentional processes in depressive disorders. *Cognitive Therapy and Research, 11*, 351–360.

Jaffe, P. G., & Carlson, P. M. (1976). Relative efficacy of modeling and instructions in eliciting social behavior from chronic psychiatric patients. *Journal of Consulting and Clinical Psychology, 44*, 200–207.

Kahneman, D. (1973). *Attention and effort*. Englewood Cliffs, NJ: Prentice-Hall.

Kanfer, F. H. (1970). Self-regulation: Research issues and speculations. In C. Neuringer & J. L. Michael (Eds.), *Behavior modification in clinical psychology*. New York: Appleton-Century-Crofts.

Kanfer, F. H. (1971). The maintenance of behavior by self-generated stimuli and reinforcement. In A. Jacobs & L. B. Sachs (Eds.), *The psychology of private events: Perspective on covert response systems*. New York: Academic Press.

Kanfer, F. H. (1975). Self-management methods. In F. H. Kanfer & A. P. Goldstein (Eds.), *Helping people change: A textbook of methods* (pp. 309–355). Elmsford, NY: Pergamon Press.

Kanfer, F. H., & Karoly, P. (1972). Self-control: A behavioristic excursion into the lion's den. *Behavior Therapy, 3*, 398–416.

Kazdin, A. E. (1974). Effects of covert modeling and model reinforcement on assertive behavior. *Journal of Abnormal Psychology, 83*, 240–252.

Kazdin, A. E. (1975). *Behavior modification in applied settings*. Homewood, IL: Dorsey Press.

Kendon, A., & Ferber, A. (1973). A description of some human greetings. In R. P. Michael & J. H. Crook (Eds.), *Comparative ecology and behaviour in primates*. London: Academic Press.

Kent, G. G., Davis, J. D., & Shapiro, D. A. (1978). Resources required in the construction and reconstruction of conversation. *Journal of Personality and Social Psychology, 36*, 13–22.

Kindness, K., & Newton, A. (1984). Patients and social skills groups: Is social skills training enough? *Behavioral Psychotherapy, 12*, 212–222.

Klerman, G. L. (1977). Better but not well: Social

and ethical issues in the deinstitutionalization of the mentally ill. *Schizophrenia Bulletin, 3*, 617-631.

Koh, S. (1978). Remembering in schizophrenia. In S. Schwartz (Ed.), *Language and cognition in schizophrenia*. Hillsdale, NJ: Lawrence Erlbaum.

Lazarus, A. A. (1981). *The practice of multimodal therapy*. New York: McGraw-Hill.

Lehman, A. F., Ward, N. C., & Linn, L. S. (1982). Chronic mental patients: The quality of life issues. *American Journal of Psychiatry, 134*, 1271-1276.

Liberman, R. P., Falloon, I. R. H., & Wallace, C. J. (1984). Drug-psychosocial interventions in the treatment of schizophrenia. In M. Mirabi (Ed.), *The chronically mentally ill: Research and services* (pp. 175-212). New York: SP Medical & Scientific Books.

Liberman, R. P., Lillie, F. J., Falloon, I. R. H., Harpin, E. J., Hutchinson, W., & Stoute, B. A. (1984). Social skills training for relapsing schizophrenics: An experimental analysis. *Behavior Modification, 8*, 155-179.

Liberman, R. P., Marshall, R. D., Marder, S. R., Dawson, M. E., Nuechterlein, K. H., & Doane, J. A. (1984). The nature and problem of schizophrenia. In A. S. Bellack (Ed.), *Schizophrenia: Treatment, management, and rehabilitation*. New York: Grune & Stratton.

Liberman, R. P., Massel, H. K., Mosk, M. D., & Wong, S. E. (1985). Social skills training for chronic mental patients. *Hospital and Community Psychiatry, 36*, 396-403.

Liberman, R. P., Mueser, K. T., & Wallace, C. J. (1986). Social skills training for schizophrenic individuals at risk for relapse. *American Journal of Psychiatry, 143*, 523-526.

Liberman, R. P., Mueser, K. T., Wallace, C. J., Jacobs, H. E., Eckman, T., & Massel, H. K. (1986). Training skills in the psychiatrically disabled: Learning coping and competence. *Schizophrenia Bulletin, 12*, 631-647.

Liberman, R. P., Nuechterlein, K. H., & Wallace, C. J. (1982). Social skills training and the nature of schizophrenia. In J. P. Curran & P. M. Monti (Eds.), *Social skills training: A practical handbook for assessment and treatment* (pp. 5-56). New York: Guilford Press.

Livesay, J. R. (1981). Inconsistent interpersonal judgement in thought-disordered schizophrenia. *Psychological Reports, 49*, 179-181.

Longin, H. E., & Rooney, W. M. (1975). Teaching denial assertion to chronic hospitalized patients. *Journal of Behavior Therapy and Experimental Psychiatry, 6*, 219-222.

Magaro, P. A. (1980). *Cognition in schizophrenia and paranoia: The integration of cognitive processes*. Hillsdale, NJ: Lawrence Erlbaum.

Magaro, P. A., Johnson, M. H., & Boring, R. (1986). Information processing approaches to the treatment of schizophrenia. In R. E. Ingram (Ed.), *Information processing approaches to clinical psychology* (pp. 285-305). New York: Academic Press.

Magaro, P. A., & West, A. N. (1983). Structured learning therapy: A study with chronic psychiatric patients and level of pathology. *Behavior Modification, 7*, 29-40.

Malm, U., May, P. R. A., & Dencker, S. J. (1981). Evaluation of the quality of life of the schizophrenic outpatient: A checklist. *Schizophrenia Bulletin, 7*, 477-487.

Mariotto, M. J. (1978). Interaction of person and situation effects for chronic mental patients: A two year follow-up. *Journal of Abnormal Psychology, 87*, 676-679.

Mariotto, M. J., & Paul, G. L. (1975). Person versus situations in the real-life functioning of chronically institutionalized mental patients. *Journal of Abnormal Psychology, 84*, 483-493.

Martinez-Diaz, J. A., Massel, H. K., Wong, S. E., Wiegand, W., Bowen, L., Edelstein, B. A., Marshall, B. D., & Liberman, R. P. (1983). *Training of generalization of conversation skills in chronic schizophrenics*. Paper presented at the World Congress on Behavior Therapy, Washington, DC.

Marzillier, J. S., & Winter, K. (1978). Success and failure in social skills training: Individual differences. *Behaviour Research and Therapy, 16*, 67-84.

McFall, R. M. (1982). A review and reformulation of the concept of social skills. *Behavioral Assessment, 4*, 1-33.

McFall, R. M., & Lillesand, D. B. (1971). Behavior rehearsal with modeling and coaching in assertion training. *Journal of Abnormal Psychology, 77*, 313-323.

McFall, R. M., & Twentyman, C. T. (1971). Four experiments on the relative contributions of rehearsal, modeling, and coaching to assertion training. *Journal of Abnormal Psychology, 81*, 199-218.

McKnight, D. L., Nelson, R. O., Hayes, S. C., & Jarrett, R. B. (1984). Importance of treating individually assessed response classes in the amelioration of depression. *Behavior Therapy, 15*, 315-335.

Meichenbaum, D. H. (1966). The effects of social reinforcement on the level of abstraction in schizophrenics. *Journal of Abnormal Psychology, 71*, 354-362.

Meichenbaum, D. H. (1969). The effects of instructions and reinforcement on thinking and language behavior of schizophrenics. *Behaviour Research and Therapy, 7*, 101-114.

Meichenbaum, D. H., & Cameron, R. (1973). Training schizophrenics to talk to themselves: A means of developing attentional controls. *Behavior Therapy, 4*, 515-534.

Miller, G. A., Galanter, E., & Pribram, K. H. (1960). *Plans and structures of behavior*. New York: Henry Holt.

Miller, I. W., Norman, W. H., Keitner, G. I. (1989). Cognitive-behavioral treatment of depressed inpatients. *Behavior Therapy, 20*, 25-47.

Mischel, W. (1968). *Personality and assessment*. New York: Wiley.

Mischel, W. (1973). Toward a cognitive social learning reconceptualization of personality. *Psychological Review, 80*, 252-283.

Monti, P. M., Curran, J. P., Corriveau, D. P., Delancey, A. L., & Hagerman, S. M. (1980). Effects of social skills training groups and sensitivity training groups with psychiatric patients. *Journal of Consulting and Clinical Psychology, 48*, 241-248.

Moos, R. H. (1969). Sources of variance in responses to questionnaires and in behavior. *Journal of Abnormal Psychology, 74*, 405-412.

Morrison, R. L., & Bellack, A. S. (1981). The role of social perception in social skill. *Behavior Therapy, 12*, 69-79.

Morrison, R. L., & Bellack, A. S. (1984). Social skills training. In A. S. Bellack (Ed.), *Schizophrenia: Treatment, management, and rehabilitation* (pp. 247-279). Orlando, FL: Grune & Stratton.

Morrison, R. L., & Bellack, A. S. (1987). Social functioning of schizophrenic patients: Clinical and research issues. *Schizophrenia Bulletin, 13*, 715-725.

Morrison, R. L., Bellack, A. S., & Mueser, K. T. (1988). Deficits in facial affect recognition and schizophrenia. *Schizophrenia Bulletin, 14*, 67-83.

Nezu, A. M. (1986). Efficacy of a social problem-solving therapy approach for unipolar depression. *Journal of Consulting and Clinical Psychology, 54*, 196-202.

Nuechterlein, K. H. (1983). Signal detection in vigilance tasks and behavioral attributes among offspring of schizophrenic mothers and among hyperactive children. *Journal of Abnormal Psychology, 9*, 24-28.

Nuechterlein, K. H., & Dawson, M. E. (1984a). A heuristic vulnerability/stress model of schizophrenic episodes. *Schizophrenia Bulletin, 10*, 300-312.

Nuechterlein, K. H., & Dawson, M. E. (1984b). Information processing and attentional functioning in the developmental course of schizophrenic disorders. *Schizophrenia Bulletin, 10*, 160-203.

Paul, G. L. (Ed.). (1986). *Assessment in residential treatment settings: Principles and methods to support cost-effective quality operations. (Assessment in residential treatment settings, part 1.)* Champaign, IL: Research Press.

Paul, G. L. (Ed.). (1987a). *The Time-Sample Behavioral Checklist: Observational assessment instrumentation for service and research. (Assessment in residential treatment settings, part 2.)* Champaign, IL: Research Press.

Paul, G. L. (Ed.). (1987b). *The Staff-Resident Interaction Chronograph: Observational assessment instrumentation for service and research. (Assessment in residential treatment settings, part 3.)* Champaign, IL: Research Press.

Paul, G. L. (Ed.). (in press a). *The Computerized TSBC/SRIC Planned-Access Observational Information System: Observational assessment instrumentation for service and research. (Assessment in residential treatment settings, part 4.)* Champaign, IL: Research Press.

Paul, G. L. (Ed.). (in press b). *The TSBC/SRIC System Implementation Package: Observational assessment instrumentation for service and research. (Assessment in residential treatment settings, part 5.)* Champaign, IL: Research Press.

Pearlin, L., & Schooler, C. (1978). The structure of coping. *Journal of Health and Social Behavior, 19*, 2-21.

Phillips, E. L. (1978). *The social skills basis of psychopathology: Alternatives to abnormal psychology and psychiatry*. New York: Grune & Stratton.

Platt, J. J., Siegel, M. J., & Spivack, G. (1975).

Do psychiatric patients and normals see the same solutions as effective in solving interpersonal problems? *Journal of Consulting and Clinical Psychology, 43*, 279.

Platt, J. J., & Spivack, G. (1972a). Problem-solving thinking of psychiatric patients. *Journal of Consulting and Clinical Psychology, 39*, 148–151.

Platt, J. J., & Spivack, G. (1972b). Social competence and effective problem-solving thinking in psychiatric patients. *Journal of Clinical Psychology, 28*, 3–5.

Platt, J. J., & Spivack, G. (1975). *The Means Ends Problem-Solving Procedure manual.* Philadelphia: Author.

Rehm, L. P. (1977). A self-control model of depression. *Behavior Therapy, 8*, 787–804.

Rehm, L. P. (1982). Self-management in depression. In P. Karoly & F. H. Kanfer (Eds.), *The psychology of self-management: From theory to practice*. Elmsford, NY: Pergamon Press.

Rehm, L. P. (1984). Self-management therapy for depression. *Advances in Behavioral Research and Therapy, 6*, 83–94.

Rehm, L. P., Fuchs, C. Z., & Roth, D. M. (1979). A comparison of self-control and assertion skills treatments of depression. *Behavior Therapy, 10*, 429–442.

Richardson, F. L., & Tasto, D. L. (1976). Development and factor analysis of a social anxiety inventory. *Behavior Therapy, 7*, 453–462.

Ross, L. (1977). The intuitive psychologist and his shortcomings: Distortions in the attribution process. In L. Berkowitz (Ed.), *Advances in experimental social psychology* (Vol. 10). New York: Academic Press.

Sacuzzo, D. P., & Braff, D. L. (1981). Early information processing deficits in schizophrenia: New findings using subgroups and manic controls. *Archives of General Psychiatry, 38*, 175–179.

Schank, R. C., & Abelson, R. P. (1977). *Scripts, plans, goals, and understanding*. Hillsdale, NJ: Lawrence Erlbaum.

Scheflen, A. E. (1964). The significance of posture in communication systems. *Psychiatry, 27*, 316–331.

Searle, J. R. (1975). A taxonomy of illocutionary acts. In K. Gunderson (Ed.), *Minnesota studies in the philosophy of language*. Minneapolis: University of Minnesota Press.

Shepherd, G. (1986). Social skills training and schizophrenia. In C. R. Hollin & P. Trower (Eds.), *Handbook of social skills training: Clinical applications and new directions* (Vol. 2, pp. 9–38). Elmsford, NY: Pergamon Press.

Siegel, J. M., & Spivack, G. (1976a). A new therapy program for chronic patients. *Behavior Therapy, 7*, 129–130.

Siegel, J. M., & Spivack, G. (1976b). Problem solving therapy: The description of a new program for chronic psychiatric patients. *Psychotherapy: Theory, Research, and Practice, 13*, 368–373.

Spencer, P. G., Gillespie, C. R., & Ekisa, E. G. (1983). A controlled comparison of the effects of social skills training and remedial drama on the conversational skills of chronic schizophrenic inpatients. *British Journal of Psychiatry, 143*, 165–172.

Spivack, G., Platt, J. J., & Shure, M. B. (1976). *The problem solving approach to adjustment.* San Francisco: Jossey-Bass.

Spring, B. J., Levitt, M., Briggs, D., & Benet, M. (1983). *Distractibility in relatives of schizophrenics*. Paper presented at the 91st Annual Convention of the American Psychological Association, Anaheim, CA.

Stiles, W. B. (1978). *Manual for a taxonomy of verbal responses*. Chapel Hill: Institute for Research in Social Science, University of North Carolina, Chapel Hill.

Stokes, T. F., & Baer, D. M. (1977). An implicit technology of generalization. *Journal of Applied Behavioral Analysis, 10*, 349–369.

Strauss, J. S., & Carpenter, W. T. (1972). The prediction of outcome in schizophrenia: I. Characteristics of outcome. *Archives of General Psychiatry, 27*, 739–746.

Strauss, J. S., & Carpenter, W. T. (1974). The prediction of outcome in schizophrenia: II. Relationships between predictor and outcome variables: A report from the WHO International Pilot Study of Schizophrenia. *Archives of General Psychiatry, 31*, 37–42.

Strauss, J. S., & Carpenter, W. T. (1977). The prediction of outcome: III. Five year outcome and its prediction. *Archives of General Psychiatry, 34*, 159–163.

Test, M. A. (1984). Community support programs. In A. S. Bellack (Ed.). *Schizophrenia: Treatment, management, and rehabilitation*. New York: Grune & Stratton.

Trower, P. (1979). Fundamentals of interpersonal behavior – a social-psychological perspective.

In A. S. Bellack & M. Hersen (Eds.), *Research and practice in social skills training*. New York: Plenum Press.

Trower, P. (1980). Situational analysis of the components and processes of behavior of socially skilled and unskilled patients. *Journal of Consulting and Clinical Psychology, 48*, 327–339.

Trower, P. (1982). Toward a generative model of social skills: A critique and synthesis. In J. P. Curran & P. M. Monti (Eds.), *Social skills training: A practical handbook for assessment and treatment*. New York: Guilford Press.

Trower, P. (1986). Social skills training and social anxiety. In C. R. Hollin & P. Trower (Eds.), *Handbook of social skills training: Clinical applications and new directions* (Vol. 2). Elmsford, NY: Pergamon Press.

Trower, P., Bryant, B., & Argyle, M. (1978). *Social skills and mental health*. London: Methuen.

Tversky, A., & Kahneman, D. (1974). Judgement under uncertainty: Heuristics and biases. *Science, 185*, 1124–1131.

UCLA Social & Independent Living Skills Series. (1990). Available from Dissemination Coordinator, Camarillo–UCLA Research Center, PO Box 6022, Camarillo, CA 93011-6022.

Ullmann, L. P., & Krasner, L. (1975). *A psychological approach to abnormal behavior* (2nd ed.). Englewood Cliffs, NJ: Prentice-Hall.

Van Dam-Baggen, R., & Kraaimaat, F. (1986). A group social skills training program with psychiatric patients: Outcome, dropout rate, and prediction. *Behaviour Research and Therapy, 34*, 161–169.

Vaughn, C. E., Snyder, K. S., Freeman, W., Jones, S., Falloon, I. R. H., & Liberman, R. P. (1982). Family factors in schizophrenic relapse: A replication. *Schizophrenia Bulletin, 8*, 425–444.

Wallace, C. J. (1982). The Social Skills Training Project of the Mental Health Clinical Research Center for the Study of Schizophrenia. In J. P. Curran & P. M. Monti (Eds.), *Social skills training: A practical handbook for assessment and treatment*. New York: Guilford Press.

Wallace, C. J. (1984). Community and interpersonal functioning in the course of schizophrenic disorders. *Schizophrenia Bulletin, 10*, 233–257.

Wallace, C. J., Boone, S. E., Donahoe, C. P., & Foy, D. W. (1985). The chronically mentally disabled: Independent living skills training. In D. Barlow (Ed.), *Clinical handbook of psychological disorders: A step-by-step treatment manual* (pp. 462–501). New York: Guilford Press.

Wallace, C. J., & Liberman, R. P. (1985). Social skills training for patients with schizophrenia: A controlled clinical trial. *Psychiatry Research, 15*, 239–247.

Wallace, C. J., Nelson, C. J., Liberman, R. P., Aitchison, R. A., Lukoff, D., Elder, J. P., & Ferris, C. (1980). A review and critique of social skills training with schizophrenic patients. *Schizophrenia Bulletin, 6*, 42–63.

Wallace, C. J., Robinson, L., & Webster, C. (1978). *Problem solving skills of schizophrenics and normals*. Unpublished manuscript, Camarillo State Hospital/UCLA Clinical Research Center for Schizophrenia and Psychiatric Rehabilitation, Los Angeles, CA.

Weinberger, D. R., Berman, K. F., & Illowsky, B. P. (1888). Physiological dysfunction of dorsolateral prefrontal cortex in schizophrenia: III. A new cohort and evidence for a monoaminergic mechanism. *Archives of General Psychiatry, 45*, 609–615.

Weinberger, D. R., Berman, K. F., & Zec, R. F. (1986). Physiological dysfunction of dorsolateral prefrontal cortex in schizophrenia: I. Regional cerebral blood flow evidence. *Archives of General Psychiatry, 43*, 126–135.

Zigler, E., & Phillips, L. (1961). Social competence and outcome in psychiatric disorders. *Journal of Abnormal and Social Psychology, 63*, 264–271.

Zigler, E., & Phillips, L. (1962). Social competence and the process-reactive distinction in psychopathology. *Journal of Abnormal and Social Psychology, 65*, 215–222.

Zubin, J., & Spring, B. (1977). Vulnerability—a new view of schizophrenia. *Journal of Abnormal Psychology, 86*, 103–126.

CHAPTER 6

SOCIAL-LEARNING PROGRAMS

Shirley M. Glynn
Kim T. Mueser

The emphasis on brief hospitalizations and increased community tenure for even the most seriously mentally ill highlights the importance of rehabilitation as a critical treatment goal for these patients. Traditional psychotherapy has failed to meet the needs of the seriously mentally ill, and alternative approaches, incorporating training in frequently deficient life skills, appropriate medication regimens, and behavioral interventions to reduce psychotic behavior, have shown great promise (Paul & Lentz, 1977). In this chapter, we present a detailed description of the most successful of these innovative programs, a comprehensive social-learning program for back ward psychiatric patients conducted by Gordon Paul and his colleagues in the late 1960s and early 1970s. Years later, this investigation still adds much to our understanding of the most efficacious treatments of the seriously mentally ill. Following a critical analysis of the therapeutic elements of the Paul and Lentz program, we present overviews of other inpatient and outpatient programs that have successfully incorporated comprehensive social-learning approaches. Finally, we discuss the current status of social-learning theory and practice pertaining to the seriously mentally ill.

PROBLEM OF THE SERIOUSLY MENTALLY ILL

The rehabilitation of long-term institutionalized psychiatric patients poses an ongoing challenge to mental health practi-

This research was supported, in part, by grant No. U10-MH-39998-02 from the National Institute of Mental Health. This chapter is based on a previous article, "Social Learning for Chronic Mental Inpatients," *Schizophrenia Bulletin, 12*, 648–668, 1986.

tioners. Almost 14 years after its publication, the comparative study of a social-learning program for chronic psychiatric patients reported by Paul and Lentz (1977) remains unmatched in both its comprehensiveness and methodological rigor (Rhoades, 1981). Social-learning procedures appear to be the most cost-effective approach to meeting the treatment needs of low-functioning, institutionalized psychiatric patients. The inadequacy of existing services for the chronically mentally ill is reflected in at least three disturbing facts: (a) many psychiatric patients are unable to maintain community tenure; (b) even "rehabilitated" chronic patients often have severe ongoing deficits in self-care and social skills; and (c) patients left in traditional institutional settings are understimulated and frequently lead barren lives.

Rehospitalization rates for psychiatric patients range from 35% to 50% within the first year postdischarge (Friedman, von Mering, & Hinko, 1966; Wolkon, Karmen, & Tanaka, 1971). About 60% of public psychiatric beds are occupied by patients who have been continuously hospitalized for more than 1 year, and as many as 90% of these patients are unresponsive to pharmacological treatment (Paul, 1984). However, even the ability to live in the community is not a guarantee of satisfactory social functioning. Psychiatric patients frequently reside in dismal social conditions in the community (Kirk & Therrien, 1975), and the functioning of many chronic patients living in community residential settings actually declines over time (Dickey, Gudeman, Hellman, Donatella, & Greenspoon, 1981; Kohen & Paul, 1976; Spivack, Siegel, Sklaver, Deuschle, & Garrett, 1983).

The inadequacy of chronic patients' social skills may limit their ability to cope with and blunt the noxious effects of stressors, making them more vulnerable to symptom exacerbations (Liberman, 1982). While social deficits of patients in the community lead to social rejection and a higher risk of rehospitalization, they are also indicative of the impoverished quality of their lives (Lehman, 1983; Lehman, Ward, & Linn, 1982). In fact, social competence is the best single predictor of successful community tenure following discharge from psychiatric facilities (Paul, 1987a). Treatment programs that strive to remediate the social deficits of chronic patients may be expected to improve their clinical condition, social adjustment, and potential for community tenure.

Just as overstimulating, stressful environments worsen the symptoms of many psychiatric patients, understimulating and unstructured environments also promote maladaptive behavior (Rosen, Sussman, Mueser, Lyons, & Davis, 1981; Wing & Freudenberg, 1961; Wong, Massel, Mosk, & Liberman, 1987). Many programs for the chronically ill include few structured activities and minimal patient-staff contact. Patient-staff interaction in state and veterans administration (VA) hospitals accounts for less than 11% of patient waking hours, and less than 15% of staff working hours (Paul, 1986a). Increased interaction of appropriate types and levels between patients and staff in structured or semistructured environments could lessen inappropriate behaviors that present obstacles to community survival (Paul, 1986b).

The high proportion of chronic psychiatric patients with severe social deficits who reside in understimulating environments that merely maintain, rather than rehabilitate, suggests the need for programs that actively seek to improve these patients' skills competency (Bellack & Mueser, 1986). The social-learning program of Paul and Lentz (1977, in preparation), because of its demonstrated efficacy and relevance to community as well as hospital-based programs for disabled chronic mental patients, deserves a renewed focus and descriptive evaluation.

PSYCHOSOCIAL PROGRAMS

The study of Paul and Lentz (1977) compared traditional hospital treatment and two comprehensive psychosocial treatment programs for psychiatric inpatients that actively sought to enhance patients' functional independence: a social-learning program, based on learning principles such as associative learning, problem solving, reinforcement, modeling, punishment, and shaping; and a milieu therapy program based on communication theory and the therapeutic community model that promotes pro-social behavior through communicating attainable expectations, stimulating patient involvement, and generating group cohesiveness. Both psychosocial programs aimed at resocializing patients by developing self-maintenance and interpersonal skills; decreasing bizarre, inappropriate behaviors; and facilitating discharge and maintenance in the community. Successful community tenure was defined as a spectrum of levels of functioning including independent living, residence in board-and-care homes, and gainful or sheltered employment. Declining-contact aftercare in the community was an important treatment component that was provided to patients discharged from traditional hospital wards as well as to those discharged from the psychosocial units. The declining-contact aftercare consultation was provided directly to discharged patients and their significant others for those living independently and to the facilities for those living in community placements.

The comparative study was conducted with chronically institutionalized, severely debilitated, aggressive, and psychotic psychiatric patients. The specific, comprehensive social-learning and milieu programs that were developed and evaluated employed the same clinical staff members, who rotated between the two programs on a daily basis to equate time and exposure. These programs engaged patients in structured therapeutic and training activities much of their waking hours (85%), unlike the traditional hospital group (5%). The psychosocial programs were conducted concurrently for $4\frac{1}{2}$ years with a minimum 18-month declining-contact follow-up while the control hospital program continued as usual with monitoring of patients for 6 years.

Patients and Staff

The patients were 18 to 55 years old, equally divided in gender, and had been residing continuously for at least 2 years in one of four state hospitals in Illinois. The great majority of patients were divorced or had never been married, and all were low in socioeconomic status. All had diagnoses of chronic process schizophrenia and had few or no friends or relatives in the community. Overall, the patient group had spent an average of 17 years—about two-thirds of their adult lives—in psychiatric hospitals. As a group, the patients demonstrated higher levels of inappropriate, "crazy" behavior and greater deficits in self-care, interpersonal, and communication skills than any previous psychiatric group that had been subject to programmatic study. This population had received many prior somatic treatments and all had received chemotherapy, although they were clearly "hard-core" chronic mental patients for whom neuroleptic medications are largely not beneficial (Paul, Tobias, & Holly, 1972). Initially, three patient groups of 28 each were equated on 16 variables and randomly assigned to the three treatment programs. "New" patients were admitted from the original chronic population to maintain 28 inpatients in each program with equation at the entry assessment for additional patients as well.

The clinical staff who implemented the social-learning and milieu programs were 20% professionals (e.g., psychologists, social workers, nurses, and occupational therapists) and 80% nonprofessionals (aide-level with a high school degree). The staffing level and staff-patient ratios were purposely equal to those in the traditional hospital treatment, and all were considerably lower than the average staffing ratios in public mental hospitals nationwide.

Treatment Setting

The two inpatient psychosocial programs were located in identical adjacent 28-bed units in a regional mental health center.

These units were coeducational and had been designed to facilitate staff–patient interaction. Unique features of the units included a kitchen, bedrooms that varied from six-bed dormitory-type rooms to private ones, a living room, a television room, a classroom-lounge, and a sunken activity pit in the center of an open area of the ward. Administrative structure and patient care services were totally decentralized to treatment units.

The regional state hospital that served as the control inpatient treatment housed approximately 1,000 residents and contained a wide variety of departments, treatment facilities, and support services, including occupational, industrial, and educational programs as well as recreational and art facilities. The 28 comparison beds and patients were located in wards that were segregated by sex and varied in size from 16 to 84 beds. The declining-contact aftercare for discharged patients from both center programs and the hospital comparison group was provided by the psychosocial staff, who traveled to the community residence of ex-patients for on-site consultations.

The social-learning and milieu therapy programs shared several features and basic aims. Both inpatient psychosocial programs used a level system where residents promoted to higher steps were gradually exposed to less structured situations, earned greater privileges, and carried added responsibility. Both programs covered all aspects of patients' lives and functioning with consistent interactional–educational conceptual models, including integrated principles, procedures, and assessments 24 hours per day, 7 days per week. Participants in the programs were referred to as "residents" rather than "patients," and an emphasis was placed on the use of descriptive, action-oriented language. A list of 10 rules (see Table 6.1) was conspicuously posted around both units to remind the residents to attend to the expected norms of behavior. Patient schedules included individual times and places for assessment and training of specific aspects of cognitive, social, and instrumental functioning. The programs stressed the importance of residents' acquiring desirable intrapersonal, interpersonal, and instrumental aspects of functioning through continuous assessment of each resident's needs and progress, modeling appropriate social interactions, teaching vocational, housekeeping, communication, problem solving, coping, and self-care skills, gradually reacquainting the residents with the outside world, and programming for generalization into the community. Both psychosocial programs were "high technology" in the sense of requiring precise specification of appropriate staff interactions with patients demonstrating a variety of behaviors in a number of settings. The factor that discriminated between the social-learning and milieu therapy inpatient programs was the specific nature and content of staff–patient interactions.

Social-Learning Inpatient Program

The social-learning inpatient program was based on a token economy motivational structure. Residents in the first three step levels earned tokens (colored strips of plastic) redeemable for goods or privileges contingent upon engaging in appropriate behaviors. Consistent verbal and nonverbal staff–patient interactions were paired with token exchanges. As patients progressed to higher steps, the number of tokens they could earn grew, as did the availability of increasingly more desirable privileges. For example, tokens could be earned by attending and participating in meetings and classes, engaging in appropriate information conversations, cleaning the unit, good mealtime behavior, maintaining one's personal appearance, and working in vocational training positions; tokens could be spent on more pleasant sleeping quarters, passes, privacy time, food, appointments with staff members, and promotion to a higher step. Throughout the program, the particular performances necessary to obtain a set number

Table 6.1. Psychosocial Program Rules

As a resident of the rehabilitation unit, you are expected to:

1. Care for yourself and present a desirable appearance
2. Perform your own housekeeping chores and share in those of the unit
3. Think, talk, and act straight (in ways that make sense to others)
4. Show gentlemanly or ladylike behavior
5. Show respect for the rights of others, for yourself, and for your property
6. Interact cooperatively and actively with residents, staff, and others
7. Attend and participate in all scheduled activities (be where you're supposed to be)
8. Acquire and demonstrate work habits and skills that will provide for an income after you leave
9. Move through the 4 step levels of the program and return permanently to the outside community
10. *Not* act "crazy"

Note: Adapted from Paul, G., & Lentz, R. (1977).

of tokens were clearly specified in objective, readily observable terms for each patient, as were the privileges for which the tokens could be exchanged. As patients were promoted, gradual delays of reinforcement were introduced to enhance internal planning and control.

Guidelines governing the operation of the social-learning program were derived from two basic learning principles: the *law of effect*, and the *law of association by contiguity*. The law of effect was applied in the social-learning program by arranging for desired behavior to be followed by social and material *positive reinforcement* or by the removal of *negative reinforcers*, and for undesired behavior to be followed by either punishment (*aversion*), loss of positive reinforcers (*response cost*), or no consequence at all (*extinction*). The law of association by contiguity was incorporated into the program in many ways: to assure that a resident's desirable or undesirable behavior was met immediately with the appropriate consequence; to develop new affective and cognitive learning and problem-solving skills; to establish social stimuli as positive or reinforcing events; and to shift or generalize new skills and coping responses from dependence on tokens to internal and verbal controls.

In addition to these laws, other learning principles were systematically integrated in the social-learning program to facilitate the acquisition of appropriate behavior, including *shaping* (reinforcing successive behavioral approximations to a criterion), *chaining* (teaching a new behavior by systematically linking components in a sequence), and *positive and negative prompts* (instructing desired performance through physical guidance, demonstration and modeling, and written or verbal means, along with verbal specification of resulting consequences). Direct verbal instruction and modeling were also incorporated in classes and therapy groups to provide new knowledge and skills.

Milieu Therapy Inpatient Program

The milieu program was based on a therapeutic community structure wherein all patients were members of 9- to 10-person living groups which were assigned the tasks of identifying problems and promoting change among individual members. Unit tasks such as meal preparation were assigned by living groups, and attempts were made to keep group members on similar daily schedules for training classes and activities. Members were also encouraged to spend free time and passes together. The major vehicle for promoting change was the social and group pressure exerted by each living group on its members. All patients and staff were also members of the unit-wide community group which, through discussion and majority vote, dealt with any decisions affecting the entire community, while an executive council with elected members from each living group was responsible for agendas.

The milieu treatment program was based on three laws: *expectancy, involvement*, and *group cohesiveness*. The *law of expectancy* was operationalized by the staff's use of *positive statements* that specified and encouraged performance of desirable behavior before it occurred, *positive feedback* that verbally acknowledged a recent desirable performance and/or the value of the person, and *negative feedback* that acknowledged and discouraged a recent undesirable act or verbalization. Clarification and interpretation of meta-communicative aspects of behavior were important. Since the use of *negative statements* could communicate to the resident an expectation that he or she would engage in an undesirable behavior, these were not used in either treatment program. Unlike the social-learning program, staff applied no nonsocial or material consequences whatsoever (except for "expelling" patients from the group to seclusion as a consequence for assaults) and contingent social consequences occurred only incidentally when positive feedback coincided with a particular patient performance. On the basis of the *law of involvement*, residents in the milieu program always assumed the maximum responsibility for making decisions and implementing them, frequently practiced problem solving, and were encouraged to engage in behaviors in which they had previously experienced failure. *Group cohesion* was enhanced by the entire community and living-group structure, encouraging an "us" and "them" attitude within the groups, and the endorsement of group pressure as a vehicle for change in group members. Milieu therapy patients and social-learning patients attended identical classes; both received verbal instruction and modeling to provide new knowledge and skills. Classes, however, were assigned by living groups rather than by individuals.

Community Aftercare Component

The inpatient psychosocial programs focused on preparing patients for community functioning by establishing minimal levels of competence in self-care, interpersonal communications, and instrumental role skills, and by reducing or eliminating psychotic manifestations and other extremely bizarre behavior. The inpatient programs also attempted to bridge the gap from residential treatment to community living by training for generalization to natural support systems and establishing living arrangements, training or vocational positions, and at least one supportive friend or relative in the community before discharge. An aftercare program involving scheduled contacts in the community on a declining basis by trained psychosocial staff was an equally important component to ensure generalization of inpatient gains and maintenance of functioning and community tenure. Early on, it became clear that social-learning principles were the most promising on which to base aftercare consultations; consequently, patients discharged from all three inpatient programs were provided with declining-contact follow-up employing social-learning principles and technology. At least 4 weekly, 5 biweekly, and 3 monthly contacts followed by semiannual contacts were scheduled, with additional contacts as needed. Declining-contact aftercare was provided for at least 2 years to each patient discharged to independent functioning and self-support, and for 18 months to board-and-care facilities that accepted community placements from any of the three inpatient programs.

Assessment and Evaluation Procedures

A comprehensive set of assessment and evaluation procedures is necessary to ensure coverage of patient, staff, and program functioning as well as to evaluate the impact of interventions in residential and community treatment (Paul & Mariotto, 1986). In the comparative study, a battery of standardized rating instruments and structured interviews was administered to all patients in all three treatment groups before and after entry to study programs, every 6 months thereafter during inpatient treatment, immediately before discharge, and every 6 months after discharge. Ongoing reliability checks were obtained for each measure. Along with demographic variables, these measures served to equate treatment groups on initial patient entry and to sample levels of adjustment during and after inpatient treatment on common instruments at identical time periods. Measures of staff attitudes, opinions, and personality characteristics were similarly obtained on all clinical staff.

In addition to the above assessments, three direct observational coding systems were continuously employed in both inpatient psychosocial programs. The *Clinical Frequencies Recording System* (CFRS) (Paul & Licht, 1987a) was an integral part of the application of both comprehensive social-learning and milieu programs. The CFRS consists of a set of standardized time-place-situation specific forms completed by clinical staff concurrent with therapeutic activity. CFRS forms provide 100% event-recording of low-frequency critical acts (e.g., assaults and other intolerable behavior) and of setting-dependent aspects of patient functioning (e.g., on time, on task, progress toward normal appearance) as well as staff responses to each patient's behavior. Higher order CFRS scores combine recordings over forms and weekly periods to provide objective data for program evaluation on the rate with which different classes of behavior were performed. The detailed daily records ensured consistent identification and monitoring of each patient's level of achievement, subtargets for clinical programming, and consistency of staff response.

Two multivariate direct observational systems employed by a small cadre of independent noninteractive observers provided continuous objective assessment of staff and patients in both psychosocial programs through stratified hourly time sampling of all patient waking hours for the entire $4\frac{1}{2}$-year inpatient phase. Full-week samples of resident and staff functioning in community board-and-care facilities were also obtained every 3 months during the follow-up period. The *Time-Sample Behavioral Checklist* (TSBC) (Paul, 1987a; Paul & Licht, 1987b) records the context of each observation as well as the presence/absence of 69 specific codes within seven content categories: Location, Position, Awake-Asleep, Facial Expression, Social Orientation, Appropriate Concurrent Activities, and Crazy Behaviors. Weekly summarization of TSBC data provides objective rates of occurrence for each individual code as well as higher order components of functioning, both appropriate (e.g., Interpersonal Interaction, Total Appropriate Behavior) and inappropriate (e.g., Cognitive Distortion, Total Inappropriate Behavior) for each patient and treatment unit as well as documenting how and where time is spent.

The *Staff-Resident Interaction Chronograph* (SRIC) (Paul, 1987b; Licht & Paul, 1987) records the context of each observation, and the nature, content, and frequency of 21 classes of staff verbal and nonverbal response to four classes of resident functioning (Appropriate, Inappropriate Failure, Inappropriate Crazy, "Straight" Requests) or staff-initiated interactive or noninteractive activity (Resident-"Neutral"). Weekly summarization of SRIC data provides objective rates of occurrence for each cell of the 5 (resident behavior) × 21 (staff behavior) matrix, and higher order scores reflecting total staff activity, total staff-resident interactions, actual resident/staff ratios and attention received by all residents in a program to document the psychosocial treatment provided. SRIC summaries for individual staff or staff groups were also used for monitoring and feedback. TSBC/SRIC observers were trained to 100% accuracy on both instruments, and the obtained data were highly reliable.

Rehabilitation Outcomes

Because the patients who participated in this study exhibited such bizarre behaviors and deficits in adaptive functioning, the relative efficacy of the social-learning and milieu programs compared to traditional hospital treatment needs to be evaluated with regard to three practical goals that are critical for such a disabled population:

- increasing patients' adaptive functioning (e.g., self-care and social skills) and decreasing patients' psychotic functioning and extremely bizarre behavior
- reducing the psychotropic medications necessary to stabilize patients
- facilitating discharge and successful maintenance in the community

In all three domains, milieu therapy resulted in greater gains than were seen in the hospital comparison group, and the social-learning program yielded strikingly better results than the milieu treatment. Furthermore, the improvement in social-learning patients was not related to any individual characteristics, pretreatment level of functioning, or diagnosis, and was obtained in the relative absence of psychotropic medication. The structured, comprehensive, and integrated procedures of the social-learning program led to the development of personal and interpersonal skills that were remarkable on an absolute level for this chronic group, the reduction of idiosyncratic and "crazy" motor and verbal behavior to fractions of initial levels, a radical decrease in the number of patients prescribed psychotropic medications, and to successful discharge or community placement without rehospitalization for the vast majority of patients.

The social-learning program treated nearly 30% more patients than either the milieu or hospital programs with essentially identical resources. Consequently, it was three to four times as cost effective as traditional programs and is thus also the treatment of choice on purely economic grounds. Within the comprehensive, constructive program the social-learning patients received fewer aversive or intrusive events than other inpatients, with the program ensuring that least-restrictive or intrusive procedures were invoked; thus, it is also the treatment of choice based on ethical and humanitarian concerns. The specificity of procedures and precision of feedback provided by the integrated observational assessment systems allowed both professional and nonprofessional staff to be trained to exceptional levels of competency in implementing the program. This resulted in nearly errorless performance in the ongoing conduct of the comprehensive procedures—it was accessible to and accepted by the levels of staff already employed in the usual public psychiatric hospital. Figure 6.1 illustrates the outcomes for the three treatment groups, including release rate, days in the community, cost per patient, weeks in the treatment program, percent on psychotropic medications, and changes on a common ward rating scale, the *Nurses Observation Scale for Inpatient Evaluation* (NOSIE-30) (Honigfeld, 1966). Declining-contact aftercare for discharged patients was successful in maintaining community tenure in more than 97% of cases, indicating unquestioned superiority of the social-learning program over the milieu and hospital comparison groups.

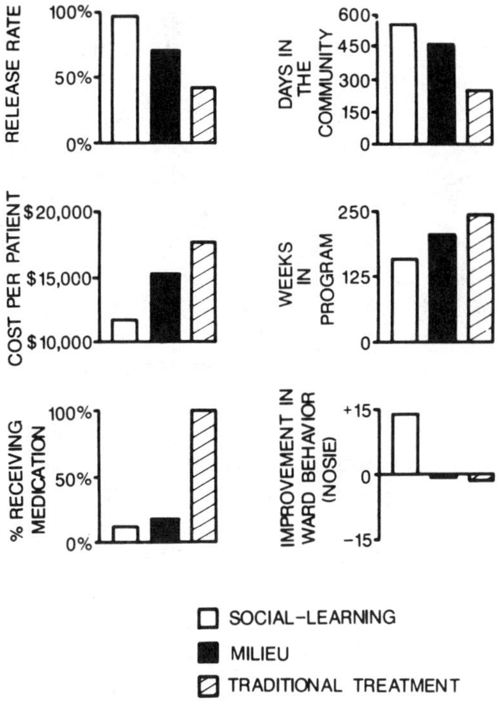

Figure 6.1. Differential treatment outcomes of patients with schizophrenia participating in the long-term comparative study. On all six dimensions, the social-learning program achieved results better than the results of the milieu program, which were better than those of the standard treatment comparison. *Note:* Adapted from Paul, G., & Lentz, R. (1977).

Increasing Adaptive Functioning and Decreasing Bizarre Behavior

Outcomes could not be clearer regarding the absolute efficacy of the social-learning program in achieving the goals of increasing patients' adaptive functioning and decreasing patients' psychotic functioning and extremely bizarre behavior, as well as its relative superiority to the milieu program conducted by the same staff. The detailed ongoing assessment of patient functioning with the TSBC and CFRS found the milieu program to produce significant reductions in all classes of bizarre and inappropriate behavior except for dangerous and aggressive acts, for which milieu procedures were ineffective. However, the social-learning program was even more effective in reducing excesses in bizarre and psychotic behavior, with all components of maladaptive functioning showing an average reduction from incidence at entry exceeding 60%. Comprehensive social-learning procedures were particularly effective in eliminating belligerence and dangerous and aggressive acts—producing an average reduction of 97% reflecting complete elimination of such behavior for all but 1 patient, whose physical condition precluded participation in those procedures known to be effective. The only area of maladaptive functioning in which the milieu therapy program was ultimately as effective as the social-learning program was in the reduction of bizarre verbal statements and inappropriate facial expressions indicative of thought disorder (e.g., delusions, hallucinations, incoherent speech); even here, the social-learning program was more efficient, producing such reductions more rapidly and consistently.

Differential effectiveness of the social-learning program was even greater for increasingly adaptive cognitive, social, and instrumental functioning. Whereas the milieu program produced an average increase in overall competent functioning of only about 25% above incidence at entry, the social-learning program was remarkably effective in overcoming the severe deficits in this chronic population, demonstrating improvements in overall competent functioning nearly 10 times the rate achieved by the milieu program. On an absolute level, the average social-learning patient increased interpersonal and communicative skills by over 1200% of their entry level.

Overall, the social-learning program produced significant improvement in functioning in every patient who was physically capable of participation, including those who had failed to improve in the milieu program. In fact, 25% of these severely disabled patients had improved to the point of being indistinguishable from the "normal" population. Sustained improvement in the milieu program was obtained for only 55% of the number improved in the social-learning program, while less than one-third that number showed any improvement in hospital programs. Further, no additional improvements were observed in milieu or hospital groups while nearly all classes of patient functioning continued to show improvement in the social-learning program until the time the inpatient units were closed. On the basis of the practical goals of increasingly adaptive functioning and decreasing bizarre behavior, the social-learning program is the clear treatment of choice.

Reducing Psychotropic Medications

Since psychotropic medications frequently have deleterious side effects, and many institutionalized patients who are refractory to neuroleptic drugs receive them on a "superstitious" basis, treatment programs that reduce the need for such medications are especially desirable. As might be expected given the chronic nature of the patients included in this study, the vast majority of all patients (91.7%) were receiving psychotropic medications at its inception. After $3\frac{1}{2}$ years of operation of inpatient programs, however, 89% of the social-learning patients and 82% of the milieu patients were not prescribed such medications, and this low level was maintained through the end of the inpatient treatment phase. This low medication rate is particularly impressive in view of the fact that medications were held constant on psychosocial programs over the last year when significant improvements in functioning were obtained, and that *none* of the patients in the hospital comparison group were medication free at the end of the inpatient period. The reader will note, of course, that both alternative psychosocial programs yielded significant reductions in prescribed medications; by this criterion, both the social-learning and milieu programs were effective, and the milieu program was nearly as effective as the social-learning program.

To assess whether psychotropic medications affected the clinical efficacy of either the social-learning or milieu treatments, Paul et al. (1972) randomly assigned half the patients in each group at pretreatment to placebo while half continued to receive neuroleptics. Physicians, staff members, and patients were blind to each patient's medication status for the following 17 weeks of the active program. The ward behavior of all patients improved over the study period, with patients in the social-learning group improving the most. After 17 weeks of the treatment, there were no differences between patients on neuroleptics and those receiving placebos. However, patients receiving neuroleptics improved at a slower rate during the first 2 months of treatment than patients receiving placebos, suggesting that medication may actually impede recovery in at least some psychiatric patients. This finding is consistent with a review of the literature by Liberman, Falloon, and Wallace (1984) who concluded that as many as half of all aged and medicated chronic schizophrenic outpatients were actually unresponsive to neuroleptics and would function just as well on very little or no medication, especially when involved in structured behavior therapy programs.

Facilitating Discharge and Community Tenure

A major goal in working with chronically institutionalized psychiatric patients is to improve functioning to a level enabling them to be successfully discharged and maintained in the community. On the basis of this criterion, the social-learning program was again established as significantly more successful than the milieu treatment and the traditional hospital comparison groups. Through the end of the common inpatient period, the social-learning program treated 40 patients, of whom 97.5% were successfully discharged with a minimum community stay of at least 90 days, as compared to 31 milieu patients with 71% discharged and 29 hospital comparison patients with 44.8% discharged. Of the original equated groups, discharge to independent living and self-support without rehospitalization was achieved for 10.7% of the social-learning patients, 7.1% of the milieu patients, and none of the hospital patients—any such discharge being astounding for the severely disabled population. All other discharges were to community board-and-care facilities with, at best, employment in a sheltered workshop. Unfortunately, about 80% of the patients discharged to board-and-care facilities were readministered psychotropic drugs once they were in the facilities, independent of the nature of level of functioning. The investigators had hoped to extend the social-learning program to community aftercare facilities, but budgeting constraints and logistical difficulties precluded the full development of this plan and responsibility for programming had to be relinquished to the facilities. The declining-contact aftercare consultation was, however, conducted for discharges to independent living and to community board-and-care placements. These social-learning aftercare procedures were successful in maintaining community tenure for more than 97% of patients discharged from all three inpatient programs, without differential rehospitalization rates from the different inpatient units. Community tenure ranged from a minimum of 18 months to more than 5 years at the end of the follow-up period. Thus, all the evaluative goals—increasing adaptive functioning and decreasing psychotic and bizarre behavior, reducing psychotropic medications, and facilitating discharge and community tenure—identify the comprehensive social-learning program as the clear treatment of choice for the severely disabled, chronically institutionalized psychiatric patient.

Practical Acceptability of Innovations

As any practitioner can attest, treatment efficacy must be evaluated on many dimensions, including its acceptability and relevance in clinical settings. The most useful treatments must result in benefits for patients, of course, but they must also be cost effective, ideologically acceptable, and manageable by staff. Even a surefire cure is of little value if it is too costly to purchase or no one can administer it. Once the success of the social-learning program in reducing symptoms and enhancing adaptive functioning among chronic mental patients is accepted, four important questions remain: (a) Is the treatment cost effective? (b) Is it acceptable on ethical and humanitarian grounds? (c) Can it be delivered consistently in the face of external pressures? (d) Is it comprehensible, manageable, and acceptable to typical public hospital staff?

Cost Effectiveness

Paul and Lentz (1977) report a detailed and conservative cost-effectiveness analysis of the comparative dollars spent and saved by the different treatment programs during the 6-year period—noting that only differential costs and savings have meaning without estimating the effects of inflation and discounting. Although staff–patient ratios were equal between psychosocial programs and the hospital comparison, staffing costs were slightly higher for the psychosocial programs as a result of including aftercare functions within inpatient staffing and a relatively greater proportion of psychologists (including Paul's consultant costs) in contrast to nurses in the psychosocial programs. However, the reduced use of psychotropic drugs in the psychosocial programs resulted in lower medication costs. Thus, the daily cost of the social-learning program for staffing and medication combined was only 1.6% higher than that of the hospital program while the cost of the milieu program was only 2% higher in these regards. All other per diem costs of the social-learning program were equal to or less than those of the milieu program, the costs of which were in turn equal to or less than those of the hospital comparison.

The greater efficiency and effectiveness of the psychosocial programs in producing successful discharge and community tenure resulted in a considerable economic gain since aftercare is much less costly than continued hospitalization. Even when the cost side of the equation is limited to the differential expense of staff and drug costs, the social-learning program returned more than three times the dollar savings for the same dollars spent compared to traditional programs during the project period, and 30% more than the milieu program when calculations include only the original equated groups. If the greater number of patients treated is considered, the social-learning program was nearly four times as cost effective as the hospital comparison and 50% more cost effective than the milieu program. Thus, purely on the basis of economic factors, both psychosocial programs were more effective than traditional hospital treatment, and the social-learning program again emerged as the treatment of choice.

Ethical and Humanitarian Concerns

The majority of social-learning procedures that are directed toward increasing patient motivation and decreasing inappropriate and bizarre behavior consist of positive reinforcement of adaptive competencies through application of both social and material consequences and constructive training in appropriate alternative behavior. However, the social-learning program also includes the use of primary reinforcement (e.g., food and sleep) as well as explicit behavior-contingent application of extinction, aversion, and response-cost procedures about which many commentators have ethical and humanitarian concerns.

Paul and Lentz (1977) provide a detailed analysis of all procedures within the social-learning program that could be considered aversive, restrictive, or intrusive by nearly any standard as well as comparative data on the frequency of such events in traditional hospital programs and in the milieu program, where the only specified negative consequence was for dangerous and aggressive acts. In the traditional hospital program, 20.9% of staff–patient interactions involved such negative components compared to 12.3% within the milieu program and only 7.5% within the social-learning program. Further detailed analyses of the absolute level of deprivation, intrusions, or punishment showed the social-learning program to be the most humanitarian of all inpatient programs in these regards. The presence of an integrated, constructive treatment program with many positive social and material consequences and few explicit and consistent negative ones further increased the effectiveness of purely verbal procedures, even for terminating ongoing inappropriate behavior (e.g., such verbal procedures increased from a low of 94% effectiveness to 98% in the social-learning program compared to the milieu program in which verbal procedures started at 75% effectiveness and declined over time to only 55%). Thus, the comprehensiveness of the program with explicit criteria and contingency rules based on ongoing objective assessment ensured almost automatically that the least restrictive or intrusive means necessary for treatment of each patient would be used. Consequently, the social-learning program also emerges as the treatment of choice on purely ethical and humanitarian grounds.

Treatment Consistency

Although social-learning treatment was clearly an effective intervention, its effectiveness was occasionally compromised by external events (e.g., a patient death, fiscal constraints, and hospital policy changes made at the state level). Each of these circumstances at least temporarily decreased improvements gained through behavioral programming. The most dramatic decrease occurred subsequent to a revision of Illinois state policy on the use of restrictive and aversive interventions. Previously, nursing staff had the option of placing highly assaultive and aggressive patients in seclusion for up to

48 hours, but the modified state policy limited the duration of this seclusion to a 2-hour maximum. A gradual increase in assaultive behavior followed in both psychosocial programs, with even nonassaultive patients demonstrating decreases in adaptive behavior and increases in inappropriate behavior. Fortunately, the new policy was eventually revised to allow longer duration in seclusion, and many treatment gains were reestablished.

While the circumstances surrounding this policy change may be specific to Illinois, the larger issues apply to all innovative treatment programs. They are uniquely sensitive to administrative fiats, budgetary constraints, and sociopolitical pressures. Thus, mental health professionals who wish to develop or implement novel treatment programs must be prepared to defend sedulously their rationale and treatment practices, and even then to be faced with external mandates for change. Consistent programming becomes especially problematical. However, the Paul and Lentz experience indicates that diligence in defending new programs can greatly facilitate their continued existence.

Program Accessibility to Staff

Public psychiatric hospitals must rely on nonprofessionals (e.g., high school graduates) with some additional training to provide most of the ongoing patient care. Consequently, alternative treatment approaches must be comprehensible and manageable by staff members lacking advanced training in the behavioral sciences. One of the greatest strengths of the comparative study reported by Paul and Lentz is the demonstration that nonprofessional staff could be taught to conduct two comprehensive and rigorous but distinct "high technology" psychosocial treatment programs. After less than 6 months of training, all trainees were regularly certified to work independently in all functional components of both the social-learning and milieu programs. Furthermore, continuous hourly time sampling on the SRIC verified that staff members were conducting the two programs differentially and with excellent fidelity to their models. After only 6 weeks of initial training, over 90% of the staff–patient interactions in the milieu program followed detailed procedures and over 98% of the staff–patient interactions in the social-learning treatment followed the social-learning procedures. After inservice training incorporated SRIC as well as CFRS data for staff feedback, the fidelity of staff execution of both psychosocial programs improved to more than 99.5% and remained there until termination (more than 2 years). It is interesting that staff opinion was somewhat divided about the alternative treatment programs. Most staff consistently judged the milieu program to be closer in ideology to their preferred form of intervention, but found the actual work on the social-learning unit to be more enjoyable and accurately judged the social-learning program to be more effective.

In summary, the social-learning program, which was the treatment choice by all other criteria, is clearly manageable, acceptable, and accessible to the types and levels of staff already employed in public psychiatric hospitals. Nevertheless, the development and implementation of social-learning programs for chronic mental patients has critical prerequisites. These include substantial administrative support and encouragement, highly specialized and competent leadership, careful extensive staff training, and an ongoing commitment to quality assurance. Only with these prerequisites satisfactorily met can a behavioral treatment program develop and flourish. The implications of implementing a social-learning program for chronic mental patients are outlined fully in Table 6.2.

Rehabilitative Characteristics of Psychosocial Programs

The focus of this section is on program characteristics that can improve the clinical outcome for institutionalized patients, draw-

Table 6.2. Implications of Implementing a Social-Learning Program for Chronic Mental Patients

PERSON TO WHOM IMPLICATIONS APPLY	IMPLICATION
On-line staff in psychiatric facilities	Even the most disordered institutionalized schizophrenics can be treated effectively, treated and discharged to community care: Work in structured/effective units is more enjoyable than that in unstructured/ineffective units
Mental health professionals	Through psychosocial programming, most institutionalized psychiatric patients can be stabilized and discharged with low doses of psychotropic medications; comprehensive programs that effectively use nonprofessional staff are more enjoyable and better than when only professionsals try to carry the treatment load
Psychiatric hospital administrators and unit directors	Nonprofessional staff can be taught to conduct a rigorous comprehensive treatment program reliably, thus increasing the effectiveness of treatment; aftercare should be integrated with inpatient programs
Mental health policy makers	Using funds to develop and implement social-learning programs at public psychiatric facilities is an investment that will be recouped by shorter hospital stays and reduced recidivism; policy decisions can have far-reaching negative effects and should be piloted carefully before they are mandated
Chronically institutionalized patients, their loved ones, and society at large	Rational, cost-effective, and humanitarian treatment programs can be implemented; the situation need not continue to be hopeless

Note: These implications were derived from results of Paul & Lentz's 1977 report.

ing on the findings from the Paul and Lentz (1977) study and other relevant findings (Paul, 1984) in the literature.

Commonalities Between the Social-Learning and Milieu Programs

Four common remediative aspects of the psychosocial programs in the long-term comparative study have also received considerable theoretical and empirical support in other literature. These features are not only necessary prerequisites to the proper implementation of a social-learning program but are likely to enhance the rationality and rehabilitative efficacy of any inpatient or residential program for all patient populations in the mental health field.

Ongoing assessment systems. The CFRS, employed by clinical staff as an integral part of the conduct of treatment programs, and the TSBC and SRIC, employed by a small cadre of independent noninteractive observers, provided ongoing moment-to-moment and hour-by-hour objective assessment of patient and staff functioning in both psychosocial programs. These instruments are not only necessary to provide the detailed information for ongoing monitoring needed to implement the treatment of choice, but a thorough analysis of sources of information and methods of assessment also found them to be prototypical primary strategies of a comprehensive assessment paradigm that would provide all the information needed for reasonable, cost-effective operation of residential treatment programs and facilities (Paul & Mariotto, 1986). These assessment strategies provide nearly all the information needed on patient, staff, and program functioning for rational, moment-to-moment, concurrent monitoring of individuals and groups, placement and disposition decisions (i.e., patient admission/assignment and discharge/transfer; staff hiring/assignment and discharge/transfer), identification of patient problems and assets, staff development and utilization, absolute and comparative program evaluation, legal and ethical regulation and documentation, need for more expensive assessment strategies such as individual interviews, and applied research.

Paul and his colleagues (Paul, 1986; Paul, in press a) have developed the TSBC and SRIC into the Computerized TSBC/SRIC Planned-Access Observational Information System to provide timely information with documented applicability to all types of residential or inpatient programs for the full range of adult patients, including mentally retarded as well as alcohol and substance abuse and acute and chronic mentally ill (Paul, 1987a, 1987b). Because of the quality and amount of useful assessment information and documentation provided by independent observers and the computer, clinical staff are freed from unnecessary paperwork with the result that four- to five-fold increases in attention received by patients from staff in the social-learning and milieu programs can be obtained without increasing existing numbers of staff–patient ratios.

Decentralized administrative structure with integrated staffing. Another common and critical aspect of the psychosocial programs in the long-term comparative study was the decentralized administrative organization to the treatment units with permanent rather than rotating staff assignments, and authority and responsibility based on demonstrated competency rather than discipline. Comprehensive psychosocial programs could be housed in a variety of physical locations, including public or private mental hospitals, inpatient units of mental health centers or general hospitals, and community residential facilities; however, the decentralized administrative and staffing organization is crucial to allow consistent staff training, monitoring, and communication as well as continuity of care—preferably extended to responsibility for postdischarge aftercare as well. Such an organization allows the maximum use of the large number of existing nonprofessional staff as direct providers of service, instead of being just caretakers while the professionals attempt to provide treatment. As demonstrated in the long-term study and elsewhere, positive attitudes, program identification, and improved performance of all levels of staff can result from such a structure with integrated staffing. This structure also helps buffer patients and staff from the vagaries and irrationalities of funding and external political events that can keep some component of any centralized administrative structure—where authority is based on disciplinary lines—in upheaval at all times. It is probably the only way in which the low staffing levels and resultant desirable cost-effectiveness ratios obtained in the long-term study could provide effective treatment in any program. In fact, Paul and Lentz argue that all program components and funding, except maintenance functions, should be decentralized to program subunits on a block-grant performance-contracting basis to ensure continuity of programs and to provide incentives for effective treatment without increasing costs.

Comprehensive educational/rehabilitative focus. The common focus of the psychosocial program on establishing minimal competencies in specific components of intrapersonal, interpersonal, and instrumental skills, reducing or eliminating extreme bizarre behavior, and bridging the gap from inpatient programs to community functioning was originally derived from a review of the literature on factors leading to hospitalization or rehospitalization. More recent literature, as well as the predictability of community functioning up to 18 months after discharge from the psychosocial programs, strongly confirms the importance of these minimal goals for any inpatient or residential program. In addition, both social-learning and milieu programs structured the daily and weekly schedule of each patient so that specific times and places ensured the opportunity for assessment and training in each component of adaptive functioning while inappropriate behavior was dealt with whenever it occurred. Comprehensive scheduling of all patient waking hours as well as the step system further ensured that all aspects of patient functioning were treated in a systematic, integrated fashion to equip patients with the skills necessary for community living and concurrently to protect patients and the community from premature discharges and revolving door episodes. Consistent with a wide range of other research, the focus on structured activities, classes, and meetings served not only to build skills, but also to produce significant decreases in many aspects of bizarre and idiosyncratic behavior for milieu patients as well as for social-learning patients.

Another important aspect of the educational and rehabilitative focus of both psychosocial programs was the use of descriptive language—"resident" versus "patient" status—and patient accountability. In traditional hospital settings, "patients" are defined as "sick" and are provided with "care" until they are "well." Such conceptualizations may be useful with physical illnesses, but they may also individually reinforce the patient for maintaining the "sick role" (Goffman, 1961). While a full discussion of this controversy is outside the scope of this chapter, it is clear that setting attainable, positive goals for change and communicating to patients that they are capable and responsible for meeting these goals is a critical first step for any effective treatment program, including ones for the chronically mentally ill.

Consistent, systematic, goal-oriented, staff–patient interactions. An important commonality between the social-learning and milieu programs allowed clear, unique, explicit rules about appropriate staff behavior in interacting with patients in a variety of settings that facilitated staff training and ongoing monitoring. This specification allowed consistent and systematic staff–patient interactions. Further, these staff–patient interactions and overall program structures were always goal-oriented. Each activity in each patient's daily schedule was included only if it served a specific purpose designed ultimately to achieve discharge to the community—including gradual reexposure to the less structured setting of the external community. Paul and Lentz present SRIC data documenting that the type, rather than the amount, of staff–patient interaction is more important for improving most classes of patient functioning; however, the greater consistency and amount of staff–patient interaction achieved in both psychosocial programs clearly allowed for more efficient use of limited staff resources and were effective in reactivating dormant skills and in reducing cognitive dysfunction and indicants of thought disorder among participants in both programs.

Uniquely Effective Ingredients of the Social-Learning Program

By attending to the commonalities between the social-learning and milieu treatments, mental health practitioners working with chronically institutionalized patients can enhance the rehabilitative efficacy of their overall programs. Further improvements in patient functioning may be accomplished by implementing the unique features of the social-learning program, which was the most effective treatment of all and the clear treatment of choice for the chronically institutionalized.

Integrated procedures emphasizing the acquisition of patient competencies. Although both milieu and social-learning programs showed higher staff–patient interactions than traditional programs, no specific class of patient behavior covaried with total staff activity or attention received by patients. Rather, staff–patient interactions following social-learning principles were more effective with both equal and fewer rates of interaction than in the milieu program. This was especially true for increasing adaptive behavior and teaching patient competencies. The specification of desired behavior, provision of opportunities to perform, and overall goal-directed staff–patient interactions resulted in substantial improvements within 1 to 2 months in both psychosocial programs;

however, milieu patients' adaptive functioning continued to show gradual and major improvements. Paul and Lentz suggest that the initial response reflected the activation of previously dormant skills, with SRIC data showing that adaptive functioning of milieu patients was maintained only when milieu procedures happened to result in the application of staff–patient interactions that also followed social-learning principles (i.e., contingent social reinforcement).

In contrast, the consistent and systematic application of individual prompts and modeling, response-contingent consequences with both social and material reinforcement, associative learning procedures, and careful decomposition of patient adaptive behavior into learnable components that successively approximated the "normal" functioning ultimately desired was remarkably effective in helping social-learning patients to acquire new self-care, interpersonal, and communications skills. These social-learning procedures, combined with brief time-out and token response costs for failures, were also exceptionally effective in increasing patients' attention span, improving their attendance at classes, meetings, and vocational training sessions, and developing other instrumental skills as well as increasing the complexity of performance in vocational areas. These social-learning procedures have shown documented effectiveness when applied independently in other studies with a wide range of functional psychotics (Wong et al., 1986). When the procedures were integrated within the comprehensive program they were uniquely powerful in developing new intrapersonal, interpersonal, and instrumental skills for even the most severely disabled patients.

Integrated procedures to reduce or eliminate extreme bizarre and inappropriate behavior. In keeping with other research findings, the active participation in alternative adaptive activities did lead to significant reductions in bizarre motoric behavior and some aspects of cognitive dysfunction (e.g., delusions and hallucinations, incoherent speech, and smiling without a stimulus). The vast majority of social-learning patients reduced extreme maladaptive behavior as a result of staff's ignoring inappropriate acts while prompting and differentially reinforcing incompatible adaptive behavior. The explicit, consistent, behavior-contingent application of time-out and token response costs was also usually effective in reducing or eliminating extreme bizarre behavior, including dangerous and aggressive acts, when these procedures were applied within the context of the overall construction focus of the social-learning program—even though the frequency of application and level of averseness were lower than procedures typically applied in most institutional programs. Overcorrection and restitution procedures were 100% effective in eliminating assaults and other dangerous behavior that did not respond to the overall programmatic procedures. Although the consistent application of such negative consequences was an important and effective component of the integrated social-learning program, its greatest value may be in increasing the effectiveness of purely verbal social-learning procedures, since verbal prompts were 94% effective in terminating ongoing bizarre behavior from the start of the program, increasing over time to 98% effectiveness. Thus, the consistency of such staff–patient interactions was critical in terminating bizarre and psychotic acts to allow positive training in alternative coping and problem-solving skills. Social-learning procedures involving graduated reinforced exposure in stressful circumstances, the provision of active solutions, information, and advice, and training in alternative adaptive skills were considerably more effective than milieu procedures in assisting patients to overcome negative emotional reactions to stress and maladaptive behavior based on conditioned anxiety reactions. Although these overall programmatic procedures were adequate in reducing such emotional reactions in the chronically mentally ill to a level allowing discharge and community tenure, the most effective social-learning procedures for treating conditioned anxiety reactions would require more professional staff for their inclusion (Paul & Bernstein, 1976), especially if large numbers of acutely admitted patients were being treated.

Token economy structure. The overall token economy motivational structure was a critical component of the social-learning program for effective treatment of the severely debilitated chronic psychiatric patient. However, Paul and Lentz caution that the "token economy" of the social-learning program may have little in common with others that do not include all the unique integrated aspects of the specific program that was found to be the treatment of choice. For severely desocialized patients, tangible tokens within a "tight economy" (preventing inflation and deflation), which includes primary reinforcers as backups, are necessary to provide the immediate consequences required for motivational purposes and to facilitate new learning by providing immediate feedback (Reynolds, 1968; Skinner, 1938). Such undersocialized patients respond to few purely social stimuli without new learning, and any time lag at all allows interference from poor attention and/or the inability to receive and process information (Wallace & Boone, 1984). The staff's consistent verbal and nonverbal interactions with patients, contingently paired with token disbursement and collection, not only make the immediate social communication salient but, over time, help patients gradually learn to value and benefit from social contact, verbal instruction, and social reinforcement alone. The token economy comes to function primarily as an efficient management system for patients as they develop internal controls and learn to value social stimuli, or for patients who are less severely disabled initially. The carefully developed and implemented token economy thus provides the immediacy of informational feedback and reinforcement with fine gradations for patients who need it, and an overall management system for all patients until they function well enough to "buy out" of the use of tangible tokens at the highest step in the program.

Consistent pacing and generalization training. Considerable research on cognitive processes in schizophrenia indicates that either understimulating environments or hyperarousal can interfere with performance and/or the reception, processing, and action on relevant versus irrelevant information. Many studies have reported deleterious effects from some intensive inpatient programs (Liberman et al., 1984). The careful structure and pacing of focused, positively reinforced concrete skills training in small steps over all waking hours, as in the comprehensive inpatient social-learning program, in addition to the application of specific principles and procedures to particular problems, may be critical to effectiveness with the severely disabled. High-demand programs with less pacing in concrete problem solving and skills building may overstimulate patients who are hyperaroused or who are too deficient in cognitive skills to benefit from new information in time-limited training periods. Low-demand programs may fail to activate patients enough to attend to external stimuli or attempt to learn from the services offered. The careful pacing incorporated within the comprehensive social-learning program also ensures generalization of patient skills across staff and situations with gradual fading of dependence on immediate token reinforcement. As patients progress in the social-learning program, treatment and consultations are systematically shifted from staff-initiated problem identification, solution, and skills training through eliciting problem solving from patients to patient-initiated problem solving and action. Paul (1984) notes that these aspects of the social-learning inpatient and aftercare programs of the long-term comparative study are common to successful community or aftercare programs, starting with less severely debilitated patients, that have been reported by more than 10 clinical research groups in different locales.

CURRENT STATUS OF SOCIAL-LEARNING TREATMENT

Because of the experimental design of the long-term comparative study reported by Paul and Lentz, it is the only study to date in the institutional literature to provide cause-effect evidence for the absolute and relative effectiveness of total treatment programs. Consequently, the comprehensive social-learning program in that study is the clear treatment of choice for the severely debilitated chronic mental patient. The findings of the long-term comparative study also provide support and clarification for the effectiveness of a number of social-learning principles and procedures reported in a wide range of research and clinical studies (Wong et al., 1986; Liberman, King & DeRisi, 1976).

Given the results of the Paul and Lentz study, it is somewhat surprising that social-learning programs are still in the minority in psychiatric facilities. Reasons for this limited implementation of intensive social-learning programs include staff resistance, reduced length of inpatient admissions, greater emphasis on community-based treatment where control over environmental contingencies is more difficult, economic constraints, and legal and ethical challenges (Glynn, 1990). Nevertheless, the importance of social-learning interventions can be seen both in the growing emphasis on patient accountability for behavior and in specialized psychiatric treatment programs for especially problematic patients.

General Incorporation of Accountability and Awareness Incentives

The principles of social learning have had at least two major effects on the current psychiatric treatment of institutionalized patients. First, holding patients accountable for their actions appears to be a common component of many programs. Level systems and earned privileges are routinely found as part of the treatment plan in most psychiatric hospitals. Even severely disorganized patients are often expected to perform simple self-care and housekeeping tasks before being given access to television, grounds, and other privileges. Second, the philosophy of positively reinforcing adaptive behavior and punishing negative behavior (behavior modification) is well known to most mental health professionals today. Behavioral programs providing access to reinforcers (e.g., cigarettes, coffee) for adaptive behavior and limiting access to such reinforcers (e.g., time-out, extinction) for maladaptive behavior are integral parts of many psychiatric treatment plans. Nevertheless, well-organized, behaviorally oriented treatment programs are the exception rather than the rule (Glynn, 1990).

Camarillo Clinical Research Unit

The clinical research unit at Camarillo State Hospital is a unique psychiatric unit that strives to adhere to the social-learning principles found effective in the study reported by Paul and Lentz. This 11-bed unit, under the joint sponsorship of Camarillo State Hospital and the UCLA Department of Psychiatry, has been in continuous operation since 1970, longer than any other social-learning unit extant. The day-to-day unit programming and token economy are similar to those reported by Paul and Lentz, with objective data on patients being collected almost continuously. All patients are expected to adhere to specified rules backed by contingencies of reinforcement. In addition, specific intervention programs are developed for problems not addressed through general unit programming (e.g., water intoxication patients earn ground privileges for 7 days of controlled liquid intake; a loud, verbally abusive patient accrues small token fines for each verbal outburst). The clinical research objectives of this unit require special equipment (e.g., computers) and higher staff–patient ratios than throughout the hospital, so additional funding is provided through National Institute of Mental Health grants, the university, and the state hospital.

The CRU serves three purposes at Camarillo State Hospital. First, it is an intensive treatment facility for some of the most intractable patients at the hospital. Patients referred to the CRU are usually long-term, multiple-admission patients with numerous behavioral excesses and deficits. A review of the data from 218 patients discharged from the CRU before July 1988 indicated that the most common patient problems included deficits in self-care and grooming, social skills, and work and leisure skills, as well as excesses in assaultiveness, property destruction, stereotyped movements and posturing, and verbal aggression. Seventy-two percent of the patients exhibited one or more of these difficulties when admitted to the CRU, but even with this chronic, refractory population, behavioral programming yielded substantial benefits. The typical patient improved by at least 50% from baseline levels on the spectrum of targeted clinical problems. Shown in Table 6.3 is the improvement rate in clinical problems of the patients, measured through direct observation of patient behavior.

This positive effect of social-learning treatment was also maintained in long-term follow-up evaluation of discharged CRU patients. Banzett, Liberman, Moore, and Marshall (1984) did a 2-year follow-up of CRU patients discharged from 1975 to 1979 and found that 80% of respondents (patient relatives, conservators, or treatment staff) reported maintenance or further improvement both in the patients' overall functional and clinical status and in their original referring problems since discharge. Fifty-two percent of ex-patients were living in noninstitutionalized settings. Although this rate of discharge and community tenure is lower than that obtained by Paul and Lentz, the patient populations and goals are not directly comparable; this discharge rate is better than that of the chronic units at Camarillo State Hospital. It is especially impressive given the exceedingly low level of patient functioning resulting from the referral of intractable patients and the presence of state-mandated policies that prohibit use of more powerful primary reinforcers (e.g., food) for patients.

The CRU serves two other purposes at Camarillo State Hospital. It is a site for a variety of research projects directed toward improving functioning of institutionalized patients. Current research includes a study on the effects of innovative behavioral and pharmacotherapies on treatment-refractory schizophrenia and studies on social-skills training (Liberman et al., 1985; Wallace & Liberman, 1985) for severely withdrawn and thought-disordered schizophrenics. Finally, the CRU staff act as consultants on behavioral programming to other hospital staff who have identified patients for whom standard hospital treatment is ineffective. By acting as consultants, the CRU staff help to disseminate behavioral techniques and encourage the development of social-learning programs throughout the hospital. In recent years, members of the CRU staff, under the auspices of the UCLA Clinical Research Center for Schizophrenia and Psychiatric Rehabilitation, have provided technical assistance and professional training to over 3,000 mental health and rehabilitation practitioners in psychiatric agencies and hospitals throughout the world.

Dissemination of the Comprehensive Social-Learning Program

Although the consulting and dissemination functions of special units such as the Camarillo CRU can be expected to increase the rehabilitative efficacy of psychiatric pro-

Table 6.3. Impact of Behavioral Treatment on the Camarillo/UCLA Clinical Research Unit[a]

PROBLEM BEHAVIOR	NUMBER OF PATIENTS WITH PROBLEM BEHAVIORS	AVERAGE[a] IMPROVEMENT LEVEL
Prader-Willi syndrome	9	1.0
Spitting and mucous smearing	4	1.0
Entering restricted areas	1	1.0
Anxiety	1	1.0
Vomiting	1	1.0
Psychogenic polydipsia	3	1.33
Self-injury	21	1.61
Peskiness, demandingness	19	1.63
Verbal aggression	40	1.70
Screaming, tantrums	4	1.75
Work and leisure skills	48	1.84
Self-care, grooming	146	1.89
Depression	13	1.92
Social skills deficit	73	1.92
Stereotypic movements and posturing	32	1.97
Antisocial behavior (stealing, disruption)	2	2.0
Sexual deviance	9	2.11
Assault and property destruction	92	2.17
Delusional speech	21	2.19
Social isolation	17	2.24
Mutism	2	2.5
Incoherent speech	2	2.5
Hallucinations, self-talk	5	2.60
Inactivity, amotivation	3	2.67
Incontinence	4	2.72
Obsessive-compulsive behavior	2	3.0
Total number of patient behaviors treated:	574	
Overall average improvement level:		1.93

[a]Levels of improvement for different categories of behavioral problems targeted for the 218 patients treated on the CRU (1970–1988). Pretreatment baseline rates of behavior were compared to the rate of the same behavior during the last 3 weeks of CRU treatment. For each subject, % change was calculated and improvement level was assigned using the following scale: marked improvement (1) = 75–100% change from baseline; moderate improvement (2) = 50–74% change from baseline; slight improvement (3) = 25–49% change from baseline; and no improvement (4) = less than 25% improvement.

grams as well as contributing new clinical-research findings, the full benefits of social-learning programs cannot be achieved by service providers without the complete implementation of comprehensive inpatient and aftercare elements, including integrated assessment systems. On the basis of their obtained rates of change, Paul and Lentz estimate that effective implementation of social-learning programs could improve the functioning of disabled chronic psychiatric patients to a level of acceptability for community placement in 26 to 30 weeks. In fact, given appropriate implementation mechanisms, social-learning programs could be conducted in community-based residential facilities as well as in hospital and mental health centers.

The major impediment to widespread dissemination of the comprehensive social-learning program has been the unavailability of the assessment systems to provide the detailed information needed for proper implementation and conduct of the program. Since Paul and his colleagues have completed the research and development for the TSBC/SRIC System to serve as the core assessment strategy for nearly any inpatient or residential program and population, the materials required to implement the TSBC/SRIC System and the social-learning CFRS will soon be available (Paul, in press b).

Community Programs

While both the Paul and Lentz and Camarillo CRU programs focus on inpatients, social-learning principles have also been utilized with success among seriously mentally ill outpatients. One of the most impressive of these efforts is the Fairweather Lodge program (Fairweather, Sanders, Maynard, Cressler, & Bleck, 1969). Fairweather and his colleagues adopted an approach that used the hospital as a base for initial training of patients in interpersonal skills, effective decision making, and group governance and cohesion. Following this training, the patients were transferred as a group to living quarters in the community. These quarters resembled a lodge and the patients were assisted in gradually assuming full responsibility for its maintenance and operation. They bought and prepared food, kept financial records of income and expenditures, and consulted community-based physicians and agencies for their medical, psychiatric, and support needs. Live-in staff gradually performed fewer tasks until the lodge residents were functioning autonomously. In addition, the patients earned money by starting a local business that provided janitorial services, yard work, general hauling, and painting. A 40-months' follow-up indicated that the patients trained to live and work in a community lodge sustained significantly greater time outside the hospital and in gainful employment.

RECENT DEVELOPMENTS IN SOCIAL-LEARNING PROGRAMS

Since the publication of the Paul and Lentz (1977) study, other researchers have continued to investigate social-learning approaches to the rehabilitation of the chronically mentally ill. In line with the work of Paul and Lentz, these authors typically find that social-learning programs result in dramatic improvements in behavior (Baker, Hall, Hutchinson, & Bridge, 1977; Fullerton, Cayner, & McLaughlin-Reidel, 1978; McCreadie, Main, & Dunlap, 1978; Nelson & Cone, 1979; Stoffelmayr, Faulkner, & Mitchell, 1979; Stone & Nelson, 1979; Turner & Luber, 1980; Wong et al., 1986; Woods, Higson, & Tannahill, 1984). Nevertheless, critical research and treatment issues remain.

One area of investigation concerns identification of the remediative elements within the token economy program. For example, Baker et al. (1977) found that both a token economy patient and one in a yoked control group improved in behavior, raising the possibility that improvement results from some factor (e.g., enriched positive reinforcements) other than contingent reinforcement. Studying a token economy program in a day hospital, researchers from the UCLA Clinical Research Center (Liberman, Fearn, DeRisi, Roberts, & Carmona, 1977) found that the specific behavioral goals and social reinforcement contingencies inherent in the economy accounted for therapeutic change rather than the tangible backup rewards. Similarly, Turner and Luber (1980) reported that patients judged feedback about performance (and not tokens) as being the most critical aspect of the program. Further research is needed to determine the relative importance of tokens in providing information and motivation. In addition, alternate explanations for the success of the token economy must be developed and tested.

A second important issue concerns generalization of improvements. Maintenance and generalization of treatment gains are, of course, critical tests of the utility of treatment interventions. For social-learning programs, the crucial question is this: Are token economies primarily prosthetic, resulting in behavioral change only when it is supported by contingent token reinforcement? Or are they therapeutic, resulting in long-term behavioral change across settings? The answers to these questions have not been fully determined. Woods, Higson, and Tannahill (1984) found that there were extreme differences among patients' maintenance of behavioral improvements when contingent tokens were changed to noncontingent tokens. Some patients showed no decrements in performance while others deteriorated almost immediately. The authors' data suggested that rapid initial rates of change when the token economy was applied predicted maintenance. These investigators suggest that some patient improvements are maintained because they are "trapped" by positive social reinforcement. Certainly, identifying patient variables that are related to the development and maintenance of improvements in functioning is an important issue that merits attention.

Finally, the extreme deficits of treatment-refractory schizophrenics raise the possibility that a social-learning program may be a necessary but insufficient condition for successful community tenure of these patients. Two recent studies (Massel et al., in press; Wallace & Liberman, 1985) offered structured, intensive social skills training to treatment-resistant schizophrenics as an adjunct to their treatment on a token economy hospital unit with encouraging results. Patients' social skills increased dramatically in both studies, and Wallace and Liberman (1985) found that participation in social-skills training actually decreased the probability of relapse during a 2-year follow-up. This addition of specialized remediation of skill deficits to a strong social-learning program maximizes patients' likelihood of behavioral improvement and may augment the benefits of behavioral rehabilitation (Liberman & Evans, 1985).

Because psychosocial interventions based on social-learning principles are effective in reducing maladaptive behavior and increasing adaptive functioning of "hardcore" institutionalized psychiatric patients, reducing medications, facilitating discharge, and maintaining community tenure, they merit continued attention, refinement, and dissemination. The comprehensive social-learning program, including the integrated assessment systems and inpatient and aftercare technologies, is the clear preferred treatment for chronically institutionalized mental patients on economic, clinical, and humanitarian grounds.

REFERENCES

Baker, R., Hall, J. K., Hutchinson, K., & Bridge, G. (1977). Symptom changes in chronic schizophrenic patients on a token economy: A controlled experiment. *British Journal of Psychiatry, 131*, 381–393.

Banzett, L. K., Liberman, R. P., Moore, J. W., & Marshall, B. D. (1984). Long term follow-up of the effects of behavior therapy. *Hospital and Community Psychiatry, 35*, 277–279.

Bellack, A. S., & Mueser, K. T. (1986). A comprehensive treatment program for schizophrenia and chronic mental illness. *Community Mental Health Journal, 22*, 175–189.

Dickey, B., Gudeman, J., Hellman, S., Donatella, A., & Greenspoon, L. (1981). A follow-up of de-institutionalized chronic clients four years after discharge. *Hospital and Community Psychiatry, 32*, 326–329.

Fairweather, G. W., Sanders, D. H., Maynard, H., Cressler, D. L., & Bleck, D. S. (1969). *Community life for the mentally ill: An alternative to institutional care*. Chicago, IL: Aldine Publishing Company.

Friedman, I., von Mering, O., & Hinko, E. N. (1966). Intermittent patient-hood: The hospital career of today's mental patient. *Archives of General Psychiatry, 14*, 386–392.

Fullerton, D. I., Cayner, J. J., & McLaughlin-Reidel, T. (1978). Results of a token economy. *Archives of General Psychiatry, 35*, 1451–1453.

Goffman, E. C. (1961). *Asylums*. Garden City, NY: Doubleday.

Glynn, S. M. (1990). The token economy: Progress and pitfalls over 25 years. *Behavior Modification, 14*, 383–407.

Honigfeld, G. (1966). *Nurses Observation Scale for Inpatient Evaluation (NOSIE-30)*. Glen Oaks, NY: Honigfeld.

Kirk, S. A., & Therrien, M. E. (1975). Community mental health myths and the fate of former hospitalized patients. *Psychiatry, 38*, 209–217.

Kohen, W., & Paul, G. L. (1976). Current trends and recommended changes in extended-care placement of mental patients: The Illinois system as a case in point. *Schizophrenia Bulletin, 2*, 575–594.

Lehman, A. (1983). The well-being of chronic mental patients. *Archives of General Psychiatry, 40*, 369–373.

Lehman, A. F., Ward, N. C., & Linn, L. S. (1982). Chronic mental patients: The quality of life issue. *American Journal of Psychiatry, 139*, 1271–1276.

Libermam, R. P. (1982). Social factors in schizophrenia. In L. Grinspoon (Ed.), *Psychiatry 1982 Annual Review* (pp. 97–111). Washington, DC: American Psychiatric Press.

Liberman, R. P., & Evans, C. C. (1985). Behavioral rehabilitation for chronic mental patients. *Journal of Clinical Psychopharmacology, 5*(Supplement), 8s–14s.

Liberman, R. P., Falloon, I. R. H., & Wallace, C. J. (1984). Drug-psychosocial interactions in the treatment of schizophrenia. In M. Mirabi (Ed.), *The chronically mentally ill: Research and services* (pp. 175–212). New York: SP Medical & Scientific Books.

Liberman, R. P., Fearn, C. H., DeRisi, W. J., Roberts, J., & Carmona, M. (1977). The credit incentive system: Motivating the participation of patients in a day hospital. *British Journal of Social and Clinical Psychology, 16*, 85–94.

Liberman, R. P., King, L., DeRisi, W. J. (1976). Behavior analysis and modification in community mental health. In H. Leitenberg (Ed.), *Handbook of behavior therapy and behavior modification* (pp. 566–603). Englewood Cliffs, NJ: Prentice-Hall.

Liberman, R. P., Massel, H. K., Mosk, M. D., & Wong, S. E. (1985). Social skills training for chronic mental hospital patients. *Hospital and Community Psychiatry, 36*, 396–403.

Licht, M. H., & Paul, G. L. (1987). The Staff-Resident Interaction Chronograph (SRIC). In M. Hersen & A. S. Bellack (Eds.), *Dictionary of behavioral assessment techniques*. Elmsford, NY: Pergamon Press.

Massel, H. K., Corrigan, P. W., Liberman, R. P., & Milan, M. A. (in press). Conversation skills training of thought disordered schizophrenics through attention focusing. *Psychiatry Research*.

McCreadie, R. G., Main, C. J., & Dunlap, R. A. (1978). Token economy, pimozide, and chronic schizophrenia. *British Journal of Psychiatry, 133*, 179–181.

Nelson, G. L., & Cone, J. D. (1979). Multiple baseline analyses of a token economy for psychiatric inpatients. *Journal of Applied Behavior Analysis, 12*, 255–271.

Paul, G. L. (1984). Residential treatment programs and aftercare for the chronically institutionalized. In M. Mirabi (Ed.), *The chronically mentally ill: Research and services* (pp. 239–262). New York: Medical and Scientific Books, Spectrum Publications.

Paul, G. L. (1986a). Net relative cost of the maximum potential utility paradigm. In G. L. Paul (Ed.), Assessment in residential treatment settings: *Principles and methods to support cost-effective quality operations. (Assessment in residential treatment settings, part 1.)* (pp. 165–190). Champaign, IL: Research Press.

Paul, G. L. (1986b). Rational operations in residential treatment settings through ongoing assessment of client and staff functioning. In D. R. Peterson & D. B. Fishman (Eds.), *Assessment for decision* (pp. 1–35). New Brunswick, NJ: Rutgers University Press.

Paul, G. L. (Ed.). (1987a). *The Time-Sample Behavioral Checklist: Observational assessment instrumentation for service and research. (Assessment in residential treatment settings, part 2.)* Champaign, IL: Research Press.

Paul, G. L. (Ed.). (1987b). *The Staff-Resident Interaction Chronograph: Observational assessment instrumentation for service and research. (Assessment in residential treatment settings, part 3.)* Champaign, IL: Research Press.

Paul, G. L. (Ed.). (in press a). *The Computerized TSBC/SRIC Planned-Access Observational*

Information System: Observational assessment instrumentation for service and research. (Assessment in residential treatment settings, part 4.) Champaign, IL: Research Press.

Paul, G. L. (Ed.). (in press b). *The TSBC/SRIC System Implementation Package: Observational assessment instrumentation for service and research. (Assessment in residential treatment settings, part 5.)* Champaign, IL: Research Press.

Paul, G. L., & Bernstein, D. A. (1976). Anxiety and clinical problems. In J. T. Spence, R. C. Carson, & J. W. Thibaut (Eds.), *Behavioral approaches to therapy* (pp. 47–87). Morristown, NJ: General Learning Press.

Paul, G. L., & Lentz, R. J. (1977). *Psychosocial treatment of chronic mental patients: Milieu versus social-learning programs.* Cambridge, MA: Harvard University Press.

Paul, G. L., & Lentz, R. J. (in preparation). *Psychosocial treatment of chronic mental patients: Milieu versus social-learning programs* (2nd ed.). Champaign, IL: Research Press.

Paul, G. L., & Licht, M. H. (1987a). The Clinical Frequencies Recording System (CFRS). In M. Hersen & A. S. Bellack (Eds.), *Dictionary of behavioral assessment techniques.* Elmsford, NY: Pergamon Press.

Paul, G. L., & Licht, M. H. (1987b). The Time-Sample Behavioral Checklist (TSBC). In M. Hersen & A. S. Bellack (Eds.), *Dictionary of behavioral assessment techniques.* Elmsford, NY: Pergamon Press.

Paul, G. L., & Mariotto, M. J. (1986). Potential utility of the sources and methods: A comprehensive paradigm. In G. L. Paul (Ed.), *Principles and methods to support cost-effective quality operations: Assessment in residential settings, part 1* (pp. 113–164). Champaign, IL: Research Press.

Paul, G. L., Tobias, L. L., & Holly, B. L. (1972). Maintenance psychotropic drugs in the presence of active treatment programs: A "triple-blind" withdrawal study with long-term mental patients. *Archives of General Psychiatry, 27,* 106–115.

Reynolds, G. S. (1968). *A primer of operant conditioning.* Glenview, IL: Scott, Foresman.

Rhoades, L. J. (1981). *Treating and assessing the chronically mentally ill: The pioneering research of Gordon L. Paul* (DHHS Publication No. ADM 81-1100). Rockville, MD: Science Reports Branch, Division of Scientific and Public Information, National Institute of Mental Health.

Rosen, A. J., Sussman, S., Mueser, K. T., Lyons, J. S., & Davis, J. M. (1981). Behavioral assessment of psychiatric inpatients and normal controls across different environmental contexts. *Journal of Behavioral Assessment, 3,* 25–36.

Skinner, B. F. (1938). *The behavior of organisms.* New York, NY: Appleton-Century-Crofts.

Spivack, G., Siegel, J., Sklaver, D., Deuschle, L., & Garrett, L. (1983). The long-term client in the community: Lifestyle patterns and treatment implications. *Hospital and Community Psychiatry, 33,* 291–295.

Stoffelmayr, B. E., Faulkner, G. E., Mitchell, W. S. (1979). The comparison of token economy and social therapy in the treatment of hard-core schizophrenic patients. *Behavior Analysis and Modification, 3,* 3–17.

Stone, M. E., & Nelson, G. L. (1979). Coordinated treatment for long-term psychiatric inpatients. *Social Work, 15,* 406–410.

Turner, S. M., & Luber, R. F. (1980). The token economy in day hospital settings: Contingency management or information feedback. *Journal of Behavior Therapy and Experimental Psychiatry, 11,* 89–94.

Wallace, C. J., & Boone, S. G. (1984). Cognitive factors in the social skills of schizophrenic patients: Implications for treatment. In W. D. Spaulding & J. K. Cole (Eds.), *Nebraska symposium on motivation, 1983* (pp. 282–318). Lincoln: University of Nebraska Press.

Wallace, C. J., & Liberman, R. P. (1985). Social skills training for patients with schizophrenia: A controlled clinical trial. *Psychiatry Research, 15,* 239–247.

Wing, J. K., & Freudenberg, R. K. (1961). The response of severely ill chronic schizophrenic patients to social stimulation. *American Journal of Psychiatry, 118,* 311–322.

Wolkon, G. H., Karmen, M., & Tanaka, H. T. (1971). Evaluation of a social rehabilitation program for recently released psychiatric patients. *Community Mental Health Journal, 7,* 312–322.

Wong, S. E., Massel, H. K., Mosk, M. D., & Liberman, R. P. (1986). Behavioral approaches to the treatment of schizophrenia. In G. D. Burrows, T. R. Norman, & G. Rubenstein (Eds.), *Handbook of studies on schizo-*

phrenia (pp. 79–100). Amsterdam: Elsevier Science Publishers.

Wong, S. E., Terranova, M. D., Bowen, L., Zarate, R., Massel, H. K., & Liberman, R. P. (1987). Providing independent recreational activities to reduce stereotypic vocalizations in chronic schizophrenics. *Journal of Applied Behavior Analysis, 20*, 77–81.

Woods, P. A., Higson, P. J., & Tannahill, M. M. (1984). Token economy programmes with chronic psychiatric patients: The importance of direct measurement and objective evaluation for long-term maintenance. *Behaviour Research and Therapy, 22*, 41–51.

CHAPTER 7

TRAINING IN COMMUNITY LIVING

Mary Ann Test

In the past 2 decades considerable progress has been made in developing and empirically validating an array of biological, psychological, and social interventions that are useful in facilitating the community tenure and psychosocial rehabilitation of persons with serious mental illnesses (Test, 1984). Yet, workers in the field of community treatment and rehabilitation need to know how to deliver these services in a way that reaches the target population in a timely fashion that optimizes the chances that clients and significant others will receive *what* they need, *when* they need it. Training in Community Living (TCL) is a service delivery model that has received substantial empirical support in this regard. A summary of this model and its relevant research findings are the focus of this chapter.

HISTORICAL OVERVIEW

The TCL model evolved from our work on the research ward of Mendota State Hospital in Madison, Wisconsin, in the late 1960s (Marx, Test, & Stein, 1973). We observed that a large number of the patients we discharged soon rotated back to the hospital, despite intensive programs to prepare them for community living, and despite our having linked them with an apparently good aftercare system. It became clear that fol-

The Training in Community Living program is funded by the Mendota Mental Health Institute of the State of Wisconsin Department of Health and Social Services. The evaluations of the program have been funded in part by the Mendota Mental Health Institute, and by grants from the National Institute of Mental Health and the University of Wisconsin. The writing of this paper was supported by grant MH40886 from the National Institute of Mental Health.

lowing discharge our patients were not receiving the services and supports they needed to remain in the community and to grow in psychosocial areas. Although most were in a state of remission on discharge, they were far from being cured of their serious mental illnesses. Hence, they continued to be extremely vulnerable to stress and to need extensive assistance.

The problems with the aftercare system were twofold. In many cases there was an underestimation and/or misconceptualization of how much and what kinds of help persons with serious mental illnesses need. An even greater problem was that existing services often were not reaching our patients. For instance, although we might link discharged patients to an outpatient therapist and perhaps to a day treatment program or sheltered workshop, many patients soon dropped out of treatment, often because of a reemergence of symptoms. When this occurred, no provider in the aftercare system made persistent attempts to reinvolve the patient or to update the treatment plan to meet current needs. Without biological or psychosocial assistance these patients deteriorated and returned to the hospital.

These experiences led us to develop in the early 1970s a new model of community care (TCL) that involved a reconceptualization of both what services or interventions persons with serious mental illnesses needed to live and grow in the community, as well as how these services must be organized and delivered to reach their intended recipients in a timely fashion.

Since the development of TCL we have implemented the model and evaluated its effectiveness in three different controlled studies. The initial project, by Arnold Marx, Mary Ann Test, and Leonard Stein, utilized TCL principles to allow patients who had been continuously hospitalized for 3 to 18 months to be discharged early and to survive in the community (Marx et al., 1973). Leonard Stein and Mary Ann Test next found that the TCL model could be implemented successfully as an alternative to the mental hospital for a relatively unselected, diagnostically mixed group of patients who were about to be admitted to a state hospital (Stein & Test, 1980). Currently Mary Ann Test, William Knoedler, and Deborah Allness are implementing and evaluating the TCL program as an ongoing, long-term community care system for young adults with schizophrenic disorders, most of whom enter the program from the community during an acute episode (Test, Knoedler, & Allness, 1985).

DESCRIPTION OF THE MODEL

The TCL model today, as modified based on our earlier research findings and clinical experience, is summarized in Table 7.1.

The Organization and Delivery of Services in TCL

In community care programs services need to be organized and delivered in a manner that optimizes continuity of care across both functional areas and time. Four aspects of TCL service organization and delivery are critical to achieve this end.

Core Services Team

The primary provider of services in TCL is a core services team. This community-based team consists of 13 interdisciplinary staff who serve as a fixed point of responsibility for 115 young adults with schizophrenic disorders. The team's function is to see that all the patient's needs are addressed in a timely fashion. *Needs* include not only mental health and rehabilitation needs but also basic needs such as housing, food, and health care. The team not only develops individualized plans with each patient to address these needs, but also provides most of the planned treatments and services itself. For instance, the team provides medications, long-term, one-to-one clinical relationships, 24-hour crisis availability, employment rehabilitation services, and assistance with housing and

Table 7.1. Elements of the Training in Community Living Model

ORGANIZATION AND DELIVERY OF SERVICES	TREATMENTS AND SERVICES PROVIDED	DESIRED PATIENT OUTCOMES
1. Core services team (continuous treatment team)	1. Direct assistance with symptom management	1. Reduced symptomatology and relapse
a. Fixed point of responsibility (all needs)	a. Medications	2. Increased community tenure
b. Primary provider of services	b. 24-hour crisis availability	
c. Continuity of care and caregivers across functional areas and across time	c. Brief hospitalization	3. Enhanced satisfaction with life
	d. Long term 1 : 1 clinical relationship	
2. Assertive outreach and in vivo treatment	2. Facilitation of an optimally supportive environment	4. Less subjective distress
3. Individualized treatment	a. Assistance with meeting basic needs (housing, etc.)	5. Improved instrumental functioning
a. Between patients		a. Employment
b. Within patients across time	b. Assistance with a supportive social environment	b. Social relations
	c. Assistance with a supportive family environment (psychoeducation)	c. Activities of daily living
4. Ongoing treatment and support		
	3. Direct assistance with instrumental functioning (work, social relations, activities of daily living)	
	a. In vivo skill teaching	
	b. In vivo support	
	c. Environmental modifications	

daily living skills. Having one team provide most of these services minimizes the notorious fragmentation of community care systems and allows for integrated clinical management. By using the same team to provide what are often called treatment and rehabilitation services, the complex interaction of symptoms and psychosocial functioning can be efficiently and effectively addressed throughout the course of the patient's illness.

Assertive Outreach and In Vivo Treatment

An essential ingredient in the way services are delivered in the TCL program is the abundant use of assertive outreach. This means that staff do not wait for patients to come to a central setting for services, but rather reach out and take both biological and psychosocial services to the patient. Indeed, the majority of treatment and rehabilitation interventions take place in the community, that is, in the patient's own place of residence and neighborhood, at employment sites scattered throughout the community, and in the same sites of recreation and leisure activities that all citizens use (e.g., parks, movie houses, and restaurants). The rationale for use of assertive outreach is to minimize patient dropout and to enable the provision of psychosocial services in vivo, right where patients need to use them. The latter factor eliminates the need for transfer of training, which has been difficult to achieve with persons with serious mental illnesses (Morrison & Bellack, 1984). A monitoring study of TCL (Brekke & Test, 1987) revealed that 76% of the time the core service team staff spend with patients occurs in the community rather than in the office which serves as a home base for staff.

Individualized Treatment

Because persons with serious mental illnesses, even within that group diagnosed as schizophrenic, are greatly heterogeneous and both person and disorder are constantly changing over time, treatments and supports must be highly individualized. Individualization of treatment across patients and across time is a central feature of the TCL program. In this regard, interventions are tailored to address the current needs and preferences of each patient rather than assigning patients to an existing group of common programs. The content, amount, timing, and form of treatments/services provided vary enormously both between patients, and within the same patient across time.

Ongoing Treatment and Support

Our earlier major controlled study (Stein & Test, 1980) showed that patients fared well while in TCL, but many relapsed or showed loss of gain following discharge from TCL. Other studies of community treatment using a variety of models have also revealed loss of gain following discharge (Test, 1981). It must be concluded that even very intensive community treatment models do not provide a cure for severe mental illnesses, but rather provide a support system within which persons with persistent vulnerabilities can live in the community and grow. It appears these supports must be ongoing rather than time limited. Additionally, for real changes in psychosocial functioning to occur it may be necessary to provide long-term treatment and services within which patients have opportunities to recompensate, consolidate gains, sometimes slip back, and then take the next steps (Strauss, Hafez, Lieberman, & Harding, 1985). Hence the current TCL model provides ongoing, long-term, rather than time-limited treatment, thus providing stable clinical relationships and continuity of care across time (Test et al., 1985).

Treatments and Services Provided by TCL

We utilize a broad biopsychosocial model of serious mental illnesses (Strauss & Carpenter, 1981) to conceptualize the treatments and services that might be helpful. Such a model suggests that programs must provide interventions in all three areas (biological, psychological, and social), focusing not only on changing the person but also on changing the environment. Additionally, programs must be attentive to the fact that symptoms, psychosocial functioning, and environmental factors are highly interactive. Thus, in TCL we make little distinction between *treatment* and *rehabilitation*, and we continually pay attention to the ongoing interactions between symptoms, psychosocial functioning, and environmental demands and supports. The interventions that the TCL program provides are grouped below into three categories that are in reality overlapping and interactive.

Direct Assistance with Symptom Management

The minimization of psychotic symptoms and the prevention of relapse is a continuing priority in our program and is not just a concern during the resolution of an acute episode. Specific interventions employed here include medications where indicated, 24-hour crisis availability, and occasional brief hospitalization. Additionally, we provide each patient with a long-term one-to-one relationship aimed at problem solving, at assisting them to learn about their illnesses, and at enhancing their own coping strategies for dealing with serious symptoms (Breier & Strauss, 1983). The latter intervention was not present in our earlier studies but is seen as particularly valuable in our current program in which we work with patients across years rather than weeks or months.

Facilitation of an Optimally Supportive Environment

We view our patients as having ongoing vulnerabilities and see most as needing not only biological but also environmental and social buffers to protect against excessive stress. At the same time we recognize that some environments (e.g., institutions) are not demanding enough; hence, our goal is to provide the patient with an optimal level of support. Numerous specific interventions are involved here and include the following:

1. *Direct assistance with meeting basic needs*. Staff help patients meet basic needs for adequate shelter, food, and health care in ways that maximize community integration and enhance patient satisfaction. For instance, staff work with patients to find "normal" kinds of housing such as apartments; few of our patients live in supervised settings. The stresses of living in the real world are buffered, however, by staff making frequent visits to patients' residences, assisting them in performing daily living skills such as food preparation, personal hygiene, and health care.

2. *Assistance with a supportive social environment*. Frequent staff contacts with patients provide a measure of social support; staff also assist patients in engaging in social and leisure activities with peers to enhance social network development. For instance, small groups of patients with staff assistance may share meals together or engage in social activities in the community. Additionally, patients may participate in groups led by staff such as a women's support or discussion group, or a group to share coping strategies for dealing with psychotic symptoms or substance use problems.

3. *Assistance with a supportive family environment*. We encourage most of our patients to live separately from their families of origin in order to allow greater independence and flexibility of options for both patients and their families. However, we view patients' families as potential systems of support for them. We provide an individualized form of low intensity, long-term psychoeducation with family members in order to facilitate the supportiveness of their interactions with their ill relatives and to assist family members in problem solving and stress reduction.

Direct Assistance with Instrumental Functioning

While research (Lieberman & Kane, 1986) indicates that symptom management and environmental support contribute substantially to the outcome goals of reduced symptomatology and sustained community tenure, for many patients these factors do not appear to make a powerful contribution to improve instrumental functioning. Research suggests that direct assistance in the areas of work, social relations, and activities of daily living may be necessary if patients are to make gains here (Test, 1981, 1984). In TCL we utilize both skill training and environmental modifications and supports in these instrumental areas. As suggested earlier, because many persons with serious mental illnesses have difficulty transferring skills learned in one setting to another (perhaps because they become overwhelmed by stress in a new setting), we carry out almost all of our interventions in "natural" work and social environments rather than in sheltered settings that require transfer of learning. Working with patients in natural environments also allows us to provide support and environmental modification as needed across time; hence, success or failure is not an all-or-none thing.

Employment plays a central role in TCL and is our major means of providing daily structure for our patients. While in our previous studies we utilized sheltered workshops to a significant extent, many of our patients found little meaning in this work and it was often difficult to individualize this approach sufficiently. Thus, in our current program we assist our patients in obtaining individualized structured employment opportunities in the real world rather than placing patients in sheltered workshops. Initially, most of these placements are part-time and many involve minimal and subsidized pay. We provide patients with active skill teaching and social support in such jobs. This involves helping both the patient and the employer on site to learn means of coping and structuring the environment so that patients are able to work in spite of what are often continuing psychotic symptoms. Our goal is that each patient be able to work at his or her optimal level. We anticipate that gradually and over the long haul this will include a number of patients working in the competitive job market for sustained periods of time.

Summary: TCL as a Continuous Treatment Team

The TCL team serves as a fixed point of responsibility for assisting the patient in meeting all of his or her needs from the day that the patient enters the program to a time extending many years into the future (Test, 1979). Torrey (1986) has suggested the term *continuous treatment team* for such an approach, and I can think of no better words to summarize what TCL is about. If the term *continuous* refers to "that which extends without interruption in either space or time," it can be seen that the TCL team provides continuous treatment across *functional areas* at any one point in time, and it provides continuous treatment across *time* itself. From what is know about the deficits in psychological and social functioning caused by serious mental illnesses, the organizational advantages of such an approach in maintaining continuity of care are enormous. For instance, dropout and falling through the cracks are minimized, integrated clinical management across functional areas is maximized, and patient and provider can plan services at any one time based on an increasing shared history and longitudinal picture of the patient's growth and setbacks.

In addition to the fact that the organization of TCL is tremendously effective in maintaining continuity of care, even more important may be Torrey's point that continuous treatment teams such as TCL also provide continuity of caregivers. The development of long-term, trusting, supportive human relationships between patient and staff are made possible. The benefits of this are compelling.

> The patient comes to rely on the team as the stable point in his or her life, the rock that is always there and that can be counted on for the future. Mental health professionals have the satisfaction of watching a patient grow and live a more normal life, in the knowledge that despite the inevitable vicissitudes over months and years, their efforts have made a difference. (Torrey, 1986, p. 1245)

RESEARCH ON THE TCL MODEL

Empirical support for the TCL model comes from controlled experimental studies in Madison, Wisconsin, conducted through the Mendota Mental Health Institute and the University of Wisconsin, and from controlled evaluations of replications and adaptations of TCL in other settings.

Use of TCL as an Alternative to the Mental Hospital

Our major previous work involved use of the TCL program as an alternative to the mental hospital (Stein & Test, 1980). An unselected group of patients (age 18 to 62) who were seeking in-hospital admission and who were of any diagnosis other than severe organic brain syndrome, mental retardation, or primary alcoholism were randomly assigned to the TCL program or to a control group which received short-term in-hospital treatment followed by aftercare in Dane County, Wisconsin. Patients assigned to TCL rarely entered the hospital but were instead taken back to the community where they were assigned to the TCL core services team. These patients received the TCL approach for 14 months; they were then discharged to the existing community programs in Dane County. All patients were followed by independent research analysts every 4 months for a total of 28 months.

The results for the TCL program during the 14 months that constituted the within-treatment phase of the study were strikingly positive (Stein & Test, 1980). Patients in the TCL group spent little time in psychiatric institutions and significantly less time in than the control patients. The TCL patients spent significantly more time than the controls in independent living situations and demonstrated significantly more favorable community adjustment than controls in the areas of employment, social relationships, symptomatology, and satisfaction with their lives.

A comprehensive economic benefit–cost study comparing the TCL with the traditional care model revealed a small overall economic advantage in favor of the TCL model (Weisbrod, Test, & Stein, 1980). A study of the relative social costs of TCL versus the traditional model revealed that the significant gains made by the TCL patients were not at the expense of additional burden to family or community members (Stein & Test, 1980).

The findings from the posttreatment follow-up phase of this study were not as positive. Many of the gains of TCL treatment were lost when patients were discharged from this special program after 14 months (Stein & Test, 1980). For instance, time spent by patients in psychiatric hospitals after their TCL treatment ended gradually increased; by the end of the 14-month posttreatment follow-up period TCL patients were spending just as much time in hospitals as the controls. Most of the advantages the TCL group had shown on the variables of symptomatology, social relationships, and increased satisfaction with life were lost following discharge. By the end of the 14-month posttreatment follow-up period, the only significant differences remaining between the TCL and control groups were in income from competitive employment and social groups attended (more by TCL than control patients).

The findings of this study provided evidence that TCL is an effective model of community treatment and rehabilitation for the "revolving door" type of patients in the study. The study findings also suggested, however, that community treatment and rehabilitation may need to be long term and ongoing. This hypothesis forms the basis for our current research.

Long-Term Treatment of Young Adults with Schizophrenia in TCL

We are currently implementing a 12-year prospective controlled study of the long-term community treatment of young adults with clearly defined schizophrenia or schizophrenia-related disorders (Test et al., 1985). Patients enter the study relatively early after the onset of their disorder. Patients assigned to TCL are then treated in an ongoing, rather than time-limited, fashion. The medium-term (2- to 10-year) courses and outcomes of young adults with schizophrenic disorders will be evaluated, as will subject, treatment, and treatment system predictors of outcome.

Patients were admitted to the study as they became available from five in-hospital and two outpatient services. Criteria for study entry were ages 18 through 30, diagnosis of schizophrenia or schizoaffective disorder (RDC) or schizotypal personality disorder (DSM-III), less than 12 months of prior (total accumulated) time in psychiatric and penal institutions, and provision of informed consent to participate in the research. Persons with mental retardation, organic brain syndrome, or a primary diagnosis of alcoholism were excluded.

Patients were randomly assigned to two different systems of progressive community treatment, the TCL program (60%), or the usual system of care in Dane County, Wisconsin (DANE) (40%). Patients remained in their respective treatment systems for the duration of the study, which ran from 1978 to 1990. One hundred twenty-two patients meeting criteria were admitted and randomly assigned (75 TCL, 47 DANE) between February 1978, and March 1985. They compose our sample for analysis. By the end of the project, these patients will have been treated and assessed in a continuing manner for between 5 and 12 years.

It is of interest in this study that the control condition, the DANE system, is also a national model for progressive community care. The DANE system operates on much the same philosophical base as TCL (Stein & Diamond, 1985) but it is organized in a different way. Rather than emphasizing one core team that provides most services across functional areas and across time, the DANE system contains many exemplary components (e.g., crisis service, psychosocial clubhouse, special living arrangements) that intervene at different times depending on the individual patient's needs. Indeed, there is even a Mobile Community Treatment team component that was initiated as a TCL-like program to provide assertive outreach to patients who drop out of treatment (Stein & Diamond, 1985).

Study patients (n = 122) represent a group that most would regard as very difficult to treat in the community. The patients are young (mean age = 23), predominantly male (67.2%), never married (86.9%), and predominantly of schizophrenic diagnoses (73.8%). Most (81.1%) had been psychiatric inpatients at some time prior to study entry; indeed these patients had accumulated a mean of 3.35 hospitalizations with a mean of 64.9 total days in institutions. Most evidence poor prior instrumental functioning. Additionally, a large segment (44.4%) had been arrested at some time prior to study entry, and many reveal significant use of street substances (Test, Wallisch, Allness, & Ripp, 1989).

All of the sample (n = 122) have now completed at least 2 years of treatment and research follow-along. Findings from patients' first 2 years indicate that the TCL model is again remarkably effective at reducing time spent in institutions. During the first 2 years, TCL patients spent little time in inpatient psychiatric hospitals (IP) and skilled nursing homes (SN), and spent significantly less time in these facilities (IP + SN) than patients being treated in the progressive DANE system. More specifically, there was a significant group effect ($p < .001$) during the 6 months after study entry, with TCL patients spending a mean of 4.89 days in IP + SN compared to 22.39 days by DANE patients. This result suggests that TCL was more successful than DANE in enabling patients to avoid hospitalization, and/or in returning patients to the community rapidly during the acute episode that brought them into the study. Then, during months 7 through 24, an 18-month period in which relapses might be expected, there was also a significant group effect for time in IP + SN, again with TCL patients spending fewer days than DANE patients (means = 5.24 vs. 44.17, respectively) ($p < .001$). The proportion of each group who spent any time in IP + SN during this 18-month period, a figure that provides some indication of relapses that required hospitalization, was 19.4% of TCL patients versus 56.10% of DANE patients ($p < .001$).

The low time spent by TCL patients in IP + SN was not offset by large amounts of time spent in jails or in shelters for the homeless. In the current study throughout the first 2 years the mean time that patients in both groups spent in these settings was small, and there were no significant group differences. While a significant number of patients spent some time in penal settings from months 7 through 24 (25% of TCL and 29.3% of DANE), the median length of incarceration was short (2 days for TCL patients, 3 days for DANE patients). Meanwhile, 6.9% of TCL and 9.8% of DANE patients spent at least a day homeless or in shelters during this period, with median times homeless or in shelters for those in these situations being 10 days for TCL patients and 21 days for DANE patients.

The goals of both treatment systems in the area of housing were to enable patients to live in normative housing whenever possible (i.e., integrated housing available on the open market), and to assist patients in moving out of their parental homes whenever this was the preference of patient and family. The results of the 2-year analyses suggest that TCL was more successful than DANE in achieving its housing goals. While there were no differences between the groups in community residential situations prior to study entry, during the initial 6 months TCL patients spent significantly more overnights in independent apartments than DANE patients ($p < .05$) and significantly less time than DANE patients living with (older generational) family members ($p < .05$). These two findings continued through months 7 through 24, with TCL patients spending more time in apartments ($p < .001$) and less time with family ($p < .05$). Indeed, considering all types of residential situations, during months 7 through 24, the greatest proportion of TCL patients (73.6%) were living in low supervision settings, primarily independent apartments, while the largest proportion of DANE patients (53.66%) were living in high supervision settings, primarily with family. Two year analyses related to psychiatric symptomatology, subjective distress, social functioning, and employment are still in progress.

For the variables analyzed thus far, results of our study in progress are similar to the findings of the within-treatment phase of the alternative to the mental hospital study. Even these early findings of our in progress study allow us to extend the conclusions from the previous study in three important ways. First, the effectiveness of TCL is generalized to a different population, that of a very difficult to treat young adult population with clearly defined schizophrenic disorders. Second and important, the gains made by patients in the current study are sustained at the 2-year point, lending support to the hypothesis that if special community supports are ongoing, positive results can be maintained. Third, the TCL program across the first 2 years of the current study is markedly more effective at reducing hospitalizations than an extremely good control community treatment system. Further study needs to be made of the reasons for this difference, but it is tempting to speculate that the organizational model of a "continuous treatment team" is more successful in minimizing dropout, maximizing continuity, and facilitating the development of long-term supportive relationships between patients and providers than is a service delivery model which consists of well-developed components of good community care but in which patients must receive services from many different providers.

Controlled Studies of Adaptations of TCL

Findings from our research program in Madison, Wisconsin, provide strong support for the internal validity of the TCL model and also contribute evidence demonstrating its generalizability across different patient populations; however, studies of the model's efficacy beyond this locale are needed to assess the model's external validity across different settings and staffs. Four controlled studies of adaptations of TCL are useful in this regard. In these studies the investigators took a number of the critical elements of TCL (see Table 7.1) and adapted them for use in the local setting. These TCL-like programs were then evaluated through random assignment of patients either to the new model or to another treatment condition which most often consisted of the existing best standard practice. The evaluations of these TCL-like programs are summarized below. The TCL adaptations are presented in the order in which they maintained fidelity to the Madison, Wisconsin, TCL model.

Kent County, Michigan

The TCL adaptation that maintained the greatest fidelity to the Madison model took place in Kent County, Michigan, in the early 1980s (Mulder, 1982). A reason for the close similarity of the Kent County program, called Harbinger, to the original model was the frequent hands-on training and feedback provided to the Harbinger staff by the TCL staff, who visited Kent County on a regular basis. The Harbinger program replicated almost all aspects of the Wisconsin model: the new Harbinger core team provided most services to patients themselves; it even maintained the emphasis on use of in vivo employment opportunities as the primary means of daily structure. The Harbinger program was initially used as an alternative to the mental hospital. In the evaluation, patients who otherwise would have been hospitalized were randomly assigned either to the Harbinger program or to the existing treatment system. Results, which cover a period of up to 30 months for part of the sample, revealed marked reductions in total days in hospitals for the experimental compared to the control program. Results regarding other variables must be accepted more cautiously because of the possibility of sampling bias and inadequate statistical tests. The findings suggest, however, that there were no differences between controls and experimentals on symptomatology, but that there were some advantages in psychosocial adjustment for the Harbinger group. Harbinger patients were more often in daily work settings and making money than the controls, and psychological tests indicated better mental and social adjustment. At 18 months, costs for control and experimental patients were about the same, but at 30 months costs per year were reported to be significantly lower for the Harbinger patients.

Sydney, Australia

Hoult and colleagues in Sydney, Australia, after reading journal reports of TCL, created and evaluated a TCL-like model in 1979–1981 and evaluated its effectiveness as an alternative to the mental hospital (Hoult, 1986; Hoult, Reynolds, Charbonneau-Powis, Weekes, & Briggs, 1983; Hoult, Rosen, & Reynolds, 1984). The TCL program consisted of a core team of seven staff and a part-time psychiatrist; this team served as a fixed point of responsibility for 60 patients. The team was available 24 hours a day and used assertive outreach and in vivo treatment; it provided biological treatments and taught patients living skills; it also provided support and education to relatives. In the Sydney project, it appears that patients were often provided with work experiences by day treatment or sheltered workshop facilities rather than by the core team itself as in the current Madison TCL model. In the evaluation, patients presenting for admission to a state psychiatric hospital were randomly assigned to traditional inpatient care and community aftercare, or to the TCL-like community-based program. Results at the end of 1 year revealed that fewer of the special TCL program patients had been hospitalized or rehospitalized, and that the TCL patients had spent markedly fewer average days in the hospital than controls (a mean of 8.4 vs. 53.5 days). On some indicators the special project patients were less symptomatic than controls. There were no group differences in employment or income statuses. The community treatment program was considered to be significantly more satisfactory and helpful by patients and by their relatives (Reynolds & Hoult, 1984), and the community program cost less than the standard care and aftercare.

Chicago, Illinois

In 1978 the TCL model was adapted for an urban environment in a program called the Bridge in Chicago, Illinois. The Bridge is a special program of Thresholds, a psychosocial center. The Bridge was developed to care for a group of patients who had not responded to the traditional Thresholds program according to a criteria of very frequent hospital use. The Bridge adopted many of the critical elements of TCL including serving as a fixed point of responsibility for its clients and providing services through assertive outreach and in vivo sites. The Bridge program differs from the Madison, Wisconsin, TCL program on the significant dimension of what proportion of services it provides itself versus what proportion is provided by others. The Bridge staff provides a smaller proportion itself and instead sees one of its major roles as that of "assertive resource coordinator." The Bridge program also differs from the Madison program in the patient population it serves since the Bridge specifically targets for service those patients who by their histories appear to be at greatest risk for frequent hospitalization.

Previously reported uncontrolled evaluations of the Bridge suggested that the new model markedly reduced patients' time in hospitals (Witheridge & Dincin, 1985). This finding has recently been supported in a controlled study conducted by Bond and colleagues (Bond et al., in press). Patients entered the study from both hospital and community settings and were persons with numerous previous hospitalizations. They were randomly assigned to either the Bridge program or to a readily accessible, low-expectation drop-in center. Across a 1-year treatment period, Bridge patients revealed significantly fewer episodes of state hospitalization and fewer state hospitalization days than did the controls. Findings on other variables must be interpreted with caution because of the possibility of sampling bias; there was greater attrition among control than experimental patients. Bridge patients reported less difficulty than controls on a self-report Areas of Difficulty Checklist. Meanwhile, there were no differences between groups on a Life Satisfaction Checklist, on mean ratings on the Global Assessment scale, or in residential patterns. It does not appear that employment outcomes were measured, though it seems unlikely that many patients in either group were employed.

Three Community Mental Health Centers

Bond and colleagues (Bond, Miller, Krumweid, & Ward, 1988) report findings from controlled studies of assertive outreach programs operating out of three urban community mental health centers in Indiana. The programs were more similar to the Bridge program than the Madison, Wisconsin, TCL model and, like the Bridge program, patients were selected based on evidence suggesting high risk of rehospitalization. The evaluation is less strong than those reported above, both because of more design problems and because the period reported covered only 6 months. Results revealed that at two of the centers those patients randomly assigned to the assertive outreach teams had fewer rehospitalizations and fewer hospital days than controls; this positive result was not found, however, at the third center. There were no differences between experimentals and controls on a self-report quality of life measure. It appears that other variables pertaining to social and employment functioning were not measured. It is reported that at one center the assertive outreach program was less costly than the control approach; at one center there were no cost differences; and at the third (the one that did not reduce hospitalizations), the assertive team was more expensive. Overall the study authors viewed their findings as being supportive of the innovative approach. They present an extensive discussion and some data that suggest the unsuccessful assertive program was not in fact a good replication of the Bridge model.

In-Progress Controlled Studies

Several other controlled studies of TCL-like programs are in progress. These include investigations by Morse and colleagues (Morse, Calsyn, Volker, Muether, & Harmann, 1988) who reported favorable early results from Morse's adaptation of the model to serve homeless persons in St. Louis, and a study by de Cangas (1989), who communicated positive preliminary results with his TCL-like program in Edmonton, Alberta, Canada. Another controlled study recently under way is being implemented by Marks and associates (Marks, Connolly, & Muijen, 1988) in London.

Summary of the Empirical Evidence

Empirical support for the effectiveness of the TCL model in markedly reducing time in psychiatric hospitals for persons with serious mental illnesses is strong. This result extends across a variety of geographic settings and staffs. It also generalizes to a number of different patient groups which include diagnostically mixed persons with serious mental illnesses who show "revolving door" type histories; persons with extensive histories of hospitalization who appear at extreme risk for rehospitalization; and young adults with clearly defined schizophrenia or schizophrenia-related disorders who as yet have spent relatively little time in hospitals. Also, the model has been used to intervene successfully at different places in the course of illness and process of service system delivery. Applications have included use as a program that allows earlier discharge for currently hospitalized patients; use as an alternative to inpatient admission at the time of acute crisis; and use as an ongoing treatment and community support system for patients who may enter the program from either hospital or community settings. In summary, it appears that the model successfully returns patients to the community earlier if they are currently hospitalized; it prevents hospitalization if patients are on the brink of entry; and it minimizes rehospitalization and/or time in the hospital over the longer-term course of the illness. Research indicates, however, that the program needs to be assertively and continuously available if patients are to reap these benefits over the long run.

Both the founders of the model (Marx et al., 1973; Stein & Test, 1980) and its current implementers in Wisconsin (Test et al., 1985) target goals for the model as going far beyond the reduction of time in hospitals. Additionally, improvements in patients' psychosocial functioning and quality of life are sought (see right column of Table 7.1). Empirical evidence regarding the impact of TCL on these variables is less clear, both because of the failure of all studies to measure a wide range of variables and because results have been more mixed among those studies which have done so. Findings, however, are promising. The model clearly aids in the reduction of symptomatology, and about half of the studies assessing this variable found greater symptom reduction through the TCL than the control program. Patient satisfaction was more favorable in the TCL program relative to the control in the majority of studies in which it was measured, and family burden was either less in TCL, or no greater than in the comparison group. Social functioning has been variously measured and findings have been mixed. Increased independent living was found in the Madison TCL studies and the Michigan replication, but not in some others. Also, the two completed Madison studies (Marx et al., 1973; Stein & Test, 1980) and the Michigan replication found more favorable employment outcomes relative to the controls; the other study that measured this variable did not (Hoult et al., 1983).

In the studies that demonstrated positive results on independent living and employment it is not clear what factors were responsible. The TCL programs that had the most success in these areas (Marx et al., 1973; Stein & Test, 1980; Test et al., 1985; Mulder, 1982), however, were ones in which the core team members themselves worked intensively in vivo with patients in these areas, rather than referring patients to other agencies (Hoult et al., 1983; Bond et al., in press; Bond et al., 1988). We hypothesize that core team involvement in these instrumental areas may be a significant contributing factor to positive results, both because greater continuity of treatment and rehabilitation is afforded and because many existing agencies may still use more passive, less intensive in-facility methods that have not been demonstrated to be successful with a large proportion of persons with serious mental illnesses.

THE ROLE OF TCL IN COMMUNITY CARE SYSTEMS

The extensive empirical support for the TCL model has stimulated widespread dissemination, adaptation, and adoption of the approach in a range of states and communities. The current interest in developing TCL-like programs makes imperative a discussion of what their role should be in a community or catchment area's total care system for persons with serious mental illnesses. In the dissemination of the TCL model three questions frequently arise: (a) Which patients with serious mental illnesses should be candidates for involvement in TCL programs? (b) Should TCL programs be additional "components" to community care systems, or should they in fact form the very heart or foundation of these systems? (c) Should the TCL core team provide most services itself, or should it play the role of "assertive case manager or resource coordinator" and link patients with existing resources while still serving as a fixed point of responsibility? More favorable psychosocial outcomes appear to be achieved when the TCL program provides most services itself.

It can be seen from the previous descriptions of the Chicago Bridge model and the Indiana programs that one adaptation of TCL principles that allows a relatively easy incorporation of the approach into an existing community care system is the development of a TCL-like team to serve those patients who very frequently drop out of existing program components, and/or who appear to be most at risk for rehospitalization (Bond et al., 1988; Bond, n.d.; Stein & Diamond, 1985; Witheridge & Dincin, 1985). In this adaptation the TCL program constitutes an additional component in a community care system that contains a number of other elements, such as outpatient therapists, a medications clinic, a psychosocial clubhouse or day treatment center, special living arrangements, and possibly a crisis team. Proponents of this kind of TCL adaptation (Stein & Diamond, 1985) believe that a community system with the components just listed, if they are held together by some kind of case management, is adequate for the large majority of persons with serious mental illnesses, but that something more is required for the very difficult patient who is often noncompliant. A TCL-like team is developed to serve these most difficult to treat patients. It provides assertive outreach and some direct services, but much of its role is that of assertive resource coordinator.

There is empirical support for the efficacy of this kind of TCL adaptation in significantly reducing hospitalization for difficult to treat patients, although favorable impact of this kind of a model on broader psychosocial outcomes has not been demonstrated (Bond et al., in press; Bond et al., 1988).

While not disputing the usefulness of such a TCL adaptation, this author and others (Test et al., 1985) believe that a different kind of community care system might offer greater benefits to persons with serious mental illnesses. Such a system would have relatively few of the components described above to serve persons with serious mental illnesses. Rather, the system would consist of one or a number of TCL core service teams, depending on the size of the community or catchment area, and virtually all patients with serious and persistent mental illnesses would be involved with a TCL team. Each TCL team would serve as a fixed point of responsibility across time for a designed group of patients, and, as in the current Madison TCL model, the team would itself provide most of the treatment and rehabilitation services that its patients needed. The type and amount of services each patient received would, of course, vary enormously among patients and within the same patient across time.

The vision of a community care system in which almost all persons with serious mental illnesses are involved with a TCL core team is based on the premises that the provision of continuity of care and continuity of caregivers is problematic, yet critical, to the success of community care for most patients with serious mental illnesses (not just for those identified as most difficult to treat), and that service provision by a TCL continuous treatment team is by far the most effective model yet developed to maximize such continuity. Widely cited 2-year relapse rates that range from 40% to 75% provide evidence that a very large proportion of patients with serious mental illnesses are at serious risk for having episodes of severe impairment. The poor success shown by traditional case management models to date (Franklin, Solovitz, Mason, Clemons, & Miller, 1987) and the existence of high relapse rates even in communities with many "model" system components and a TCL-like team to serve the most difficult to treat (Test et al., 1985) suggest that a large proportion of persons with serious mental illness may require the kind of assertive outreach and continuity provided by a TCL core team. Further, not only is a TCL team effective in preventing negative experiences from occurring (e.g., relapse); it also appears to be one of the most promising approaches for facilitating growth (e.g., independent living, employment). Hence, while perhaps best known for its use with the most difficult to treat patient, TCL in fact offers better functioning patients choices that are very appealing to them, such as support in normative living and employment settings (Leete, 1988).

If a community care system is established with TCL teams as its foundation, questions arise as to what role, if any, other kinds of rehabilitation programs would play, and how they would be related to the TCL core teams. Since TCL core team staff-to-patient ratios need to be high, most resources would be expended here and it is unlikely that large amounts of funds would be left to support additional programs. This would not pose a formidable problem, however, since the TCL teams would be providing most services themselves. Indeed, it might be recommended that the fewer the services provided by programs outside the core teams, the better for the patient in order to maximize continuity of care. Thus, program elements should be added to a TCL-based system only if they provide opportunities for treatment and rehabilitation which the TCL core teams themselves cannot provide, and only if they are supported by empirical research.

The psychosocial rehabilitation center, or clubhouse, provides an example of a program component that could potentially enhance a TCL-based service delivery system for a selected group of clients. This well-known model, which evolved from Fountain House in New York City, is primarily facility based and group oriented, and places a heavy emphasis on client empowerment. "Members" participate in work units in the clubhouse; they gain prevocational experiences, daily structure, and a strong sense of community and social support. Two controlled studies demonstrate the model's effectiveness in reducing hospitalization (Beard, Malamud, & Rossmann, 1978; Dincin & Witheridge, 1982). Only one of these studies considered broader outcomes; results suggested that while the psychosocial center led to the development of stronger social networks, it did not result in greater employment, more participation in leisure time activities, or less symptomatology relative to controls (Dincin & Witheridge, 1982). Also of relevance is a study by Bond and Dincin (1986) which examined employment rehabilitation methods. This study revealed that accelerated participation in in vivo supported employment was more efficacious than transitioning through clubhouse prevocational activities.

While the psychosocial rehabilitation center has yet to demonstrate a significant effect on some important rehabilitation variables, one might hypothesize that some clients, in some phases of their illness and life course, might show less frequent relapse and greater satisfaction from participation in the clubhouse minicommunity, with its strong client empowerment themes and greater structure, than from the highly individualized, community integration approach to treatment and rehabilitation of TCL. If research supports this view and can identify "who needs what, when" a TCL core team could selectively refer certain patients to a psychosocial rehabilitation clubhouse during the most appropriate phases of their long-term course, all the while, however, continuing to provide the client with other necessary services (e.g., medications, crisis intervention, housing) as well as maintaining its fixed point of responsibility role, which is so vital to the provision of continuity of care.

The Fairweather Lodge is another example of a program component that might enhance a TCL-based delivery system because it provides opportunities quite different from those of TCL. This model, developed in the 1960s by George Fairweather, consists of a kind of business-commune in which clients live together and also run their own business (Fairweather, Sanders, Cressler, & Maynard, 1969). While sharing the rehabilitation focus of TCL, the Lodge model differs from TCL in ways similar to the clubhouse approach—that is, its group focus and emphasis on client empowerment. The Lodge is effective in reducing time in hospitals and also has demonstrated impressive employment outcomes as long as members remain in the Lodge program. Again, comparative research examining more specifically what kinds of clients benefit most from this approach relative to the more individually oriented TCL approach, and at what costs, would provide useful information to a TCL core team responsible for seeing that its clients get the best possible treatment in the most cost-effective manner.

Along with considering the potential utility of additional programs, TCL core teams need to be open to the integration of different methods of rehabilitation into their repertoire of intervention strategies if future research demonstrates that such methods would enhance the established results of TCL, or perhaps enable similar results at a lower cost. The carefully developed skills-training modules of Liberman and colleagues (Wallace & Liberman, 1985) provide an example. It would be interesting to train TCL core team staff in some of these methods and then to investigate whether their integration into the TCL model enhanced social functioning beyond current results and allowed some clients to survive in the community with increased self-management and less frequent ongoing contacts from TCL. In an era obsessed with cost containment, investigations, such as the proposed one, that seek to determine which methods of service delivery are most effective and most streamlined for various groups of patients are critical.

Finally, the task of establishing a community care system which has TCL teams as its foundation is far more difficult to do than to propose. It is perhaps an easier task in rural areas (Allness, Knoedler, & Test, 1985) or in communities that have few existing service elements in place. It is much more difficult in locales that have already established a number of service components, since rearranging roles and responsibilities in an existing service system is an extremely difficult undertaking. Nonetheless, a TCL-based model might be well worth considering since few other approaches offer such promise.

CONCLUSION

An overview of the TCL approach to the community care of persons with serious mental illnesses has described how the model evolved, its conceptual tenets and current implementation, and its growing base of empirical support. The model's demonstrated effectiveness has resulted in its widespread dissemination and has generated interest in questions regarding the most useful role for the TCL approach in a total community care system. Sophisticated service system research is now needed to examine these issues. While the basic question—Is this effective?—must continue to be asked about each treatment and rehabilitation model, it is perhaps a sign of progress that the field must now move rapidly forward to inquire also about the relative advantages, disadvantages, and costs of various programs and system configurations. For consumers, providers, and researchers of community care, there is certainly no lack of challenge.

Acknowledgment: Co-developers with the author of the Training in Community Living model were Dr. Leonard Stein and the late Dr. Arnold Marx. Co-investigators with the author of the current long-term research project are Dr. William Knoedler and Ms. Deborah Allness. Dr. Knoedler has served as the clinical director of the program since its inception, and he and Ms. Allness are responsible for much of the "hands on" dissemination of the program. Also critical has been the commitment of the program's competent clinical staff and dedicated research personnel; the work of Ms. Suzanne Senn Burke, a research associate for almost twenty years, is particularly acknowledged.

REFERENCES

Allness, D. J., Knoedler, W. H., & Test, M. A. (1985). The dissemination and impact of a model program in process: 1972–1984. In L. I. Stein & M. A. Test (Eds.), *The training in community living model: A decade of experience* (pp. 17–27). New Directions for Mental Health Services, no. 26. San Francisco: Jossey-Bass.

Beard, J. H., Malamud, T. J., & Rossman, E. (1978). Psychiatric rehabilitation and long-term rehospitalization rates. *Schizophrenia Bulletin, 4*, 622–635.

Bond, G. R., & Dincin, J. (1986). Accelerating entry into transitional employment in a psychosocial agency. *Rehabilitation Psychology, 31*, 143–145.

Bond, G. R., Miller, L. D., Krumweid, R. D., & Ward, R. S. (1988). Assertive case management in three CMHC's: A controlled study. *Hospital & Community Psychiatry, 39*, 411–418.

Bond, G. R., Witheridge, T. F., Dincin, J., Wasmer, D., Webb, J., & De Graaf-Kaser, R. (in press). Assertive community treatment for frequent users of psychiatric hospitals in a large city: A controlled study. *American Journal of Community Psychology*.

Breier, A., & Strauss, J. S. (1983). Self-control in psychiatric disorders. *Archives of General Psychiatry, 40*, 1141–1145.

Brekke, J. S., & Test, M. A. (1987). An empirical analysis of services delivered in a model community support program. *Psychosocial Rehabilitation Journal, 10*(4), 51–61.

de Cangas, J. P. (1989). *A study of a comprehensive community living treatment program for the chronically mentally ill.* Unpublished master's thesis. University of Alberta, Edmonton, Alberta, Canada.

Dincin, J., & Witheridge, T. F. (1982). Psychiatric rehabilitation as a deterrent to recidivism. *Hospital & Community Psychiatry, 33*, 645–650.

Fairweather, G. W., Sanders, D. H., Cressler, D. L., & Maynard, H. (1969). *Community life for the mentally ill.* Chicago: Aldine.

Franklin, J. L., Solovitz, B., Mason, M., Clemons, J. R., & Miller, G. E. (1987). An evaluation of case management. *American Journal of Public Health, 77*, 674-678.

Hoult, J. (1986). Community care of the acutely mentally ill. *British Journal of Psychiatry, 149*, 137-144.

Hoult, J., Reynolds, I., Charbonneau-Powis, M., Weekes, P., & Briggs, J. (1983). Psychiatric hospital versus community treatment: The results of a randomized trial. *Australian and New Zealand Journal of Psychiatry, 17*, 160-167.

Hoult, J., Rosen, A., & Reynolds, I. (1984). Community oriented treatment compared to psychiatric hospital oriented treatment. *Social Science and Medicine, 11*, 1005-1010.

Leete, E. (1988). A consumer perspective on psychosocial treatment. *Psychosocial Rehabilitation Journal, 12*, 45-52.

Lieberman, J. A., & Kane, J. M. (Eds.). (1986). *Predictors of relapse in schizophrenia*. Washington, DC: American Psychiatric Press.

Marks, I., Connolly, J., & Muijen, J. (1988). The Maudsley daily living programme: A controlled cost-effectiveness study of community based versus standard in-patient care of serious mental illness. *Bulletin of the Royal College of Psychiatrists, 12*, 22-24.

Marx, A. J., Test, M. A., & Stein L. I. (1973). Extra-hospital management of severe mental illness. *Archives of General Psychiatry, 29*, 505-511.

Morrison, R. L., & Bellack, A. S. (1984). Social skills training. In A. S. Bellack (Ed.), *Schizophrenia: Treatment, management, and rehabilitation* (pp. 247-279). New York: Grune & Stratton.

Morse, G., Calsyn, R. J., Volker, M., Muether, R. O., & Harmann, L. (1988, May). *Community services for the homeless: Preliminary experimental results*. Paper presented at the 141st Annual Meeting of the American Psychiatric Association, Montreal.

Mulder, R. (1982). *Final evaluation of the Harbinger Program as a demonstration project*. Unpublished manuscript.

Reynolds, I., & Hoult, J. E. (1984). The relatives of the mentally ill: A comparative trial of community-oriented and hospital-oriented psychiatric care. *Journal of Nervous and Mental Disease, 172*, 480-489.

Stein, L. I., & Diamond, R. J. (1985). A program for difficult-to-treat patients. In L. I. Stein & M. A. Test (Eds.), *The training in community living model: A decade of experience* (pp. 17-27). New Directions for Mental Health Services, no. 26. San Francisco: Jossey-Bass.

Stein, L. I., & Test, M. A. (1980). Alternative to mental hospital treatment, I. Conceptual model, treatment program, and clinical evaluation. *Archives of General Psychiatry, 37*, 392-397.

Strauss, J. S., & Carpenter, W. T. (1981). *Schizophrenia*. New York: Plenum Press.

Strauss, J. S., Hafez H., Lieberman, P., & Harding, C. M. (1985). The course of psychiatric disorder, III: Longitudinal principles. *American Journal of Psychiatry, 142*, 289-296.

Test, M. A. (1979). Continuity of care in community treatment. In L. I. Stein (Ed.), *Community support systems for the long-term patient*. New Directions for Mental Health Services, no. 2. San Francisco: Jossey-Bass.

Test, M. A. (1981). Effective treatment of the chronically mentally ill: What is necessary? *Journal of Social Issues, 37*, 71-86.

Test, M. A. (1984). Community support programs. In A. S. Bellack (Ed.), *Schizophrenia: Treatment, management, and rehabilitation* (pp. 347-373). New York: Grune & Stratton.

Test, M. A., Knoedler, W. H., & Allness, D. J. (1985). The long-term treatment of young schizophrenics in a community support program. In L. I. Stein & M. A. Test (Eds.), *The training in community living model: A decade of experience* (pp. 17-27). New Directions for Mental Health Services, no. 26. San Francisco: Jossey-Bass.

Test, M. A., & Stein, L. I. (1980). Alternative to mental hospital treatment: III. Social cost. *Archives of General Psychiatry, 37*, 1243-1247.

Test, M. A., Wallisch L., Allness D., & Ripp, K. (1989). Substance use in young adults with schizophrenic disorders. *Schizophrenia Bulletin, 15*(3), 465-476.

Torrey, E. F. (1986). Continuous treatment teams in the care of the chronically mentally ill. *Hospital and Community Psychiatry, 37*, 1243-1247.

Wallace, C. F., & Liberman, R. P. (1985). Social skills training for patients with schizophrenia: A controlled clinical trial. *Psychiatry Research, 15*, 239-247.

Weisbrod, B. A., Test, M. A., & Stein, L. I.

(1980). Alternative to mental hospital treatment: III. Economic benefit-cost analysis. *Archives of General Psychiatry, 37*, 400–405.

Witheridge, T. F., & Dincin, J. (1985). The Bridge: An assertive outreach program in an urban setting. In L. I. Stein & M. A. Test (Eds.), *The Training in Community Living model: A decade of experience* (pp. 65–76). New Directions for Mental Health Services, no. 26. San Francisco: Jossey-Bass.

CHAPTER 8

SEX AND AIDS EDUCATION

David Lukoff
J. Greer Sullivan
Robert M. Goisman

Normal sexual functioning is a legitimate and important goal of a comprehensive rehabilitation program for patients with serious mental illnesses. While many treatment programs for physically disabled (Madorsky & Dixon, 1983) and ill (Golden, 1986) people now include sexual rehabilitation as part of comprehensive care, the sexual functioning of mentally ill people continues to be ignored (Wasow, 1980). The Sex Education and Information Council of the United States, which operates a clearinghouse for sex education materials, recently noted: "There are no sex education resources, such as curricula or booklets, at this time for either the mentally ill themselves or educators working with them" (SIECUS [Sex Information and Education Council of the U.S.], 1986, p. 4). Computer-assisted searches of the literature uncovered no studies on the outcome of sex education with schizophrenic patients, and only a handful of anecdotal reports describing programs with the seriously mentally ill of all diagnoses. Not one published report of an acquired immunodeficiency syndrome (AIDS) education program for the chronically mentally ill was found despite their high risk for AIDS.

Several factors contribute to these oversights. Since at least the early 1900s, sexual activity has been linked with mental illness. Von Krafft-Ebing in 1904 maintained that sexual excesses, particularly masturbation, caused insanity (Von Krafft-Ebing, 1904). Even as recently as 1972, a survey of 18 psychiatrists found that most believed sexual

A portion of this chapter is based on a previous article by D. Lukoff, D. Gioia-Hasick, G. Sullivan, & K. N. Nuechterlein, 1986, Sex Education and Rehabilitation with Schizophrenic Male Outpatients, in *Schizophrenia Bulletin, 12*, 669–677.

activity might have contributed to the development of anxiety, depression, and schizophrenia (Pinderhughes, Grace, & Reyna, 1972). Furthermore, those surveyed thought that sexual activity could retard recovery in one- to two-thirds of schizophrenic patients. Customarily, staff at mental health facilities view patients with serious mental illnesses as incapable of managing their sexuality in appropriate ways (Sadow & Corman, 1983). Although no empirical findings support such beliefs, these stereotypes continue to influence the expectations and behavior of mental health professionals. In addition to these biases, mental health professionals report discomfort when having to deal directly with patients about sexual topics (Withersty, 1976; Wolfe & Menninger, 1973).

Despite these obstacles, there are ample reasons for including sexual functioning as a component in rehabilitation programs for patients with serious mental illnesses. In Table 8.1 is summarized the rationales discussed in this chapter for making sex and AIDS education a priority in programs of psychiatric rehabilitation. In this chapter, the authors review research on the sexual behavior of seriously mentally ill patients, summarize the effects of antipsychotic medication on sexual dysfunction, suggest guidelines for reducing dysfunction, and report on two programs—sex education for schizophrenic patients and AIDS prevention for seriously mentally ill patients.

Table 8.1. Rationales for Making Sex and AIDS Education a Priority in Psychiatric Rehabilitation Programs

1. The seriously mentally ill may be at particular risk for AIDS.
2. Most patients with serious mental illnesses are sexually active and the recognition and validation of their sexuality is an important quality of life issue.
3. The incidence of sexual dysfunction in patients on antipsychotic medication is high—estimated at between 30% and 60%.
4. Noncompliance with medication among some patients has been attributed to complaints about medication-induced side effects of sexual dysfunction.
5. Worry and concern over having a sexual dysfunction can be a stressor leading to the exacerbation of symptoms or relapse.
6. Training chronic mental patients in intimacy skills and motivating them to develop sexual relationships could help them to overcome social isolation, a known risk factor in relapse.
7. Inappropriate sexual behaviors, sexual fears, and delusions of some patients may be major obstacles to their integration into the community.
8. Many of the pregnancies among seriously mentally ill women are unwanted, and unplanned, suggesting that awareness and/or use of birth control are lacking. Moreover, the birth of an unwanted child, when the mother is neither prepared for the child nor capable of rearing him or her, can be stressful and provoke a relapse.
9. Schizophrenic women are at high risk for sexual abuse.

SEXUAL BEHAVIOR OF SERIOUSLY MENTALLY ILL PATIENTS

Psychiatry, in contrast to other medical specialties, has generated little data about the sexual behavior of patients suffering from the various mental disorders (Friedman & Harrison, 1984). The few existing studies on the sexual behavior of schizophrenic patients suggest that their behavior is both qualitatively and quantitatively different from the norms of the general population. Data inTable 8.2 describe a survey of young male schizophrenic outpatients (Lukoff, Gioia-Hasick, Sullivan, & Nuechterlein, 1986) and show that all were sexually active, with most activity being autoerotic. Only 19% reported having a current sexual partner. The median number of sexual partners during their lifetimes was three, considerably below average for a group of males in their mid-20s. Studies with hospitalized male schizophrenic patients have also found that their sexual activity is generally lower than that of the general population and that autoerotic activity is the main outlet. Even premorbidly, schizophrenic males are more likely to have autoerotic activity as their primary sexual activity and to be less sexually

Table 8.2. Frequency of Sexual Activity of Recent-Onset Male Schizophrenic Patients ($n = 16$)

SEXUAL ACTIVITY		EVERY DAY	SEVERAL TIMES A WEEK	ONCE A WEEK	ONCE A MONTH	ONCE EVERY SEVERAL MONTHS	ONCE A YEAR	NEVER
Masturbation	%	19	38	31	6	0	6	0
	n	3	6	5	1	0	1	0
Sexual intercourse	%	6	6	0	6	19	13	50
	n	1	1	0	1	3	2	8

active than nonpatients (Nestros, Lehman, & Ban, 1981).

Among schizophrenic women, the incidence of sexual activity is higher than for men and their number of partners more nearly approaches the norms for the general population (Test, Knoedler, & Allness, 1988). Thus, for both men and women with schizophrenia, sexual activity is an important behavior and issue in their quality of life (Golden & Golden, 1980). The more frequent sexual activity with partners among the women patients may be due to the later onset of schizophrenia and consequent higher levels of social functioning among women; additionally, the traditionally more reactive and submissive role of women in sexual encounters may compensate for the negative syndrome and lack of social initiative that is associated with schizophrenia. Perhaps for these same reasons, schizophrenic women have been found to be at high risk for sexual abuse (Friedman & Harrison, 1984). Another area of concern is the increasing incidence of unplanned and unwanted pregnancies, suggesting that knowledge and/or use of birth control is lacking in this group (Abernethy, Grunebaum, & Clough, 1976).

Both men and women with schizophrenia and other serious mental illnesses may be at particular risk for AIDS. Some male patients report having frequent sex with multiple, anonymous partners (Lyketos, Sakka, & Mailis, 1983; Verhulst & Schneidman, 1981). Male schizophrenic patients also report infrequent use of condoms (Nestros, Lehman, & Ban, 1981). Some female patients with mania, psychosis, and severe personality disorders report engaging in multiple sexual encounters which place them at increased risk for infection with the human immunodeficiency virus (HIV). The literature reports cases of women who developed AIDS when their only risk factor for acquiring HIV was their hypersexuality during manic and psychotic episodes (Gerwitz, Horwath, & Cournos, 1988). The seriously mentally ill may also lack certain skills or attributes thought to be needed for successful risk reduction, such as good self-esteem (Ross, 1985), the ability to refuse sexual overtures (Cowell, 1986; Kelly & St. Lawrence, 1986, 1987; Solomon, 1988), and the ability to see cause-effect relationships between risky behaviors and onset of symptoms (Friedman, DesJarlais, & Soteran, 1986; Kelly & St. Lawrence, 1986). Some studies (Klaf & Davis, 1960; Lyketos, Sakka, & Mailis, 1983; Verhulst & Schneidman, 1981), but not all (Lukoff, Gioia-Hasick, Sullivan, & Nuechterlein, 1986) have found that schizophrenic men may also engage in homosexual behavior more frequently than nonschizophrenic men.

ANTIPSYCHOTIC MEDICATION AND SEXUAL DYSFUNCTION

Most persons with serious mental illness take antipsychotic medication, if not for the majority of their adult life, then for lengthy portions of it. Superimposed on the "natural history" of sexual activity in mentally ill persons is the effect these medications may have on sexual functioning. Antipsychotic medication side effects influence a patient's medication compliance and can cause depression, anxiety, and other problems that have a detrimental impact on the patient's quality of life (Marder et al., 1984; Van Putten, 1974). In males the sexual dysfunctions known to be associated with antipsychotic medications include delayed, retrograde, spontaneous, and total inhibition of ejaculation (Blair & Simpson, 1966; Keitner & Selub, 1983; Mitchell & Popkin, 1982); difficulties in achieving and maintaining erections (Kotin, Wilbert, Verberg, & Soldinger, 1976); decreased sexual desire (Witton, 1962); painful orgasms (Berger, 1979); non-painful sustained erections (Gold & Justino, 1988); and priapism, a prolonged painful erection (Moleny, Elliot, & Johnson, 1976) which has required emergency surgery in several cases (Gottlieb & Lustberg, 1982; Griffith & Zil, 1984). Certain antipsychotic medications have been associated with specific dysfunctions—for example, retrograde ejaculation with thioridazine and mesoridazine (Kotin et al., 1976; Shader, 1964; Singh, 1961; Witton, 1962). Although the impact of antipsychotic medications on women has been studied less, orgasmic dysfunction (Ghadirian, Chouinard, & Annable, 1982; Shen & Park, 1982), decreased libido (Degean, 1982; Kotin et al., 1976), menstrual irregularities and amenorrhea (Ghadirian et al., 1982; Sandison, Whitelaw, & Currie, 1960) have all been reported.

The prevalence of sexual dysfunction among persons taking antipsychotic medications is considerably higher than the 10% to 20% rate in the general population (Frank, Anderson, & Rubinstein, 1978). In a recent survey of 109 recently admitted male schizophrenic patients, 46% reported that their medication interfered with their sexual functioning. In the same study, 12% of a similar group of 33 female patients indicated the presence of sexual dysfunction (Sullivan, 1989). However, most studies have reported rates of dysfunction for both male and female patients on medications to be in the 30% to 60% range (Bartholomew, 1972; Blair & Simpson, 1966; Ghadirian et al., 1982; Kotin et al., 1976; Nestros et al., 1981; Witton, 1962). Men seem to be more vulnerable to the sexual side effects of antipsychotic medications, while women report a high incidence of menstrual irregularities or amenorrhea (90% reported these problems in one study [Ghadirian et al., 1982]).

Antipsychotic medications are believed to influence sexual functioning by their effect on the peripheral nervous system, the central nervous system, or both (Buffum, 1982). The dopamine-blocking effect of these medications may also play a role in generating sexual dysfunction by increasing prolactin levels that are related to many types of dysfunction (Drago, 1984). The antiparkinsonian medication prescribed to reduce the extrapyramidal side effects of medication may also be related to sexual dysfunctions.

Some patients discontinue their antipsychotic medication because of complaints about sexual dysfunctions (Carlson & Sadoff, 1971). Unfortunately, many studies on the causes of noncompliance have not considered sexual side effects, and these may be greatly underreported in the literature. Even patients who engage in autoerotic activity as their primary or sole activity might be very disturbed by sexual dysfunctions during masturbation. Sexual dysfunction and its attendant worries can be stressors for any individual. Within the vulnerability-stress-coping-competence model of the course of schizophrenia, sexual dysfunction could be a contributing stress factor leading to the exacerbation of symptoms or relapse (Liberman, 1988). Thus, exacerbations related to sexual dysfunction can impair coping skills and competence necessary for rehabilitation; on the other hand, satisfying sexual activity can contribute to the social competence of an individual and protect against relapse.

For these reasons, it is important to attend to sexual dysfunctions among seriously mentally ill patients. The incidence of dysfunction seems to be dose dependent, at least in males (Shen & Park, 1982). Thus, lowering

Table 8.3. Guidelines for Evaluating Sexual Dysfunction with Patients on Antipsychotic Medication

1. Be aware of the wide range of sexual dysfunctions that may occur as side effects of antipsychotic medications.
2. Ask patients routinely about possible side effects. It is unlikely that this information will be spontaneously volunteered. Patients at greatest risk are males, those on relatively high medication dosages, and those taking thioridazine.
3. Try to determine whether the dysfunction is medication-induced by taking a careful history of the dysfunction and its relationship to medication type (including antiparkinsonian medications) and dose. It is important to determine whether the patient has dysfunction in autoerotic sexual activity as well as in sexual activity with partners. For example, a male who easily has erections while masturbating but cannot obtain an erection with a partner is not likely to be suffering from medication-induced dysfunction.
4. When a sexual dysfunction is reported, find out how bothersome the dysfunction is for the patient.
5. Check for a high prolactin level, which may be suggestive of a medication-induced sexual dysfunction in males and menstrual irregularities in females.
6. Once you have decided that a dysfunction is likely to be medication-induced and that the patient is sufficiently concerned to warrant intervention, refer the patient for a medication evaluation. Be sure to include your history and other pertinent information so that the prescribing psychiatrist can make appropriate adjustments in type or dosage of medications.

the dose or changing the type of medication can reduce the occurrence and intensity of dysfunction. By providing sex education and keeping open the channels of communication about sexuality, the rehabilitation worker can play a role in monitoring and reducing medication-induced sexual dysfunction. Guidelines for evaluating sexual dysfunction in patients taking antipsychotic medications are presented in Table 8.3. Although there are detrimental side effects of antipsychotic medications on sexual functioning, the overall effect of these medications on the sexual lives of mentally ill persons may be beneficial because of their efficacy in alleviating psychotic anxiety, thought disorganization, and fear of physical intimacy with potential partners.

A SEX EDUCATION PROGRAM FOR SCHIZOPHRENIC PATIENTS

The decision to introduce a sex education program at the UCLA Schizophrenia Aftercare Clinic, a specialty clinic for 40 young schizophrenic patients, followed several incidents of inappropriate sexual behavior among the patients. For example, two female receptionists complained that two male patients from the Aftercare Clinic were constantly asking them for dates and making inappropriate sexual remarks to them. One male patient almost lost his placement at a board-and-care facility following his first experience of sexual intercourse by disruptively insisting that he and his partner needed to get married since her baby was his child. One patient had the delusion that little children were being placed in front of him to tempt him to molest them. One female patient underwent a pregnancy scare that caused her great distress, and one male patient was told not to return to his health club because several of the women complained that he touched them and made sexual remarks to them in the jacuzzi. In addition, several patients complained during therapy sessions about sexual dysfunctions, their lack of an active sex life, and guilt over masturbation.

The following goals of sex education guided the creation of the curriculum (George & Behrendt, 1985): (a) to increase participants' knowledge and comfort about their sexuality, (b) to help participants identify and clarify their values and attitudes about sexuality, (c) to help participants acquire decision-making skills regarding sexual activity, (d) to overcome medication-related sexual dysfunctions, (e) to prevent deterioration of sexual functioning, and (f) to improve intimacy skills.

The attentional and cognitive deficits of schizophrenic patients required that educational materials be simple and graphic (Liberman, Nuechterlein, & Wallace, 1982). Sexually explicit videos were shown including the *Sensate Focus* films (Bozanian,

1972) and *Tenderness* (Serber & Laws, 1980), which show a couple engaging in and then discussing mutually pleasurable exercises, and *Active Partners* (Silverman & Lenz, 1979), a documentary about a spinal cord injured male's relationship with his girlfriend and their sexual activities. These videos served as ice breakers, giving the patients permission to explore their own sexual needs, fears, and difficulties. The sessions also included training in rudimentary intimacy skills including role plays and discussions on finding appropriate partners, initiating sexual encounters, and communicating about sex with partners. Thus, the course was more explicit than is usual for programs conducted in public educational settings and similar to programs developed for persons with physical disabilities who are at risk for loss of sexual functioning (Madorsky & Dixon, 1983). A community representative from Planned Parenthood presented one session on contraception and safe sex. Table 8.4 shows the outline of lesson plans used in the sex education program (Lukoff et al., 1986).

Ten male patients attended the eight 1-hour sessions co-led by a male psychologist and a female social worker. During the group sessions, exercises introduced to facilitate sharing of experiences and exploring of attitudes were effective in stimulating active participation. Over the course of the program, the atmosphere in the group became lighter with appropriate joking, sharing of personal sexual frustrations, and asking of questions. One patient wanted help in dealing with parental disapproval of his sexual behavior. Another asked whether masturbation could cause mental illness, and another whether all orgasms were the same. A patient expressed the fear that his medication might cause birth defects in the future. He was reassured that this issue had been investigated and no evidence existed to link antipsychotic medication ingestion by males with a subsequent increase in birth defects. However, the group was also informed that for women the usual practice was to discontinue antipsychotic medication during pregnancy if the patient's condition allowed it. The impact of sex education with schizophrenic patients was positive with favorable attitudes by patients and no evidence of sexual acting-out nor symptomatic exacerbations. These positive outcomes mirror similar experiences offering sex education to the mentally ill or developmentally disabled (Demetral, 1981; Wolfe & Menninger, 1973).

AN AIDS EDUCATION PROGRAM FOR PATIENTS WITH CHRONIC MENTAL ILLNESS

A particularly important type of sex education for patients identified as chronically mentally ill is AIDS risk reduction and prevention (Baer, Dwyer, & Lewitter-Koehler, 1988; Baer, Holm, & Lewitter-Koehler, 1987; Lauer-Listhaus & Watterson, 1988). A three-session curriculum for patients in the Continuing Care Service of a university-affiliated public inpatient and outpatient facility covered basic sex education, AIDS education, and instruction in proper condom use (Kent, 1987; Kent, Goisman, & Montgomery, 1988). A behavioral approach was followed in developing a curriculum focused on repetitive safety messages (Solomon, 1988; Rehabilitation Research and Training Center in Mental Illness, 1986) and provision of specific information regarding high-risk behaviors and self-management skills (Kelly & St. Lawrence, 1986).

Because the literature indicated that staff members often have serious reservations about the ability of patients to tolerate exposure to sex education programs without decompensating or acting out (Mindek, 1974; Pepper, 1988; Pinderhughes, Grace, & Reyna, 1972; Withersty, 1976), the Continuing Care Service program directors were consulted during the development of the curriculum. Soliciting, listening to, and responding to their input allowed a cooperative, nonadversarial relationship to develop

Table 8.4. Content of Sex Education Sessions Held with Schizophrenic Patients

Session 1. Your sexual identity and self-esteem

Brief discussion on the importance of sex in everyone's life.

Exercise: Make a collage of your sexual identity. Magazines (*Playboy, Time, Sports Illustrated*, etc.), scissors, glue, crayons, and string were available for this exercise. Presentation and discussion by each person of the meaning of his or her drawing.

Session 2. Thinking of your sexual partner as a person

Exercise: List and then share three characteristics of someone you would like to meet and go on a date with. Group brainstorming session of places where one might meet potential dating partners. Role plays of introducing yourself to someone at a party.

Session 3. A. Male reproductive anatomy
B. Your strengths as a partner

Slide show of male reproductive anatomy including information on the size and functioning of the penis.

Exercise: Write a classified ad about yourself for a singles magazine. Discussion of each person's assets as a potential partner in a relationship.

Session 4. A. Female reproductive anatomy
B. Dating behavior

Slide show of female reproductive anatomy including the relationship of menstruation and lubrication to sexual intercourse.

Exercise: Share personal experiences of dates, e.g., who initiated the date and how; what did you do on the date; how did the date move into sexual intimacy; how did you feel during the different sexual phases?

Session 5. Pleasure not performance as the focus in sex

Viewing of *Sensate Focus and Tenderness* which show a couple engaging in the Masters and Johnson sensate focus exercises. Discussion of the importance of communication between partners about what is pleasurable during sexual activities.

Exercise: Each person was given a navel orange and asked to explore and report on the sensory processes of seeing, feeling, smelling, peeling, and eating the orange.

Session 6. Birth control and the prevention of sexually transmitted diseases

Presentation from a Planned Parenthood educator on the alternative forms of birth control, their proper use, and rates of effectiveness. Discussion of which birth control techniques the members of the group had employed in the past, what their personal preferences were, and what plans they had for use of birth control in the future.

Session 7. Open communication with sexual partners

Viewing of the movie *Active Partners* concerning a spinal-injured male's relationship with his girlfriend and their sexual activities. Discussion of the obstacles to living full and rewarding sexual lives experienced by the patients as the result of their schizophrenic illness, ways of overcoming them, and the diversity of possible sexual activities for achieving pleasure.

Session 8. Human sexual response and sexual dysfunction

Presentation on the four phases of the sexual response cycle, the effects of neuroleptic medication on sexual functioning, types of dysfunction, how to tell whether the dysfunction might be medication-related, and steps to take if you suspect that the dysfunction is medication-related. Patients encouraged to ask questions.

Table 8.5. Teaching Materials and Objectives for a Three-Session AIDS Education Curriculum

SESSION	MATERIAL/EQUIPMENT	OBJECTIVES
I. Sex Education	• Tape recorder • Picture booklets • Tape recording: "Sex Education" • Written script	• Clients will know and name body parts involved in sexual activities related to transmission of AIDS • Clients will recognize the sexual activities related to the transmission of AIDS
II. AIDS Information	•VCR • Video cassette: "Drugs, Sex, and AIDS" • Pamphlets: "AIDS, Sex, and You" "AIDS: The Facts" "Safer Sex for Men and Women Concerned About AIDS" • "AIDS: A Basic Fact Sheet"	• Clients will know what AIDS is • Clients will know how AIDS is transmitted • Clients will know how to avoid infection by AIDS virus • Clients will begin to discuss their feelings about AIDS and its impact on their life
III. Proper Use of a Condom	• Model of erect penis • Condoms • VCR • Video cassette: "The Proper Use of a Condom"	• Clients will understand function of condom • Clients will demonstrate proper use of condoms • Clients will know where to acquire condoms

between the educators and the program staff and minimized staff members' concerns about untoward reactions to the AIDS education (Withersty, 1976).

The curriculum is described in Table 8.5. Classes were limited in size to 6 same-sex patients and 1 leader, and the sessions were generally 1 hour long and 1 week apart. Patients were placed in homogenous groups in terms of level of functioning. Audiocasettes, picture books, videocasettes, handouts, brief lectures, group discussion, a pre- and posttest, and an anatomical model of a penis with condoms on which to practice were all used as educational techniques; thus, the format was educational rather than psychotherapeutic (Friedman, 1975; Liberman et al., 1986). An emphasis was made on incremental acquisition of small amounts of socially reinforced knowledge in a multimedia format, similar to the behaviorally oriented social-skills training approaches of Liberman and colleagues (Liberman et al., 1986).

Assessment instruments employed included a sexual history questionnaire, a pre- and posttest of knowledge regarding sexuality and AIDS, and three quantitative indicators of patient functioning and mental status. Evaluation of these tests indicated that the program did increase knowledge of sexuality, AIDS, and risk reduction, even among more impaired patients. There were no incidents of symptomatic exacerbation or acting out caused by the educational experience. Most important, a number of patients asked staff members how to obtain condoms following the completion of the program.

CONTRAINDICATIONS

Little is known about contraindications for participation in sex and AIDS education by seriously mentally ill patients. Some mental health professionals have expressed the fear that the intensity of intimate sexual relationships—or orgasm itself—might precipitate exacerbation of symptoms (Knoepfler, 1982). Indeed, there are case reports of decompensation during sex therapy with schizophrenic patients (Kaplan, 1983). However, exacerbation of symptoms is a risk in all types of rehabilitation programs. For example, an intensive vocational and sociotherapy program that produced benefits for many patients also precipitated relapses among some patients (Goldberg, Schooler, Hogarty, & Roper, 1977). Of course, patients who show an exacerbation of symptoms during a sex education program should be evaluated immediately to determine whether the treatment should be postponed.

Patients who are highly symptomatic or who are recuperating from a recent decompensation might be excluded from educational programs until their clinical condition stabilizes. On the other hand, good premorbid patients who enjoyed relatively normal social and sexual functioning and had good intimacy skills before becoming ill would be particularly appropriate candidates for programs incorporating sex education. Such programs might help overcome the social isolation often observed with the seriously mentally ill and known to be a risk factor in the onset of relapse (Sokolovsky, Cohen, Berger, & Geiger, 1978). Patients whose inappropriate sexual behaviors, sexual fears, and delusions are obstacles to their integration into the community might also be targeted for sex education (Akhtar & Thompson, 1980). When AIDS prevention is the focus of intervention, perhaps all patients should be included, with the exception of those having active sexual delusions or thought disorder, which could disrupt the sessions.

Patients should be free to choose whether or not to participate. Some may have religious values that preclude open exploration of sexuality, and some may simply prefer an asexual existence. Although the two programs discussed in this chapter used same-sex groups, the most effective format might include a follow-up session for men and women to practice communication skills jointly and explore sexual myths that interfere with heterosocial and heterosexual functioning.

CONCLUSION

The first step in reducing risky behaviors—both sexual and intravenous (IV) drug-related—is providing sex and AIDS education for the seriously mentally ill in the rehabilitation milieu. In addition, treatment plans should specifically address sexual behavior, especially high risk behavior for infection with HIV, and assess the patient's level of knowledge about AIDS. Ideally, condoms could be made available or, at a minimum, the patients informed as to the location of resources in the community for free condoms. For patients who are IV drug abusers, treatment for chemical dependency should be incorporated into the program or appropriate referrals made for treatment in other mental health settings.

The information provided in sex and AIDS education programs should be tailored to fit patients' idiosyncratic sexual preferences and behaviors. For example, at the San Francisco VA Day Treatment Center, AIDS education covered specific precautions patients should take when visiting massage parlors, a common sexual outlet among this population. For both AIDS and sex education, lectures on risky behavior, birth control, or reproduction are probably not effective interventions (Stout & Rivara, 1989). The use of a model erect penis on which to practice the proper placement of condoms, a part of the AIDS prevention program, is an example of the explicitness required in educating the seriously mentally ill. A precedent exists for such explicitness in sex education with the physically disabled. Rehabilitation of sexual functioning with physically handicapped persons has even included the services of surrogates for patients who do not have sexual partners (Tapley, 1985).

While there may be some high-functioning schizophrenic patients who could also benefit from the "hands-on" training services available from surrogates, the most effective and efficient method for rehabilitating sexual functioning with seriously mentally ill patients has yet to be determined. However, it seems evident that most patients require explicit information, ideally presented in a multimedia format to facilitate comprehension and retention (Vincent, Clearie, & Schlachter, 1987; Wallace, Boone, Donahoe, & Foy, 1985). Training in intimacy skills via social skills training (Liberman, Jacobs, & Boone, 1986) can also improve outcomes. We know from work with the developmentally and physically disabled that when professionals can communicate openly and provide information about sexual issues, their patients benefit. In the case of AIDS, such education can be life saving.

REFERENCES

Abernethy, V., Grunebaum, H., & Clough, L. (1976). Family planning during psychiatric hospitalization. *American Journal of Orthopsychiatry, 46*, 154–162.

Akhtar, S., & Thomson, J. A. (1980). Schizophrenia and sexuality: A review and a report of twelve unusual cases–Part II. *Journal of Clinical Psychiatry, 41*, 166–174.

Baer, J., Holm, K., & Lewitter-Koehler, S. (1987). Challenges in developing an inpatient psychiatric program for patients with AIDS and ARC. *Hospital and Community Psychiatry, 38*, 1299–1303.

Baer, J., Dwyer, P., & Lewitter-Koehler, S. (1988). Knowledge about AIDS among psychiatric inpatients. *Hospital and Community Psychiatry, 39*, 986–988.

Bartholomew, A. A. (1972). Experience of two year's use of a long acting phenothiazine: Fluphenazine enanthate. *Medical Journal of Austin, 2*, 22–25.

Berger, S. (1979). Trifluoperazine and haloperidol: Sources of painful ejaculation. *American Journal of Psychiatry, 136*, 350.

Blair, J., & Simpson, G. (1966). Effect of antipsychotic drugs on reproductive functions. *Diseases of the Nervous System, 27*, 645–647.

Bozanian, R. (1972). *Sensate focus.* San Francisco: EDCOA Series on Sexual Counseling.

Buffum, J. (1982). Pharmacosexology: The effect of drugs on sexual function. *Journal of Psychoactive Drugs, 14*, 5–41.

Carlson, B., & Sadoff, R. (1971). Thioridazine in schizophrenia. *Journal of the American Medical Association, 217*, 1705.

Cowell, S. (1986). Emerging risk factors for acquired immune deficiency syndrome and risk reduction education. *American Journal of College Health, 34*, 216–219.

Degean, K. (1982). Sexual dysfunction in women using major tranquilizers. *Psychosomatics, 23*, 959–961.

Demetral, G. (1981). Does ignorance really produce irresponsible behavior? *Sexuality Disability, 4*, 151–160.

Drago, F. (1984). Prolactin and sexual behavior: A review. *Neuroscience and Biobehavior Review, 8*, 443–439.

Erlenmeyer-Kimling, L., Nicol, S., & Rainer, J. (1969). Changes in fertility rates of schizophrenic patients in New York State. *American Journal of Psychiatry, 125*, 916–927.

Frank, E., Anderson, C., & Rubinstein, D. (1978). Frequency of sexual dysfunction in "normal" couples. *New England Journal of Medicine, 299*, 111–115.

Friedman, M. (1975). Family life-sex education as an adjunct to psychiatric treatment. *Family Coordinator, 24*, 297–302.

Friedman, S., DesJarlais, D., & Soteran, J. (1986). AIDS health education for intravenous drug users. *Health Education Quarterly, 13*, 383–393.

Friedman, S., & Harrison, G. (1984). Sexual histories, attitudes, and behavior of schizophrenic and "normal" women. *Archives of Sexual Behavior, 13*, 555–567.

George, K., & Behrendt, A. (1985). Research priorities in sex education. *Journal of Sex Education and Therapy, 11*, 56–60.

Gerwitz, G., Horwath, E., & Cournos, F. (1988). Patients at risk for HIV. *Hospital and Community Psychiatry, 39*, 1311–1312.

Ghadirian, A., Chouinard, G., & Annable, L. (1982). Sexual dysfunction and plasma prolactin levels in neuroleptic-treated schizophrenic outpatients. *Journal of Nervous and Mental Disorders, 170*, 463–467.

Gold, D. D., & Justino, J. D. (1988). 'Bicycle Kickstand' phenomenon: Associated with antipsychotic agents. *Southern Medical Journal, 81*, 792–794.

Goldberg, S., Schooler, N., Hogarty, G., & Roper, M. (1977). Prediction of relapse among schizophrenic outpatients treated by drug and sociotherapy. *Archives of General Psychiatry, 34*, 171–184.

Golden, J. (1986). Sexual problems of cancer patients. *Medical Aspects of Human Sexuality, 20*, 70–76.

Golden, J., & Golden, M. (1980). Cancer and sex. In J. Vaeth (Ed.), *Frontiers of radiation therapy and oncology: Body image, self-esteem and sexuality in cancer patients*. New York: Karger.

Gottlieb, J. L., & Lustberg, T. (1982). Phenothiazine-induced priapism: A case report. *American Journal of Psychiatry, 134*, 1445–1446.

Griffith, S. R., & Zil, J. S. (1984). Priapism in a patient receiving antipsychotic therapy. *Psychosomatics, 25*, 629–631.

Kaplan, H. S. (1983). *The evaluation of sexual disorders*. New York: Brunner/Mazel.

Keitner, G., & Selub, S. (1983). Spontaneous ejaculation and neuroleptics. *Journal of Clinical Psychopharmacology, 3*, 34–36.

Kelly, J. A., & St. Lawrence, J. S. (1986). Behavioral intervention and AIDS. *The Behavior Therapist, 6*, 121–125.

Kelly, J. A., & St. Lawrence, J. S. (1987). *Behavioral prevention of AIDS*. Paper presented at the Annual Meeting of the Association for the Advancement of Behavior Therapy, Boston, MA.

Kent, A. B. (1987). Unpublished material. Boston, MA: Vinfen Corporation, and CCS, Massachusetts Mental Health Center.

Kent, A. B., Goisman, R. M., & Montgomery, E. C. (1988). *AIDS education for patients with chronic mental illness*. Unpublished manuscript. Boston, MA: Massachusetts Mental Health Center.

Klaf, F. S., & Davis, C. A. (1960). Homosexuality and paranoid schizophrenia: A survey of 150 cases and controls. *American Journal of Psychiatry, 116*, 1070–1075.

Knoepfler, P. (1982). Sexuality and psychiatric disability. *Sexuality and Disability, 5*, 14–27.

Kotin, J., Wilbert, D. E., Verberg, D., & Soldinger, S. (1976). Thioridazine and sexual dysfunction. *American Journal of Psychiatry, 133*, 82–85.

Lauer-Listhaus, B., & Watterson, J. (1988). A psychoeducational group for HIV-positive patients on a psychiatric service. *Hospital and Community Psychiatry, 39*, 776–777.

Liberman, R. (Ed.). (1988). *Psychiatric rehabilitation of chronic mental patients*. Washington, DC: American Psychiatric Association Press.

Liberman, R., Jacobs, H., Boone, S., Foy, D., Donahoe, C., Falloon, I., Blackwell, G., & Wallace, C. (1986). New methods for rehabilitating chronic mental patients. In J. Talbot (Ed.), *Our Patients' Future in a Changing World*. Washington, DC: American Psychiatric Association Press.

Liberman, R. P., Nuechterlein, K. H., & Wallace, C. J. (1982). Social skills training and the nature of schizophrenia. In J. P. Curran & P. M. Monti (Eds.), *Social skills training: A practical handbook for assessment and treatment* (pp. 5–56). New York: Guilford Press.

LoPiccolo, J., & LoPiccolo, L. (Eds.). (1980). *Handbook of sex therapy*. New York: Plenum.

Lukoff, D., Gioia-Hasick, D., Sullivan, G., & Nuechterlein, K. N. (1986). Sex education and rehabilitation with schizophrenic male outpatients. *Schizophrenia Bulletin, 12*, 669–677.

Lyketsos, G. C., Sakka, P., & Mailis, A. (1983). The sexual adjustment of chronic schizophrenics: A preliminary study. *British Journal of Psychiatry, 143*, 376–382.

Madorsky, J., & Dixon, T. (1983). Rehabilitation aspects of human sexuality. *Western Journal of Medicine, 139*, 174–176.

Marder, S., Van Putten, T., Mintz, J., Labell, M., McKenzie, J., & Faltico, G. (1984). Maintenance therapy in schizophrenia. In J. Kane (Ed.), *Drug maintenance strategies in schizophrenia* (pp. 31–49). Washington, DC: American Psychiatric Press.

Mindek, L. (1974). Sex education on a psychiatric unit. *American Journal of Nursing, 74*, 1865–1868.

Mitchell, J. E., & Popkin, M. K. (1982). Antipsychotic drug therapy and sexual dysfunction in men. *American Journal of Psychiatry, 139*, 633–637.

Moleny, P., Elliot, G., & Johnson, H. (1976). Experiences with priapism. *Journal of Urology, 116*, 51–53.

Nestros, J., Lehman, H., & Ban, T. (1981). Sexual behavior of the male schizophrenic: The impact of illness and medications. *Archives of Sexual Behavior, 10*, 799–812.

Pepper, E. (1988). Sexual awareness groups in a psychiatric day treatment program. *Psychosocial Rehabilitation Journal, 11*, 45–52, 1988.

Pinderhughes, C. A., Grace, B. B., & Reyna, L. W. (1972). Psychiatric disorders and sexual functioning. *American Journal of Psychiatry, 128*, 1276–1283.

Rehabilitation Research and Training Center in Mental Illness. (1986). *Social and independent living skills: Medication-management module trainer's manual*. Los Angeles: Author.

Ross, M. W. (1985). Interventions to minimize AIDS. *Medical Journal of Austin, 142*, 279–280.

Sadow, D., & Corman, A. (1983). Teaching a human sexuality course to psychiatric patients. *Sex and Disability, 6*, 47–53.

Sandison, R. A., Whitelaw, E., & Currie, J. D. (1960). Clinical trials with Mellaril in the treatment of schizophrenia. *Journal of Mental Science, 106*, 732–741.

Serber, M., & Laws, E. (1980). *Tenderness*. Video available from Psychiatric Rehabilitation Consultants, Box A, Camarillo, CA 93011.

Sex Information and Education Council of the U.S. (1986). *The SIECUS notebook*. New York: Author.

Shader, R. I. (1964). Sexual dysfunction associated with thioridazine. *Journal of the American Medical Association, 188*, 1007–1008.

Shen, W. W., & Park, S. (1982). Thioridazine-induced inhibition of female orgasm. *Psychiatric Journal of the University of Ottawa, 7*, 249–250.

Silverman, M., & Lenz, R. (1979). *Active partners*. San Francisco: Multi-Focus.

Singh, H. (1961). A case of inhibition of ejaculation as a side effect of Mellaril. *American Journal of Psychiatry, 117*, 1041–1042.

Sokolovsky, J., Cohen, C., Berger, D., & Geiger, J. (1978). Personal networks of ex-mental patients in a Manhatten S.R.O. hotel. *Human Organization, 37*, 5–15.

Solomon, L. J. (1988). Prevention of the spread of AIDS: An interview with Jeffrey A. Kelly. *Journal of Primary Prevention, 8*, 125–141.

Stout, J. W., & Rivara, F. P. (1989). Schools and sex education: Does it work? *Pediatrics, 83*, 375–379.

Sullivan, G. (1989). *Predicting hospital recidivism in a population of schizophrenics*. Unpublished manuscript. Santa Monica, CA: RAND-UCLA Center for Health Policy Study.

Tapley, L. (1985). Sex surrogates and handicapped people. *Disabled USA, 4*, 18–20.

Test, M. A., Knoedler, W. H., & Allness, D. J. (1988, May). *Gender relevant community care of young adults*. Paper presented at the 141st annual meeting of the American Psychiatric Association, Montreal, Canada.

Van Putten, T. (1974). Why do schizophrenic patients refuse to take their drugs? *Archives of General Psychiatry, 31*, 67–72.

Verhulst, J., & Scheidman, B. (1981). Schizophrenia and sexual functioning. *Hospital and Community Psychiatry, 32*, 259–262.

Von Krafft-Ebing, R. (1904). *Textbook of insanity*. Philadelphia, PA: F. A. Davis.

Vincent, M. L., Clearie, A. F., & Schlachter, M. D. (1987). Reducing adolescent pregnancy through school and community-based education. *Journal of the American Medical Association, 257*, 3382–3386.

Wallace, C. J., Boone, S. E., Donahoe, C. P., & Foy, D. (1985). The chronically mentally disabled: Independent living skills training. In D. H. Barlow (Ed.), *Clinical handbook of psychological disorders* (pp. 462–501). New York: Guilford Press.

Wasow, M. (1980). Sexuality and the institutionalized mentally ill. *Sex and Disability, 3*, 3–16.

Withersty, D. (1976). Sexual attitudes of hospital personnel: A model for continuing education. *American Journal of Psychiatry, 133*, 573–575.

Witton, K. (1962). Sexual dysfunction secondary to Mellaril. *Diseases of the Nervous System, 23*, 175.

Wolfe, S., & Menninger, W. (1973). Fostering open communications about sexual concerns in a mental hospital. *Hospital and Community Psychiatry, 24*, 147–150.

CHAPTER 9

FAMILY MANAGEMENT

Angus Strachan

Interest in the aftercare and rehabilitation of persons with schizophrenia has shifted over the last decade toward a greater focus on providing family support, education, and treatment. As a consequence of the movement to deinstitutionalize the mentally ill and the sparseness of financial support for community residential and outpatient programs, the burden of dealing with schizophrenia has increasingly fallen on the shoulders of their families. Goldman and Gattozzi (1981) estimate that 60% of psychiatrically disabled people now live at home with other family members.

With these sociopolitical changes as background, rehabilitation workers have become increasingly interested in helping the family. In the last 10 years, there has been a tremendous change in public advocacy for the mentally ill and their families. Voluntary self-help groups and organizations have spread rapidly, foremost among them being the Alliance for the Mentally Ill, which has had a meteoric growth in membership. During the Carter years, Rosalynn Carter championed the cause of the mentally ill and brought important rehabilitation issues into the open; at the same time, the Presidential Commission on Mental Illness issued its report (Parloff, Wolfe, Hadley, & Waskow, 1978). All these developments led to an increase in the public's awareness of the plight of the mentally ill and their families.

Meanwhile, there have been important

This work was supported in part by National Institute of Mental Health grants MH 30911 and MH 08744 and by a research project grant from the John D. and Catherine T. MacArthur Foundation Research Network on Risk and Protective Factors in the Major Mental Disorders.

This chapter is based on a previous article, "Family Intervention for the Rehabilitation of Schizophrenia: Toward Protection and Coping," *Schizophrenia Bulletin, 12*, 678–698, 1986.

scientific developments. The diagnosis of schizophrenia has been made more systematic and reliable with the introduction of the *Diagnostic and Statistical Manual of Mental Disorders* ([DSM-III], American Psychiatric Association, 1980). Surveys of the relatives of the mentally ill have provided more information about what family members want from mental health professionals (Hatfield, 1981; Spaniol, Jung, Zipple, & Fitzgerald, 1987). Finally, important research on the relationship between family affective climate and the course of schizophrenia (Leff & Vaughn, 1985) has stimulated a series of systematic outcome studies of interventions with families (Falloon et al., 1982, 1985; Goldstein, Rodnick, Evans, May, & Steinberg, 1978; Hogarty et al., 1986; Leff, Berkowitz, Shavit, Strachan, Glass, & Vaughn, 1989, 1990; Leff, Kuipers, Berkowitz, Eberlein-Fries, & Sturgeon, 1982, 1983; Leff, Kuipers, Berkowitz, & Sturgeon, 1985; Tarrier et al., 1988, 1989). These in turn have provided more practical information on how family members can cope and help their mentally disabled relative. All these scientific developments mean that, now more than ever, there is the possibility of helping family members and patients with psychoeducational family intervention programs.

RELATIVES' COPING AND NEEDS

A number of investigators have surveyed relatives of the mentally ill to determine their coping patterns and what they need from mental health professionals. In some early research, Freeman and Simmons (1963) argued that relatives were most upset by severe psychiatric symptoms because the emergence of symptoms was the best predictor of rehospitalization, which suggested that the symptoms overwhelmed relatives. Later, Creer and Wing (1974) and Doll (1976) found that family members tolerated a surprisingly high amount of psychiatric symptomatology, but this tolerance was at the expense of a great deal of internal distress and family burden—physical, financial, and emotional.

Another focus has been on the patterns of coping used by relatives. For example, Hatfield (1978) surveyed the emotional reactions of relatives of the mentally ill and found a variety of patterns varying from resentment and frustration to sadness and denial. In a later study, Hatfield (1981) explored the coping styles of relatives. Because the sample volunteered from a local family support organization, they were of higher socioeconomic status, which may limit the generalizability of the findings. She distinguished between "effective" and "ineffective" copers. Effective copers actively sought out information, were realistic in their expectations of the patient, and were able to enjoy activities separate from the patient. Ineffective copers, by contrast, did not plan ahead but reacted only to crisis, felt unable to handle the patient, and had fewer interests which were separate from the patient. This survey approach to the study of coping has some conceptual problems (see below), but the surveys do illustrate the range of coping mechanisms used—emotional, cognitive, and behavioral—which have an impact on the patient and family member.

Another area of interest has been what family members want from mental health professionals and what they actually receive. Creer and Wing (1974) reported that relatives wanted information and practical advice from psychiatrists and social workers but were often ignored or given vague information. Hatfield (1981) further found that relatives perceived that the treatment offered, such as individual therapy, was not useful. Holden and Lewine (1982) reported that relatives wanted more specific information about symptoms and the effect of drugs, practical help from the treatment team about accommodation and support for the patient, and emotional support for themselves. Instead, many relatives felt that they were met with vagueness and even implied criticism. Another more recent survey of the needs and coping behaviors of the relatives of the mentally ill has been conducted by Spaniol, Jung, Zipple, and Fitzgerald (1987) who surveyed members of the Alliance of the Mentally Ill. They found that nearly half the relatives were dissatisfied with the mental health services they received. They wanted more support, more information and input to medication management, and more help with their own stress and coping abilities. The same investigators also surveyed mental health professionals, who felt that families were satisfied with the services provided. This gap between the views of professionals and family members appeared to indicate a lack of empathy for family members' viewpoints.

Recent family intervention programs have attempted to change this misfit of perceptions by altering professionals' responses to family members. Instead of ignoring or blaming relatives, these programs have given relatives the best information about schizophrenia available and have enlisted their aid in helping their disabled relative.

TOWARD AN INTEGRATIVE CONCEPTUAL FRAMEWORK

Many of the problems in the treatment of relatives by mental health professionals have been caused by overly simplistic models of the cause and treatment of schizophrenia. Too often professionals adopt a one-sided view of the etiology of schizophrenia: Either they assume schizophrenia is caused by biological factors that are passed on genetically and can be cured only by medication; or they assume schizophrenia is caused by psychological factors rooted in defects in the family that can be cured only by individual therapy away from the noxious family environment, or family therapy to change the interactional patterns assumed to cause or maintain schizophrenic symptomatology.

Thus, for professionals with a biological viewpoint, relatives are perceived as useful for describing symptoms and history but not useful in treatment; as a result, relatives may feel ignored. Professionals with an individual therapy viewpoint assume that it is important to keep family members away from the patient while he or she undergoes individual therapy; consequently, relatives often feel shunned. Professionals with a family therapy viewpoint assume it is important to involve family members and to change their interaction with the patient; as a result, family members may feel responsible and blamed (Terkelson, 1983). Thus, any simplistic model of the cause and treatment of schizophrenia can lead to family members' feeling left out or blamed.

There are other reasons that mental health professionals may be reluctant to talk with relatives about diagnosis and treatment. First, diagnoses are not always clear, and mental health professionals may be reluctant to give relatives incorrect information. Second, professionals may fear the stigmatizing impact of labeling someone as "schizophrenic" (Berkowitz, Eberlein-Fries, Kuipers, & Leff, 1984). Unfortunately, giving no information to relatives or remaining vague about diagnosis seems to compound the problem: Relatives become increasingly frustrated, fearful, or guilty. Indeed, withholding diagnostic information may even reinforce the stigma staff wish to avoid. When there is doubt about the diagnosis, professionals could be clear and direct about the lack of decisiveness, educate the patient and relative about the reasons for the ambiguity, and suggest how the diagnostic decision might be clarified (e.g., more interviews, letting time pass).

Accumulated scientific developments in schizophrenia are now leading to a more integrated conceptual framework than "either/or" models: Genetic predispositions lead to varying degrees of biological vulnerability that interact with the stresses and strains of life in causing a schizophrenic episode (Nuechterlein & Dawson, 1984). Evidence for this view comes from more sophisticated genetic research (Kessler, 1980) as well as research sparked by the finding that antipsychotic medication was not a cure-all: While phenothiazines significantly reduced the length of hospitalization of most patients, 35% of patients relapsed within 2 years even though they were maintained on medication, and the psychotic symptoms of 7% to 23% of patients remained untouched (Brown, Birley, & Wing, 1972; Leff & Wing, 1971). Similarly, Hogarty, Goldberg, and Schooler (1974) found that, over a 2-year period following discharge from the hospital, 30% of schizophrenic patients who continued on oral medication relapsed, in comparison with 68% of those who received a placebo. To investigate whether the 30% relapse rate was due to noncompliance with medication, a further study was mounted to compare long-acting injectable medication (in which compliance is assured) with oral medication. Hogarty and colleagues (Hogarty et al., 1979, 1974) found the 2-year relapse rates to be very similar: 50% for the long acting injectable; 55% for the oral medication. Thus, relapse on medication is not due to noncompliance.

Findings such as these led researchers to investigate stress factors that contribute to relapse. One body of research has suggested that for patients on medication, stressful life events play a triggering role in the onset of a schizophrenic episode (Brown & Birley, 1968; Leff, Kuipers, Berkowitz, Vaughn, & Sturgeon, 1983; Pederson-Hardesty, Falloon, & Shirin, 1985; Ventura, Nuechterlein, & Lukoff, 1986). Another body of research has examined the impact of stressful family emotional environments and has found that patients who return to live with family members who show high levels of "expressed emotion" are significantly more likely than patients who return to low expressed emotion environments to have relapses of their symptoms within 9 months and at 2-year follow-up (Brown, Birley, & Wing, 1972; Vaughn & Leff, 1976; Leff & Vaughn, 1981; Vaughn, Snyder, Jones, Freeman, & Falloon, 1984). Thus, short-term life-events and more ambient family pressures are both stressors that interact with biological predispositions and the protective effect of medication in precipitating the recurrence of schizophrenic symptomatology. Because the body of research on expressed emotion (EE) has had such an impact on the family programs that are the focus of this article, some observations about this construct are offered below.

EE Is Rated From an Interview

EE is measured from a semistructured interview with the relative about the patient's behavior over the previous 3 months. The interview is usually conducted shortly after the patient is hospitalized. The critical comments made about the patient are counted, and the level of emotional overinvolvement displayed toward the patient is rated from an audiotape of this interview. If the relative rates high on either or both of these measures, the relative is said to be high on expressed emotion.

EE Fluctuates

The level of EE changes with the course of the illness. Thus, Brown, Birley, and Wing (1972) showed that 30% of relatives in a British sample were high EE at admission, but only 14% were so ranked at 9-month follow-up. Similarly, Kottgen, Sonnichsen, Mollenhauer, and Jurth (1984a) showed that 52% of relatives in a German sample were high EE at admission, but only 27% at 6 months and 15% at 18 months.

Relatives Express EE

Several studies in the United States and England have shown that relatives do express emotional attitudes congruently in direct interaction with the patient (Miklowitz, Goldstein, Falloon, & Doane, 1965; Kuipers, Sturgeon, Berkowitz, & Leff, 1982; Valone, Norton, Goldstein, & Doane, 1983; Strachan, Leff, Goldstein, Doane, & Burtt, 1986). Critical attitudes correlate with critical interaction; supportive attitudes correlate with supportive behavior.

Our UCLA group has recently produced data suggesting that EE may tap a transactional process involving the patient. Strachan and colleagues (Strachan, Feingold, Goldstein, Miklowitz, & Nuechterlein, 1989) have shown that patients interacting with low-EE relatives show significantly more statements of autonomy and fewer criticisms than patients interacting with high-EE relatives. This suggests that EE is indexing a complex interplay of both relatives' and patients' responses to each other.

EE Measured at Admission Predicts Relapse

Several studies have shown that EE measured at admission predicts relapse. Thus, in a British sample, schizophrenic patients who returned to homes with one or more high-EE relatives were found to have 9-month relapse rates of 51%, whereas those who returned to homes with low-EE relatives were found to have relapse rates of only 13% (Vaughn & Leff, 1976). These results have been replicated at 2-year follow-up (Brown et al., 1972) and in several U.S. samples (Jenkins et al., 1986; Moline, Singh, Morris, & Meltzer, 1986; Nuechterlein et al., 1986; Vaughn et al., 1984). Of three purported nonreplications, the study by Kottgen et al. (1984a) had methodological problems; the one by MacMillan, Gold, Crow, Johnson, and Johnstone (1986) claimed that EE was not a significant factor in predicting relapse, but in the study by Mintz, Mintz, and Goldstein (1987) it was, in fact, shown to be a significant factor; and in the study by Parker, Johnson, and Hayward (1988) psychopathology was not assessed regularly through the aftercare period, which may account for some differences in results. Thus, patients who return to households with low-EE attitudes expressed at the time of admission are protected from relapse. That the admission rating is predictive suggests that relatives' reactions during the acute episode are good predictors of the tension level in the household after discharge.

Patient Disturbance Correlates with EE

Brown, Birley, and Wing (1972) did a careful analysis of the relationship between patient disturbance and EE levels. They found that EE was not correlated with symptoms, but it was highly correlated with impairment at work and disturbed behavior (.84). In a further study of 205 American and British relatives, Miklowitz, Strachan, Goldstein, Doane, and Burtt (1986) showed no relation between EE and chronicity.

EE Predicts Over and Above Patient Disturbance

Brown, Birley, and Wing (1972) showed that EE relates strongly to relapse (.75), and patient impairment does so but less strongly (.47). When patient impairment is partialed out, however, EE still strongly predicts relapse (.63). In other words, patient factors have little effect on relapse in comparison with the effect of EE. Thus, these data support the findings that an interactional process exists between patient characteristics and family attitudes on the course of schizophrenia.

While the EE construct has been successful in its impact on the scientific and professional community, it has been something of a public relations disaster in its impact on the relatives of the mentally ill and is in danger of creating a backlash if not properly understood. It is unfortunate that the name of the construct stresses the negative instead of emphasizing positive qualities of relatives. As a result, some relatives feel that, yet again, scientists and professionals are blaming them. It is important to note, however, that many relatives have low EE ratings and therefore have a positive effect on the course of the illness. The EE research does not indict relatives as causing relapse, but rather suggests that some emotional environments provide better protection of the patient against stress than others. Further, it implies that family members can control their attitudes and behavior and can change the way they express themselves, thus providing an emotional environment that could be conducive to the protection of the patient. The conceptual framework can be expanded to assume that the family environment can be a potential stressor, but it can also provide protection and "buffer" the schizophrenic against outside stressors.

The final aspect of the framework is that many schizophrenic patients are deficient in the coping skills required to deal with situations brought on by life events or stressful family environments. They may therefore experience greater distress than other people because they lack the coping abilities to solve problems and enlist social supports (Lukoff, Snyder, Ventura, & Nuechterlein, 1984). It is important to make a conceptual distinction between coping—the process of reacting to events—and the outcome of that coping; that is, how successful the coping is in affecting the patient's actual social competence (Folkman, Dunkel-Schetter, DeLongis, & Gruen, 1986). As noted above, some previous investigators have confounded these two aspects of coping when examining coping by relatives. Current work is investigating the relationship between relatives' EE and their coping styles (Strachan & Dunkel-Schetter, 1985).

EARLY FAMILY INTERVENTION WITH SCHIZOPHRENIA

Before systematic studies of family intervention with schizophrenia, psychoanalysts such as Federn (1952) thought that psychodynamic individual psychotherapy could cure schizophrenia. Later, after the discovery of the phenothiazines, other psychoanalysts thought that psychoanalytic psychotherapy in combination with neuroleptics could improve the outcome of patients with schizophrenia. However, a major study reported by May and Tuma (1976) has not supported this contention. Random assignment of patients to drug treatment, psychotherapy, drug treatment plus psychotherapy, milieu therapy, or electroconvulsive therapy, showed that an ego-supportive, reality-oriented psychodynamic therapy was neither as effective as medication, nor added to its effectiveness. More recently, a major study by John Gunderson and the Boston group (Gunderson, Frank, & Katz, 1977; Stanton et al., 1984) has shown that there were minimal outcome differences between exploratory insight-oriented therapy and reality-adaptive-supportive therapy, both given to individuals in addition to maintenance pharmacotherapy.

Subsequently, family systems theory emerged, principally from observations of families of schizophrenics viewed through lenses tinted by the historical zeitgeist of interest in the social, economic, or ecological context of a phenomenon. Thus, for example, Laing and Esterson (1964) suggested that people become schizophrenic because their families "mystified" them with their confusing communication. Esterson, Cooper, and Laing (1965) reported the results of therapy aimed at families of schizophrenics. They emphasized the importance of taking psychotic symptoms seriously and of understanding the meaning of hallucinations and delusions in relation to family communication. They took an existential approach with the patient and a demystifying approach with the family, trying to unravel the disguised family communication. Although this was not a randomized study, the authors compared 1-year rehospitalization rates in their sample of 42 families with rehospitalization rates in a matched sample of 374 provided by the Medical Research Center Social Psychiatry Unit in London. The rehospitalization rate in the treatment group was 17% compared with 52% in the comparison group, a highly significant difference.

Another early family therapist, Bowen (1978) described work in which he hospitalized whole families of schizophrenic patients for observation and treatment.

Bowen worked intensively with such families attempting to "differentiate" family members from "the undifferentiated family ego mass." This work was "intensive" in terms of the use of interpretation and insight.

In the 1960s and 1970s, the work of Weakland, Fisch, Watzlawick, and Bodin (1974) and of Palazzoli, Boscolo, Cecchin, and Prata (1978) focused on the communication of families in "schizophrenic transition." They saw the psychotic behavior of the identified patient as a symptom of a disturbed pattern of transactions in the family. Weakland et al. (1974) described the results of 96 cases (only some containing schizophrenics) who were seen for an average of seven sessions and reported that 72% were significantly improved. Palazzoli et al. (1978) also claimed success for their methods in which they saw families of schizophrenics about once a month and focused on "positive connotation" of the psychotic behavior and the prescription of therapeutic paradoxes.

At about the same time, Liberman and his colleagues were developing behavioral approaches to the families of schizophrenics. After early case studies by Liberman, Falloon, and colleagues (Liberman, 1970, 1972; Liberman, DeRisi, & King, 1973; Falloon & Liberman, 1983), they developed a comprehensive, behavioral skills-based intervention focused on changing the inappropriate communication of needs, desires, and feelings (Falloon, Liberman, Lillie, & Vaughn, 1981). These interventions also included social-skills training for the patient. This was followed by a randomized study of social-skills training and behavioral family therapy in comparison with "holistic therapy" and supportive family therapy (Snyder & Liberman, 1981; Wallace & Liberman, 1985). Significant differences were found in the social functioning of patients, favoring the skills-based therapies.

Unfortunately, while all of the above approaches represent intriguing methods of inducing change in the family system, none employed randomized assignment designs to compare outcomes of family therapy and aftercare. The more recent controlled studies had as their major focus improving the aftercare of patients discharged from the hospital by involving the family in treatment. This new focus reflects two trends, one theoretical and one pragmatic. Theoretically, these programs rely on a diathesis-stress model of schizophrenia. Pragmatically, the focus of therapy has moved from curing the patients of their psychotic symptoms to seeing what impact family therapy can have on their social functioning and resistance to stress-induced relapse once the major tranquilizers have reduced acute psychotic symptoms.

SYSTEMATIC FAMILY TREATMENT STUDIES OF SCHIZOPHRENIA

This review focuses on five recent systematic studies of the impact of family treatment on schizophrenia (see Table 9.1). Each study had a randomized experimental design with at least one comparison condition that included little or no family contact. Each study also had rigorous procedures for selecting participants according to research diagnostic criteria. The timing and pacing of treatment varied from study to study but all provided family treatment in the months immediately following hospital discharge. Most patients had previous admissions, with the exception of those in the Goldstein study, most of whom were first admissions.

Table 9.2 shows relapse rates for the family therapy condition versus one of the comparison groups. As depicted in Figure 9.1, five studies had a strong positive impact in decreasing the relapse rates at 6 or 9 months. Two studies have produced longer term follow-up data: Falloon et al. (1985) reported 2-year relapse rates of 17% for the family treatment compared with 83% for the individual treatment; Leff et al. (1985) reported 2-year relapse rates of 33% for the

Table 9.1. Comparison of Recent Family Therapy Programs with Schizophrenics

STUDY OF TREATMENT PROGRAM	COMPARISON TREATMENT GROUPS USED IN STUDY	SCHEDULE OF FAMILY MEETINGS[a]	PLACE OF MEETINGS	PATIENTS		
				NUMBER	MEAN AGE	PERCENTAGE FIRST ADMISSIONS
Goldstein et al. (1978)	2 × 2 factorial: Low and medium drug dose plus family crisis therapy; same drug dose without family therapy	6 weekly family meetings	Clinic	96	23	69%
Leff et al. (1982, 1985)	Group therapy and education for relatives vs. standard aftercare	18 biweekly relatives' group meetings plus 6 individual family meetings (average)	Group at clinic; family at home	24	35	30%
Falloon et al. (1982, 1985)	Family education and behavioral family therapy vs. individual case management	Weekly for 3 months, biweekly for 3 months, monthly for 3 months	Home	36	25	36%
Hogarty et al. (1986)	2 × 2 factorial: Family intervention plus patient social skills training vs. family intervention only vs. social skills training only vs. normal outpatient care	Twice a week during hospitalization, then every 2 or 3 weeks	Clinic	103	27	23%
Tarrier et al. (1988)	Behavioral family therapy vs. education only vs. normal outpatient care	Education plus 11 sessions of stress management and goal setting	Clinic	83	35	30%

[a]During hospitalization and the first 9 months after discharge.

Table 9.2. Relapse Rates from Five Randomized Studies of Family Therapy with Schizophrenics

		FAMILY THERAPY GROUP		COMPARISON GROUP	
STUDY	FIRST FOLLOW-UP	TYPE	RATE	RATE	TYPE
Goldstein et al. (1978)	6 months	Moderate dose medication and family therapy	0%	48%	Low dose medication, no family therapy
Leff et al. (1982, 1985)[a]	9 months	Relatives' group and education	8%	50%	Normal outpatient care
Falloon et al. (1982, 1985)[b]	9 months	Family education and behavioral family therapy	6%	44%	Individual education and case management
Hogarty et al. (1986)	9 months	Family therapy with or without social skills training	9%	28%	Individual social skills training or medication only
Tarrier et al. (1988)	9 months	Family education and behavioral family therapy	12%	53%	Normal outpatient care

[a]At 2 years, relapse rates were 33% for family cases compared with 75% for individual cases.
[b]At 2 years, relapse rates were 17% for family cases compared with 83% for individual cases.

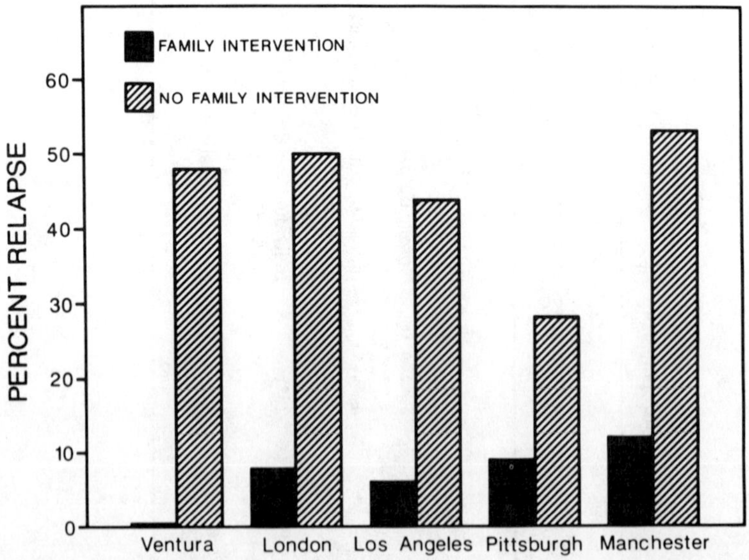

Figure 9.1. Nine-month relapse rates from five studies of family intervention with schizophrenic patients (all on continuous medication) at London, England (Leff et al., 1982), Los Angeles, California (Falloon et al., 1982), Pittsburgh, Pennsylvania (Hogarty et al., 1986), Manchester, England (Tarrier et al., 1988), and (for 6 months only) Ventura, California (Goldstein et al., 1978).

family treatment compared with 75% for normal outpatient care.

Crisis-Oriented Family Therapy

Goldstein et al. (1978) reported the first random assignment study of family therapy as used in aftercare. They examined the impact of a short-term, crisis-oriented family therapy aftercare program in combination with various levels of drug dosage.

The sample consisted of 96 first and second admissions (mean age 23 years) who received independent diagnoses of schizophrenia from ratings on the New Haven Schizophrenia Index. Of these, 69% were first admissions and 31% were second admissions who had all been admitted within the year.

Patients were assigned to one of four conditions by a stratified random method. Their premorbid sociosexual adjustment was measured on the UCLA Social Adjustment Scale, and median splits were used to stratify males and females separately into good and poor premorbid groups. Then patients were randomly assigned to cells in a 2 × 2 factorial design. One factor was the presence or absence of family therapy. The other factor was the level of medication. All patients were given long-acting injections of phenothiazines. The low-dose group received what was judged to be a minimally therapeutic dose of fluphenazine (0.25 ml); the moderate dose group received 1 ml.

The family therapy was of short duration and very concrete. Based on crisis intervention theory, the therapy was designed to help the family understand the events around the psychosis and to improve future coping. Family therapy sessions with two cotherapists were held weekly in the outpatient clinic for the 6 weeks following discharge. In the first stage of treatment, each family member, including the patient, was asked about the events before and during the patient's psychotic break. Many mental health professionals avoid dealing with this event, letting patient and relatives "seal over" emotions or feel hidden shame about the psychotic break. Goldstein and Kopeikin (1981) reported that both patient and relatives experienced a great deal of relief in talking about the breakdown, and they also became aware of its serious nature. During this initial discussion, the therapists helped the family identify stressful events that preceded the breakdown and make links between these precipitating events and the breakdown.

The second stage of therapy identified the two or three situations that were currently most stressful to the patient. The third stage developed strategies for avoiding or coping with these stressful situations. During the week, the family carried out these methods of coping and reported back at the next meeting. In the final stage, plans were made to anticipate future crises and develop stress prevention and coping mechanisms in advance of such crises. Of major importance was the discussion of the possible emergence of psychiatric symptoms. Other topics might be resuming employment, making friends, or future living arrangements. In summary, the family meetings revolved around identifying current potential stressors and planning coping mechanisms for the patient and relatives to use.

Results on Course of Illness

At the end of 6 weeks of treatment, 10 of the 96 patients had deteriorated clinically so that they had to be rehospitalized or have their medication increased dramatically. This was an overall relapse rate of only 10%, considerably less than the 31% found previously. At 6-month follow-up, the rate of relapse was 0% for the moderate dose family therapy group but 48% for the low dose no therapy group. The other two groups were in between: Moderate dose no therapy had a relapse rate of 14%; low dose no therapy was 21%. There was a significant effect of drug dosage ($p < .01$) and family therapy ($p < .05$), and the extreme groups differed very significantly ($p < .001$).

The symptomatic status of the patient was examined using behavior ratings on Overall and Gorham's Brief Psychiatric Rating Scale (BPRS, 1962). The most significant effects were for the family therapy: At 6 weeks, family therapy had a significant overall effect on symptoms, particularly on social withdrawal and blunted affect. Thus, the family therapy seemed to prevent the patient from withdrawing socially and becoming less emotionally responsive. At 6 months, only withdrawal was significantly related to treatment group: The effect of therapy at this point was found only in the group with the higher drug dosage.

It can be concluded that the 6 weeks of moderate drug dosage and short-term family therapy had significant effects on relapse rates and social withdrawal up to the 6 month follow-up. A long-term follow-up was conducted on those patients still in the area after 3 to 6 years. There were no longer any effects. In other words, the effect of the 6-week intervention ceased to be significant as its impact diminished in comparison with that of later events.

Education, Relatives' Support Group, and Family Therapy

Growing out of the research relating EE to relapse, Leff and his colleagues in London decided to examine the effect of family education and relatives' groups on relapse (Leff et al., 1982, 1985, 1983).

Consecutive admissions to several London hospitals were screened for the presence of the following: (a) continuous residence with relatives for at least 3 months before admission, (b) a diagnosis of schizophrenia according to the Present State Examination (PSE) criteria, and (c) a high level of face-to-face family contact, more than 35 hours per week. Subsequently, each relative with high face-to-face contact was given the Camberwell Family Interview (CFI) and their EE level assessed. Twenty-four high-EE families were randomly assigned to an experimental treatment group or a comparison treatment-as-usual group. Both groups received identical assessment at intake and 9-month follow-up: a PSE with the patient, a CFI, and a structured interview about their knowledge of schizophrenia with each relative. Most patients were on long-acting injections of phenothiazines. The mean age was 35 years and 30% were first admissions. This was therefore an older, more chronic group than the subjects in the Goldstein study. Sixteen low-EE families were also randomly assigned to treatment or comparison groups, but data were not reported because of dropouts from these groups.

The intervention package had three components (Berkowitz, Kuipers, Eberlein-Fries, & Leff, 1981). First, an education program was given to relatives in their homes. This consisted of four short lectures covering possible causes, symptoms, likely course, and treatment. Relatives were encouraged to ask questions. The patient's condition was explicitly described as *schizophrenia*.

The second component was a relatives' group composed of both high- and low-EE relatives. The group was led by two professionals and met every 2 weeks. Practitioners had observed previously that low-EE relatives had more effective coping mechanisms for dealing with their schizophrenic relative; this phenomenon had the dual effect of decreasing pressure on the patient and eliciting more support for themselves. Thus, the initial hope was that low-EE coping mechanisms would "rub off" on the high-EE relatives. This turned out to be overly optimistic because most of the low-EE relatives simply stopped attending. In response, the group leaders became more active in helping the relatives find better coping mechanisms.

The third component, family meetings in the home, was developed to include the patient and to deal with family dynamics. The approach was pragmatic, varied, and flexible.

Most relatives in the treatment group received the educational component and attended the group about once a month. Every family had at least one family meeting at home with an average of five. Nine months after discharge, the PSE and CFIs were repeated. A further follow-up PSE on those who had not already relapsed was repeated at 2 years.

Results on Course of Illness

Relapse was defined as the reappearance of schizophrenic symptoms that did not exist at discharge, or the exacerbation of symptoms that had stabilized at discharge (Leff et al., 1982). At 9-month follow-up, only 1 out of 12 patients in the treatment group (8%) had relapsed compared with 6 out 12 in the treatment-as-usual comparison group (50%), a significant difference (Fisher's exact test $p = .03$). During this time, two patients stopped taking medication, and one of the two relapsed. At 2-year follow-up (Leff et al., 1985), 4 out of the 12 in the treatment group (33%) had relapsed compared with 9 out of 12 in the comparison group (75%), again a significant difference (Fisher's exact test $p = .04$).

However, five patients stopped taking medication during the 2 years, two in the treatment group and three in the comparison group. To analyze the effect of treatment without the confounding effect of medication compliance, the analysis was repeated without these subjects. Only 20% relapsed in the treatment group compared with 78% in the comparison group ($p = .02$).

Further analyses examined the impact of the social interventions on EE, the focus of treatment and an indicator of the family emotional environment. The CFI was administered at admission and at 9-month follow-up. I conducted a reanalysis of the data and found that for the 11 treatment families who were initially very critical and who had both initial and follow-up data, the mean number of critical comments decreased from a mean of 17.6 to 6.9; for the 6 comparison patients with both sets of data, the mean number of critical comments decreased from 13.3 to 10.7. The ranked change scores were highly significantly different ($F = 9.6$, $df = 3/12$, $p < .001$). Changes in ratings of emotional overinvolvement were not significant, however.

Berkowitz et al. (1984) examined the impact of the education sessions on knowledge about schizophrenia. They found that high-EE attitudes were associated with disbelief that an illness caused the problems and reluctance to change from a blaming stance, whereas relatives with low-EE attitudes were less blaming and accepted the notion of an illness more easily.

In overview, these data suggest that the combination of medication and social interventions with the families of schizophrenics has a significant effect on the likelihood of relapse at both 9-month and 2-year follow-ups. Further, the analysis of EE (and knowledge) data suggests that this success is associated with relatives' developing less critical attitudes toward the patient, which is probably related to their changing attributions about the causes of the patient's behavior, the group support, the direct education, and the clear focus in family meetings on changing the way emotion was expressed.

Behavioral Family Management

The program of Falloon et al. (Falloon et al., 1985; Leff et al., 1982) differed from the previous two in several respects. First, medication was given orally and flexibly, at the minimum level possible. This design followed findings that long-acting intramuscular medication may impair social functioning more than oral medication (Falloon, Watt, & Shepherd, 1978) despite similar effects on relapse rates. Furthermore, it was assumed that flexible, minimal dosages would mean better responses to psychosocial intervention.

Second, a short educational program was given to each family. In contrast to the Leff program, however, the patient was included and made an expert on his or her own symptoms by the clinician, thus unbalancing the status hierarchy in the family.

Third, the main focus of intervention was behavioral family management with the whole family. On the basis of previous work by Falloon and Liberman (Liberman, 1970; Falloon et al., 1981, 1983), the model views the family as an effective resource for community rehabilitation. Further, the goal of the family management was to improve the family's ability to cope with stress by enhancing family problem-solving and communication skills through behavioral training techniques and structured tasks. All family sessions were conducted in the home for the first 9 months of treatment. The first two sessions were spent educating the patient and the family about the nature of schizophrenia and the rationale for combining drug and psychosocial interventions. Thereafter, family meetings were held weekly for the first 3 months, biweekly for the next 3 months, and monthly for the next 3 months. After that, families were invited to multi-family groups held monthly at the hospital.

The family meetings focused on problem solving, and thus the family was trained to pinpoint a problem, generate solutions, evaluate potential consequences, agree on a best strategy, implement the strategy, and then review results. The therapist taught the model and then coached the family, expecting them to take responsibility for problem solving between meetings. The therapist also focused on communication training, encouraging the family to communicate clearly by active listening, being specific about requests, and expressing positive and negative feelings clearly. The aim of the intervention was not to stifle emotion but to channel its expression in more constructive ways.

Behavioral family management was compared with individual case management of the patient. Therapists saw an equal number of patients in family and individual treatment. The individual program consisted of education about schizophrenia followed by supportive therapy focused on the problems of everyday living. Thirty-six schizophrenic patients were randomly assigned to individual or family management. As in the Leff program, all patients were living with families with high-EE attitudes or significant family tension. The sample had a mean age of 25 years and 36% were first admissions.

Results on Course of Illness and Cost Effectiveness

The assessment of relapse was done systematically with a variety of measures of exacerbation: PSE interviews were given at 0, 9, and 24 months; and monthly ratings were made of key schizophrenic symptoms and global BPRS scores. At 9-month follow-up, only 1 out of 18 (6%) in the family management group had had a major exacerbation of schizophrenia compared with 8 out of 18 (44%) in the individual treatment group, a highly significant difference (Fisher's exact test $p < .01$). At the 2-year follow-up, only 3 out of 18 (17%) in the family management group had had a major exacerbation compared with 15 out of 18 (83%) in the individual management group, again a highly significant difference (Fisher's exact test $p < .0001$). This higher rate of exacerbations was also associated with longer and more numerous hospital admissions.

A feature of Falloon's study was the comprehensive assessment of change, particularly in social and family functioning. Whereas the previous studies focused on psychopathology, Falloon, Boyd, & McGill (1984) reported outcome data on the social and economic benefits of their program. Multiple outcome measures were used, including the Social Behavior Assessment Schedule (Platt, Weyman, Hirsch, & Hewett, 1980), which assessed both subjective and objective measures of social functioning. Data showed enhanced functioning in the treatment group both at 9 and 24 months, as indicated by fewer hospitalizations, less behavioral disturbance, better reported family relationships, and more friends. Informants reported greater satisfaction with the patients' social behavior and less family burden. Over the 24 months, family cases were involved in full- or part-time work or education for an average of 12.6 months compared with 7.2 months for individual cases.

Examining direct interactions between family members, analyses were also performed to investigate changes in family communication and problem solving. Doane, Goldstein, and Miklowitz (1985) showed that the total number of critical and intrusive remarks made by parents was significantly lower after 3 months of family therapy compared with individual treatment. Further, parental criticism and intrusiveness were associated with relapse in the individual treatment. Using a coding scheme for recording instances in which family members adopted recommended problem-solving strategies, Doane, Falloon, Goldstein, and Mintz (1985) showed that decreases in critical or intrusive remarks were associated with increases in problem-solving statements. They concluded that problem-solving behavior had replaced negative affective interaction, although they could not determine what happened first.

A cost-benefit and cost-effectiveness analysis was performed to assess whether the home-based family management was more or less expensive (Cardin, McGill, & Falloon, 1985). All direct and indirect costs of community management to the patients, families, and health, welfare, and community agencies were recorded throughout the 2 years. Cost-benefit analysis of the 12-month data showed that total costs for family management were 19% less than those of individual management, despite the added expense of time to travel to the patients' homes for the family sessions. The greater cost effectiveness of family management was due mainly to the increased need for crisis intervention and hospitalization for the individually managed patients. The cost-benefit analysis weighed the effectiveness of treatment on clinical, social, and family functioning, against the total cost of services. Family management showed double the effectiveness at 58% less cost.

Thus, this program seems to have been extremely effective in reducing exacerbations of schizophrenia and in improving social and role functioning. Further, these were made at lower cost to society than traditional individual case management. There was some evidence that individually treated patients complied with medication less, but this effect was not strong enough to explain the large differences in the rates of exacerbation. There was a (nonsignificant) trend for family cases to have lower doses of neuroleptics prescribed and ingested than in individual cases. In conclusion, behavioral family management may allow lower drug dosages for patients and thus reduce side effects while improving social functioning.

Family Psychoeducation and Survival Skills

Hogarty et al. (1986) reported the 1-year effects of a large study of family treatment and social-skills training in conjunction with pharmacotherapy. After hospital admission, 103 patients living with high-EE relatives who met Research Diagnostic Criteria for schizophrenia or schizoaffective disorder were randomly assigned to four conditions of a 2-year aftercare study. Twenty-three percent of the patients were first admissions. Their mean age was 27 years.

The study examined the additive effect of two different treatment methods on maintenance antipsychotic medication: psychoeducational family treatment and individually oriented social-skills training. The four conditions of the study were thus (a) medication only; (b) family treatment and medication; (c) social-skills training and medication; and (d) family treatment, social-skills training, and medication.

The family treatment (Anderson, Hogarty, & Reiss, 1980; Anderson, Reiss, & Hogarty, 1986) in this study was predicated on two assumptions: that the emotionally laden atmosphere in the home should be reduced and that reasonable expectations of the patient's performance be maintained. The family treatment provided family members with education about schizophrenia and strategies for managing the patient, with the immediate goal of forming an alliance with the family.

The family treatment had four phases: In phase 1, the emphasis was on forming a good working alliance with the family and involved two sessions per week during the brief hospitalization or acute phase. During these sessions with the relatives, the therapist connected with the family members and enlisted their cooperation with the program. The therapist was empathic and, through discussion of the recent episode, aimed to decrease the guilt, frustration, and anxiety often experienced by relatives. Additionally, the family therapist acted as a mediator with the hospital and treatment system.

Phase 2 of treatment was unique to this program. Psychoeducation about schizophrenia was provided in a one-day "survival skills" workshop in which four or five families with a recently hospitalized member met to receive information about schizophrenia, concrete management suggestions, and encouragement to have lives of their own. An important aspect of this workshop was the informal interaction with other people in similar predicaments, which promoted togetherness and the beginning of a support network.

The next stage of the program involved the whole family, including the patient, meeting every 2 weeks for 6 months. The basic goal of this phase was to apply the general strategies from the survival skills workshop to the particular family. This involved reinforcing the boundaries between the patient and other family members and building connections with friends and the community. The patient was encouraged to resume responsibility gradually. Often relatives expected patients to return to work quickly and to live on their own. The family therapist encouraged relatives to lower their expectations initially, to be patient, and to help the patient accomplish small steps toward independence.

In the final phase of treatment, the family members made one of two choices. Either they continued in family therapy to improve family communication and to deal with unresolved conflict, or they decreased involvement with the treatment team. Sessions become decreasingly frequent and served to reinforce the lessons learned earlier. The clinical team remained available to families for maintenance sessions or crisis management. Thus, the family treatment was most intensive for the first year after the acute episode, becoming less frequent thereafter (Anderson et al., 1980).

The social-skills training used with the patients was similar to previous efforts with schizophrenics (Wallace et al., 1980; Liberman, Massel, Mosk, & Wong, 1985) but focused in particular on improving the patient's social skills in dealing with family members. Initially, patients were taught (through a process of instruction, modeling, role play, feedback, and assigned homework) to avoid conflict and criticism of family members, the goal being to prevent the patient from eliciting high-EE behaviors, and instead to elicit favorable responses from the family. Thus, this approach attempted to change the family emotional environment by working with the patient only.

The comparison "no treatment" condition was a combination of medication and biweekly individual supportive therapy.

For inclusion in the study, patients had to live with at least one high-EE relative. Families were rapidly inducted into treatment within a week or two of hospitalization. Patients were said to have relapsed if there was a return of schizophrenic symptoms that were not present at discharge, or if there was an exacerbation of symptoms persisting at discharge. Of the 103 patients, 90 stayed in treatment, 11 relapsed during the early process of engagement, and 2 received only minimal treatment. These latter 13 cases were designated as "partial treatment takers." Relapse was monitored for 12 months, at the end of which a repeat CFI was obtained.

Results on Course of Illness

At 1-year follow-up, the medication comparison group had a relapse rate of 41% (consistent with previous findings), whereas the group that received both family and social skills treatments had a relapse rate of 0%. The group that received only family treatment had a relapse rate of 19%, and the group that received only social-skills training had a relapse rate of 20%. Comparable figures at 9 months were 28%, 0%, 9%, and 10%, respectively. The main effects of family treatment and social-skills training were both statistically significant, but the interaction was not, suggesting that the effects were additive. Similar effects were found when partial takers were included. When only those patients who were consistently compliant in taking medication were considered, family treatment had a significant effect, and the effect of social-skills training was only marginally significant. This result appeared to come from the higher rate of noncompliance in the medication-only comparison group (24%) compared with 5% to 10% in the three psychosocial treatment groups. Sixty-six percent of these noncompliers relapsed, reducing the effect sizes.

A feature of this study was the careful measurement and analysis of EE at intake and 1-year follow-up. All patients at intake lived within high-EE households. The most interesting findings were (a) that there were *no* patient relapses in any household that changed from high to low EE, independent of treatment condition; and (b) that in households that stayed high in EE only the combination of family treatment and social skills training prevented relapse. In fact, there were no relapses in this group. These striking results suggest that reductions in the family tensions are associated with improvements in patient outcome, however the reductions are achieved. Further, family treatment may be the most effective in this regard because changes in EE level were most pronounced in the two family therapy conditions.

These findings also supported data from an earlier study designed by Liberman, Falloon, and Aitchison (1984). They used an eight-session multifamily behavioral family treatment in conjunction with social-skills training with 14 patients from high-EE families. In comparison with a contrast group from a similar population that received supportive family therapy plus holistic health therapy, 9-month relapse rates were 21% versus 56%, with a concomitant drop in EE.

In conclusion, the Hogarty study provided important information on combining medication, family treatment, and individual social-skills training. Note that the combination of these three treatments led to the best outcome. Of particular pertinence was the fact that social-skills training had an effect additive to the antipsychotic medication and psychoeducational family therapy.

Family Behavioral Intervention Versus Education Only

Inspired by the protective effects of family intervention generated by the studies described above, a clinical research team from Manchester, England, led by Tarrier designed a study to investigate two issues: (a) whether behavioral family treatment has an effect over and above that of providing relatives with educational information about schizophrenia; and (b) whether a participative form of family treatment in which family members are actively involved in role-playing differs from treatment in which the same skills are taught through lecture and discussion (Tarrier et al., 1988; 1989).

Schizophrenic patients who had lived with their family for 3 months prior to their hospitalization and who intended to return there were recruited. Eighty-three families participated, 64 of whom were high-EE households. Of these patients, 30% were experiencing first episodes; therefore, this sample was similar in composition to the Leff, Falloon, and Hogarty samples.

Patients from high-EE families were assigned in a stratified, random manner to one of four groups, while the patients from low-EE families were assigned to one of two groups. Ten families dropped out of treatment leaving 73 in the study. Most patients received depot injections; some received oral medication. The high-EE families were assigned to four groups; behavioral intervention inactive; behavioral intervention symbolic; education only; and routine treatment. Both behavioral groups had similar content in terms of the skills that were taught. They differed, however, in that the inactive condition involved active practice of the content skills taught in both conditions inside and outside the sessions. Both groups received two sessions of education, three sessions of stress management, and eight sessions of goal-setting over the 9-month period. The education-only group received two family sessions of education about schizophrenia. The routine treatment was normal outpatient psychiatric care with no special family interventions. Finally, low-EE families were assigned to either education only or routine treatment.

Results on Course of Illness

As shown in the previous studies, relapse rates for high-EE families in the two behavioral family treatment groups combined together (12%) were significantly less than the relapse rate in the routine treatment group (53%; $p < .02$). The relapse rate in the education-only group (43%) was not significantly different from that in the routine treatment group, but there was a trend ($p < .08$) for it to differ from the two behavioral family treatment groups. Relapse rates in the two low-EE groups were not significantly different: routine treatment (20%); education only (22%). However, as has been found in most previous naturalistic studies, the relapse rate in the two low-EE groups combined (21%) was significantly lower than the relapse rate in the high-EE routine treatment group (53%; $p < .05$).

Thus, the main findings reinforced the other studies in showing the effectiveness of adding a family component to normal outpatient medication. Further, this study supported the notion that brief educational interventions are *in*effective in forestalling relapse: Family intervention is effective in reducing rate of relapse only when education about schizophrenia is provided with an opportunity to discuss and to practice skills learned over a period of months. There is an urgent need to replicate these tentative findings since many clinical sites are introducing brief psychoeducational interventions for families that may not be effective.

Comparisons were also made between the two behavioral interventions to assess their differential effectiveness. Contrary to the expectations of the investigators, the inactive behavioral intervention with its focus on active behavioral involvement of relatives through role-playing, practice, and corroborated out-of-session practice did not produce larger effects on EE or relapse than did the symbolic behavioral intervention that involved instruction and discussion without a focus on behavioral practice. However, differential effects of family intervention may emerge when the results are reported on social functioning of the patients, and on 2-year relapses rates.

A feature of this study was that the CFI was repeated at 4½ months and 9 months. The main finding was that both the high-EE symbolic ($p < .05$) and high-EE inactive ($p < .01$) groups showed significant changes from high to low EE at 9 months, with most of the change taking place in the first 4½ months. In terms of the components of EE, levels of criticism, emotional overinvolvement, and (surprisingly) warmth all decreased significantly. Further, the behavioral intervention groups had significantly fewer high-EE relatives at 9 months than did the high-EE education and routine treatment groups. (These findings should be treated with some caution because the statistical analyses were conducted using multiple Z tests instead of appropriate analysis of variance.) However, none of these effects could be attributed to differences in medication compliance or contact with psychiatric services.

Family Therapy Versus a Relatives Group

Building on the Leff et al. (1982, 1985, 1986) study of customary care compared with family therapy *and* relatives' groups, Leff, Berkowitz, and colleagues (Leff et al., 1989; 1990) compared the impact on schizophrenics from high-EE families of *either* individual family therapy *or* a relatives group led by a professional. Relatives in the family therapy stream ($n = 12$) received a median of 17 sessions in the first 9 months, with only one patient refusing further visits after 4 months. By contrast, adherence to the relatives group was not so good, with five of the 11 families failing to attend a single group. The remaining six families attended a median of 4½ times. The data were analyzed separately for those attending and those not attending the group.

At 9-month follow-up, the patients in the family therapy condition had a relapse rate of 8%; patients whose relatives attended the group had a relapse rate of 17%; and patients whose relatives did not attend the group had a relapse rate of 60%. Further, there were significant reductions in criticism and rises in warmth in both conditions. These data suggest that both family therapy and relatives' groups had an impact on changing the family emotional atmosphere, *if* relatives attended.

COMMON FEATURES OF FAMILY INTERVENTION PROGRAMS

The new generation of family intervention programs has different emphases: Goldstein et al. (1978) stressed family crisis intervention but did not offer psychoeducation; Leff et al. (1982) stressed multifamily group support and skill sharing; Falloon et al. (1982) stressed problem solving and communication training; Hogarty et al. (1986) stressed survival skills and management of the patient; and Tarrier et al. (1988) stressed a comparison of behavioral family treatment and education.

Nevertheless, these programs share a number of common features that may explain their greater effectiveness than previous psychosocial programs for persons suffering from schizophrenia. Some of these common features are so-called nonspecific therapy factors that transcend particular techniques (Gurman & Razin, 1977). Others are specific techniques.

Family Therapy Techniques

In general, the therapists in all five programs were warm, empathic, and concrete in their focus on helpful management strategies. None of the programs used traditional psychodynamic (intensive, exploratory, uncovering, insight-oriented) therapy with families (Boszormenyi-Nagy, 1965). Interpretive family therapy can be overstimulating for patients and can lead to psychotic regression. For example, depth interpretations of internal motivations can lead to patients' thinking the therapist can read their minds and can play into delusional thinking. Thus, Kottgen, Sonnichsen, Mollenhauer, and Jurth (1984b) described a program in which patients and relatives met separately in analytically oriented psychotherapy groups. These groups, which used an uncovering, insight-oriented approach, did not reduce the likelihood of patient relapse, presumably because they were overstimulating and lacked the practical, learning-based focus of the new generation of family interventions.

In contrast, the five successful programs used some or all of the following processes of connecting with relatives and patients, reframing their intentions, focusing on current transactions, focusing on communication, problem solving, psychoeducation, and improving drug compliance.

Connecting with Relatives and Patients

The initial evaluations of patients and relatives were conducted using research interviews with a model of respectful inquiry (the Present State Examination or the Schedule for Affective Disorder and Schizophrenia for patients; the Camberwell Family Interview [CFI] for relatives). Relatives are asked to describe in detail the problems that *they* have experienced in relation to the patient's behavior while patients' experiences with their symptoms are solicited in a concerned manner. Relatives often report that the interview itself was cathartic and helpful. These respectful interviews help build a respectful relationship between the clinician and family members.

Second, investigators from three psychoeducational programs report that the educational sessions in particular help with the process of connecting with the families and patients in a therapeutic alliance. The relatives often described great relief in finally getting answers to their questions about the patient's illness and treatment. Cozolino and Nuechterlein (1986) report that even a single, limited educational session had salutary effects on the therapeutic relationship and alliance between relatives and professionals.

Finally, because of the legal requirement for obtaining informed consent, clear contracts were negotiated at the outset with each patient and his or her family. The aims, structure, and length of the program were explained fully, including randomization to treatment conditions and follow-up procedures.

Reframing

Relatives often feel that their contribution to helping the patient is not appreciated by clinical staff. They may also feel blamed for the patient's problems, especially if they hear the phrase "family therapy." Thus, they may react defensively and reject any attempt at "treatment." Further, their guilt and anxiety can lead them to behave toward the patient in counterproductive ways.

Therefore, it is often useful to talk not of "family therapy" but of "family meetings," or "family education," expressions that do not imply there is something wrong with family members. Other terms more acceptable to relatives of the mentally ill are "psychoeducation," "family coping," or "family skills training." Furthermore, relatives can often be engaged in treatment by appealing to their altruism and asking them to come "so we can help you help (the patient)."

Once the joining process has taken place, the intentions of relatives and patient might be positively reframed. Depth interpretations that can imply criticism and induce guilt are avoided. Rather, every effort is made to see the problem from each person's point of view and to reframe intentions positively. Thus, parents can be described as making their best efforts to be helpful, as being "protective" rather than "emotionally overinvolved," as "encouraging independence" rather than being "hostile and critical."

Focus on Current Transactions

The focus of treatment in the currently effective family programs was on the current transactions between family members. Therapists focused neither on the historical development of the family nor on the development of personality, but on present-day coping, on how the patient and relatives deal with stress, and how they react to each other. Very quickly, the focus was moved away from "What is wrong with the patient and how can he be cured?" at one extreme, or "What is wrong with the relatives and how can they be tamed?" at the other. Instead, therapists and family members conjointly examined family interaction to generate alternative methods of coping that could be used to deal more effectively with the inevitable stressors of life, compounded by managing the burdens of a disabled mentally ill person in the family circle.

Focus on Communication

Effective family intervention programs focused on having clear communication between family members and improving the family's emotional atmosphere. However, there were different emphases. Goldstein and his associates, for example, focused on the patient's and relatives' communication about what happened during the acute episode, what experiences the patient had (often never revealed to family members), the reactions of relatives, and the meaning of the precipitant to the family. The other programs focused more explicitly on reducing the "emotional temperature" in these families, which were selected as high-risk environments because relatives were rated as being high on EE. Although EE attitudes are indirect measures of relatives' behavioral responses to the patient, they have been shown to relate to the quality of emotional interaction in the family (Strachan, Goldstein, & Miklowitz, 1986).

The programs of Leff and Hogarty focused explicitly on reducing high EE in the relatives. In contrast, the Falloon and Liberman approach did not focus explicitly on the goal of reducing EE. Instead, they assumed that high EE was an index of emotional distress in a relative, which was a reaction to lack of conflict-resolution. Relatives were not expected to reduce the intensity of their emotional expression but rather to express their feelings more clearly, differentiating their personal reactions from other people's internal motivations. In fact, even though there was not a focus on reducing emotional expression, the redirection of expression led to a reduction in the number of criticisms and intrusions directed at the patient in direct interaction with treatment (Doane, Falloon et al., 1985; Goldstein & Strachan, 1986).

Focus on Concrete Problem Solving

All of the new generation of family intervention programs focused explicitly on structured techniques for problem solving, practical issues of management, and concrete coping strategies. Except for the Leff and Goldstein groups, all the family programs concentrated on specific and directive skill building, both in terms of communication and problem solving or goal setting. It could be that such a behavioral skill-building focus may be particularly beneficial to the many schizophrenic patients who have deficits in social skills, resulting in the more favorable social and occupational rehabilitation outcomes in follow-up studies of behavioral family management (Snyder & Liberman, 1981; Falloon et al., 1985).

Psychoeducation

Each program stressed the importance of facing the psychotic experience directly, although each treated this slightly differently: Goldstein focused on understanding the precipitants of the psychotic episode without talking about schizophrenia explicitly; Falloon, Anderson, Tarrier, and Leff all had structured education programs about schizophrenia that were given to families; Falloon and Goldstein included the patient whereas Anderson and Leff did not.

It is interesting that the education, although short, seems to be very powerful and helpful, particularly for relatives of people who have had several hospitalizations over the years (Cozolino & Nuechterlein, 1986). They may have been asking what was wrong over the years and received only vague answers from mental health professionals. They may have recognized that medication helped but had no idea what it did. They may have felt guilty, particularly if hospital staff had told them to stay away because their visits upset the patient. And, perhaps most important, the fantasy may have developed that there was something terribly wrong, fueled by the vague answers of mental health professionals, just as people guess they have cancer from the growing wall of silence around them: "Maybe my relative is mad and will only get worse and worse. Maybe he (or she) has even got the dread disease 'schizophrenia.'"

The educational program seems to burst this bubble and leads to relief instead of despair. Knowing at last that their relative has schizophrenia and hearing explanations of its likely course and response to treatment (which most relatives experience as better than their worst fantasies), they tend to be much more optimistic (Cozolino & Nuechterlein, 1986). Paradoxically, they feel more in control. They are more realistic and now have a better idea of what they can expect and what is and is not possible for them to do to help.

Improving Drug Compliance

It has been argued that family therapy may have a beneficial effect on relapse by increasing compliance with medication. Falloon et al. (1982) noted that more reliable tablet-taking was found in their family treatment group and suggested that even if family treatment only leads to greater compliance with medication and hence less symptom exacerbation, the family treatment approach is indeed a step forward. However, in the Leff, Tarrier, and Goldstein studies, medication compliance was excellent in both the treatment and comparison groups, and the family approach still reduced relapse rates. In the study of Hogarty et al., the effects of family treatment were apparent whether all patients were considered or just those who were compliant with medication. Thus, family treatment, while improving medication compliance, has an effect beyond that of increased compliance.

IMPLICATION FOR A CONCEPTUAL FRAMEWORK FOR SCHIZOPHRENIA

It is assumed that persons with schizophrenia have a biopsychological *vulnerability* that makes them particularly susceptible to *stressors* and that reductions in external stressors and/or increases in personal *coping* can lead to increased *competence*. The vulnerability of schizophrenic patients seems to be manifest as a sensitivity to their social environment (even when they are not experiencing symptoms) such that either an overstimulating or an understimulating social environment may lead to a return of positive or negative symptoms and increased arousal (Wing & Brown, 1970).

The focus of the new and effective family programs has been on reducing overstimulation from the natural environment: by buffering the patient against the stress of external, independent life events (Brown & Birley, 1968); by improving family coping; and by decreasing stress from the family (Leff & Vaughn, 1980; Doane, West, Goldstein, Rodnick, & Jones, 1981; Goldstein, 1985; 1987).

However, as Hogarty and associates have pointed out (Hogarty et al., 1986), overstimulation can also occur in the therapeutic environment. Thus, overenthusiastic attempts to rehabilitate long-stay patients can inadvertently lead to the return of symptoms that had been absent for years (Brown et al., 1972). For example, one ambitious psychosocial rehabilitation program, termed Major Role Therapy (MRT), appeared to have had expectations of role performance that were too high and thus too stimulating for some patients (Hogarty et al., 1974). Thus, MRT helped patients who were free of symptoms but increased relapse in more symptomatic patients (Goldberg, Schooler, Hogarty, & Roper, 1977). Similarly, the disappointing results of the Kottgen et al. (1984b) program appear to have been due to the overstimulating nature of their interpretive interventions.

Somewhat forgotten in the push to reduce overstimulation has been the deleterious effect of *understimulation*. Thus, as Wing and Brown (1970) observed, an understimulating "back ward" may lead to withdrawal and a lack of external social stimulation and support. Internal stimuli may therefore come into the foreground and lead either to increased negative symptoms or relapse. This understimulation can occur in natural environments as well as therapeutic environments. Thus, some overprotective family environments may neglect or shelter the patient from social stimulation to the extent that internal stimuli come to the fore, thereby precipitating a relapse or interfering with social functioning. In other words, the level of expectation of the patient can be reduced too far below that of the high expectations of the critical relative.

These programs suggest that increasing the problem-solving and communication abilities of families that include a person with schizophrenia protects and buffers the sick relative from external life stressors and reduces stress from family conflict. Further, it is argued that both therapeutic and natural environments can be overstimulating and can increase stress, or understimulating and thus provoke social withdrawal.

Models that focus directly on the social skills of the patient as well as family members may have additive effects on the long-term social functioning of the patient. The programs designed by Liberman and Falloon, Anderson and Hogarty, and Tarrier had directive skill building and "enactment" for the patient in the family context. These direct interventions with the patients may lead to better social functioning at outcome than a purely psychoeducational approach. Improvements in patients' coping with the associated improvements in social competence may decrease the impact of an underlying vulnerability and decrease the number of life events caused by the patients' lack of competence.

CONCLUSIONS

Family psychoeducational treatment programs in conjunction with antipsychotic medication substantially improve the prognosis of schizophrenic patients. Despite varied methods of intervention with families, all of these programs when combined with neuroleptic medication have demonstrated very significant decreases in relapse rates; some have also demonstrated improvements in social and role functioning. This review has illustrated the consistent effectiveness of structural and educational programs that, despite differences in where the family is seen, which family members are seen, and the format and timing of sessions, share the common features of respectful inquiry, the provision of information, and concrete management strategies. These characteristics differentiate them from more traditional, interpretive, insight-oriented family therapy. Further, the improvements in symptomatic, social, and psychological functioning of the patients and the relatives are particularly associated with reductions in the intensity of negative emotional family interaction.

1. *Family psychoeducational treatment programs reduce costs.* As the Falloon study showed, even though a family approach requires additional time and money in the short term, it is cost-effective and saves money in the long term because of fewer rehospitalizations and less use of crisis facilities, as well as improved role functioning in the community.

2. *All kinds of families may benefit from a psychoeducational family treatment approach.* The three later psychoeducational programs selected patients living in highly charged emotional atmospheres (high-EE families) as being most at risk for relapse. However, practitioners are now beginning to recognize that patients who live in neutral and/or supportive emotional atmospheres (low-EE families) are also at risk for relapse (albeit less so) due to the stress of life events or noncompliance with medication (Leff et al., 1985; Hogarty et al., 1986). Furthermore, the selection of patients living with high-EE relatives has led to a preponderance of unmarried males living with parents in these studies. There is little doubt that married and unmarried female schizophrenics could also benefit from such programs. Thus, all types of families can benefit from education about schizophrenia and improved family coping.

3. *Psychoeducation cannot stand alone.* The information provided to relatives about the symptoms, likely course, causes, and treatment of schizophrenia reduce guilt feelings and blame, factors that can exacerbate the patient's problem. However, the psychoeducational family programs have been successful in the context of provision of maintenance antipsychotic medication, long-term support to families, and the integration of medical and community services with the family approach. The family approach is neither a panacea nor a substitute for community facilities such as residential rehabilitation programs, crisis residential facilities, group homes, and back-up psychiatric day hospitals and inpatient units. Family programs are but one link in a comprehensive system of care.

4. *Family programs should be tailored to the family.* Probably the most important variables affecting the family's response to family-based treatment are the number of previous admissions and the length of the illness. Anderson (1983) noted that relatives of long-term patients usually respond with relief to the survival-skills workshop whereas relatives of recent-onset patients can be shocked by information about schizophrenia and its likely course; they find the prognosis to be pessimistic and grim. In fact, the prognosis for a one-time admission is much better than for a repeat admission; it is entirely possible, albeit unlikely, that the patient will never experience another psychotic break.

Thus, it may be most appropriate in the case of recent-onset patients to talk with the family about the "psychotic experiences" of the patient, possible precipitants, and future ways of coping in the brief crisis-oriented approach pioneered by Goldstein and his associates. If further admissions occur, it may then be appropriate to talk directly about schizophrenia and its implications, and to involve the family in a long-term program of aftercare.

5. *Family treatment may allow reduced or intermittent medication.* In Falloon's study of behavioral family management, medication compliance was better, but also patients were prescribed and ingested lower

dosages. This suggests that behavioral family intervention may subserve a reciprocal protective benefit with medication, thereby lowering the risk of long-term side effects while allowing greater improvement in social functioning.

The drawbacks of continuous long-term medication have been noted by clinical researchers for some time: Many patients develop tardive dyskinesia or an exacerbation of the "deficit" syndrome. Several investigators have experimented with targeted medication in which patients are followed drug free until prodromal signs of an impending relapse appear (Carpenter & Heinrichs, 1983; Herz, 1985; Carpenter, 1986). Medication is then started to prevent an exacerbation and stopped when the patient restabilizes. However, this approach depends upon the cooperation of people who interact with the patient to respond to prodromal signs. Because of the nature of their illness, patients are less likely to be able to monitor prodromal signs. Therefore, targeted intermittent antipsychotic drug therapy has been applied in the context of psychoeducational programs for families. Early results from these drug-psychosocial programs suggest that medication can be reduced significantly without increasing psychopathology (Carpenter, 1986; Carpenter & Heinrichs, 1983; Herz, 1985).

6. *Supportive, skill-oriented treatment can help, too.* The Hogarty and Anderson research team showed that a supportive program of social-skills training, when focused on improving communicational skills with the family, significantly improves patients' prognoses, particularly when given in conjunction with family treatment. This suggests that there is a role for individual or group treatment of schizophrenic patients, if it is practical and skills-oriented, and proceeds at an appropriate pace.

Docherty (1984) suggested that the sequencing of treatment is important. A family approach is most critical during the first year posthospitalization; social-skills training may have an effect in the beginning of the second year; and a subgroup of patients may benefit from a supportive form of psychotherapy thereafter. Future research should determine whether behaviorally oriented skills training is necessary for patients to attain higher levels of social and occupational outcomes.

Treatment of patients without their relatives may be the only choice available for certain patients because of the large number of chronic patients who have become estranged from their families. Platman (1983) cites a New York state study which showed that of patients who had been hospitalized more than 6 months, only 23% returned to private residences, compared with 63% hospitalized less than 6 months. For these patients, a family approach cannot be used and work can be done only with the individual or in groups of peers. However, psychoeducational programs could still be mounted in nonfamilial settings such as foster and board-and-care homes.

7. *Family psychoeducational programs may generalize to other populations.* It has now been shown that the family emotional atmosphere predicts the outcome of disorders other than schizophrenia. Hooley, Orley, and Teasdale (1986) showed that depressed patients have poorer outcomes if they live with high-EE, critical spouses. Similarly, Miklowitz et al. (1988) showed that turbulent family atmospheres, indexed by EE and affective style, predict relapse of bipolar-manic patients living with parents. These naturalistic studies suggest that family intervention may be applicable to the treatment of other disorders as well.

In an example of such a generic family intervention program, Glick et al. (1985) worked with both schizophrenic and affectively disordered inpatients and their relatives. Preliminary results showed that global outcomes at discharge were better for good premorbid schizophrenics, marginally better for patients with major affective disorders, but not better for poor premorbid schizophrenics, when compared with customary hospital care. That effects were not more pronounced may have been due to the brevity of the family intervention, and, in particular, that it did not extend after discharge. Nevertheless, such a program provides some optimism about the generalization of family psychoeducational approaches to other disorders.

8. *Further research is required to distinguish the active ingredients of family treatment.* It is unclear what the active ingredients of these family treatments are. Some active ingredients may be specific treatment approaches while others may be nonspecific therapist factors. I have outlined presumed ingredients above, but these remain speculative. Additionally, although decreases in relapse are particularly associated with decreases in the intensity of emotional atmospheres in the home, it has not been proved that decreasing emotional temperature is the cause of a better outcome. Doane, Falloon, Goldstein, and Mintz (1985) showed that a negative parental affective style is associated with poor problem solving. It is as plausible to argue that Falloon's family program improved problem solving which displaced negative emotion as it is to argue that decreases in conflict allowed improved problem solving. It is important therefore in future research to study both stressful and protective aspects of family process.

9. *Good science can be poor politics.* The social scientists who innocently coined the term *high expressed emotion* to describe the expression of critical attitudes, hostility, and overinvolvement knew little of the storm of reactions from relatives of the mentally ill that would emerge two decades later (Brown, Monck, Carstairs, & Wing, 1962). Relatives of the mentally ill have felt unfairly blamed for precipitating relapses, that their contributions to helping remain unacknowledged, and that the burden of coping remains on their shoulders: The scientists are out to get the family again.

There is more than a grain of truth to the charge that mental health professionals focus on the negative side of people and look for what is wrong. A major part of their training as diagnosticians is to find out what is wrong. However, this does not invalidate the scientific research that has been completed. An important body of research has accumulated that shows the prognostic importance of EE. That low EE may index useful coping strategies such as self-control, good problem solving, and emotional distancing rather than confrontation has not been investigated—and certainly not publicized to relatives.

There has been a public relations gap. Managers in the private sector know well about "staying close to the customer" and "management by wandering around" (Peters & Austin, 1985). They study how to market their products. It seems that in the case of EE, social scientists have been poor politicians, communicating with their peers but forgetting the real "customers"—patients and their relatives (Imber-Mintz, Liberman, Miklowitz, & Mintz, 1987). Nevertheless, there are still opportunities for research scientists to recast their findings on EE more positively, for family members to understand the EE research better, and for administrators to recognize that the family intervention programs spawned by this research provide the possibility of adding one important cost-effective component to the long-term care of people with schizophrenia.

REFERENCES

American Psychiatric Association. (1980). *Diagnostic and statistical manual of mental disorders-III* (3rd ed.). Washington, DC: Author.

Anderson, C. M. (1983). *Psychoeducational family interventions: Suggested modifications for specific subgroups of schizophrenic patients.* Paper presented at the Max Planck Institute International Conference on Young Schizophrenic Patients, Bavaria, West Germany.

Anderson, C. M., Hogarty, G. E., & Reiss, D. J. (1980). Family treatment of adult schizophrenic patients: A psychoeducational approach. *Schizophrenia Bulletin, 6,* 490–505.

Anderson, C. M., Reiss, D. J., & Hogarty, G. E. (1986). *Schizophrenia in the family: A prac-*

titioners guide to psychoeducation and management. New York: Guilford Press.

Berkowitz, R., Eberlein-Fries, R., Kuipers, L., & Leff, J. P. (1984). Educating relatives about schizophrenia. *Schizophrenia Bulletin, 10*, 418–429.

Berkowitz, R., Kuipers, L., Eberlein-Fries, R., & Leff, J. (1981). Lowering expressed emotion in relatives of schizophrenics. In M. J. Goldstein (Ed.), *New developments in interventions with families of schizophrenics*. London: Jossey-Bass.

Boszormenyi-Nagy, I. (1965). A theory of relationships: Experience and transaction. In I. Boszormenyi-Nagy, & J. L. Framo (Eds.), *Intensive family therapy*. New York: Harper & Row.

Bowen, M. (1978). *Family therapy in clinical practice*. New York: Jason Aronson.

Brown, G. W., & Birley, J. L. T. (1968). Crises and life changes and the onset of schizophrenia. *Journal of Health and Social Behavior, 9*, 203–214.

Brown, G. W., Birley, J. L. T., & Wing, J. K. (1972). Influence of family life on the course of schizophrenic disorders: A replication. *British Journal of Psychiatry, 121*, 241–258.

Brown, G. W., Monck, E. M., Carstairs, G. M., & Wing, J. K. (1962). Influence of family life on the course of schizophrenic illness. *British Journal of Preventative and Social Medicine, 16*, 55–68.

Cardin, V. A., McGill, C. M., & Falloon, I. R. H. (1985). An economic analysis: Costs, benefits, and effectiveness. In I. R. H. Falloon (Ed.), *Family management of schizophrenia*. Baltimore: Johns Hopkins University Press.

Carpenter, W. T. (1986). Early targeted pharmacotherapeutic intervention in schizophrenia. *Journal of Clinical Psychiatry, 47*, 23–29.

Carpenter, W. T., Jr., & Heinrichs, D. W. (1983). Early intervention, time-limited, target pharmacotherapy of schizophrenia. *Schizophrenia Bulletin, 9*, 533–542.

Cozolino, L., & Nuechterlein, K. (1986). A pilot study of the impact of a family education program of relatives of recent onset schizophrenic patients. In M. J. Goldstein, I. Hand, & K. Hahlweg (Eds.), *Treatment of schizophrenia: Family assessment and intervention*. Heidelberg: Springer-Verlag.

Creer, C., & Wing, J. K. (1974). *Schizophrenia at home*. London: Institute of Psychiatry.

Doane, J. A., Falloon, I. R. H., Goldstein, M. J., & Mintz, J. (1985). Parental affective style and the treatment of schizophrenia. *Archives of General Psychiatry, 42*, 34–42.

Doane, J. A., Goldstein, M. J., & Miklowitz, D. J. (1985). The impact of individual and family treatment on the affective climate of families of schizophrenics. *British Journal of Psychiatry, 148*, 279–287.

Doane, J. A., West, K. L., Goldstein, M. J., Rodnick, E., & Jones, J. E. (1981). Parental communication and affective style: Predictors of subsequent schizophrenia-spectrum disorders in vulnerable adolescents. *Archives of General Psychiatry, 38*, 679–695.

Docherty, J. P. (1984). O tempora, O mores: Directions in research on the psychotherapeutic treatment of schizophrenia. *Schizophrenia Bulletin, 10*, 621–623.

Doll, W. (1976). Family coping with the mentally ill: An unanticipated problem of deinstitutionalization. *Hospital and Community Psychiatry, 27*, 183–185.

Esterson, A., Cooper, D. G., & Laing, R. D. (1965). Results of family oriented therapy with hospitalized schizophrenics. *British Medical Journal, 2*, 1462–1465.

Falloon, I. R. H., Boyd, J. L., & McGill, C. W. (1984). Family care of schizophrenia: A problem-solving approach to the treatment of mental illness. New York: Guilford Press.

Falloon, I. R. H., Boyd, J. L., McGill, C. W., Razani, J., Moss, H. B., & Gilderman, A. M. (1982). Family management in the prevention of exacerbations of schizophrenia. *New England Journal of Medicine, 306*, 1437–1440.

Falloon, I. R. H., Boyd, J. L., McGill, C. W., Williamson, M., Razani, J., Moss, H. B., Gilderman, A. M., & Simpson, G. M. (1985). Family management in the prevention of morbidity of schizophrenia: Clinical outcome of a two-year longitudinal study. *Archives of General Psychiatry, 42*, 887–896.

Falloon, I. R. H., & Liberman, R. P. (1983). Behavioral family interventions in the management of chronic schizophrenia. In W. R. McFarlane (Ed.), *Family therapy in schizophrenia*. New York: Guilford Press.

Falloon, I. R. H., Liberman, R. P., Lillie, F. J., & Vaughn, C. E. (1981). Family therapy for relapsing schizophrenics and their families: A pilot study. *Family Process, 20*, 211–221.

Falloon, I. R. H., Watt, D. C., & Shepherd, M. (1978). The social outcome of patients in a trial of long-term continuation therapy in schizophrenia: Pimozide vs. fluphenazine. *Psychological Medicine, 8*, 265–274.

Federn, P. (1952). *Ego psychology and the psychoses*. New York: Basic Books.

Folkman, S., Dunkel-Schetter, C., DeLongis, A., & Gruen, R. J. (1986). The dynamics of a stressful encounter: Cognitive appraisal, coping, and encounter outcomes. *Journal of Personality and Social Psychology, 50*, 992–1003.

Freeman, H. E., & Simmons, O. G. (1963). *The mental patient comes home*. New York: Wiley.

Glick, I. D., Clarkin, J. F., Spencer, J. H., Haas, G. L., Lewis, A. B., Peyser, J., DeMane, N., Good-Ellis, M., Harris, E., & Lestalle, V. A. (1985). A controlled evaluation of inpatient family intervention: I. Preliminary results of the six-month follow-up. *Archives of General Psychiatry, 42*, 882–886.

Goldberg, S. C., Schooler, N. R., Hogarty, G. E., & Roper, M. (1977). Prediction of relapse in schizophrenic outpatients treated by drug and social therapy. *Archives of General Psychiatry, 34*, 171–184.

Goldman, H. H., & Gattozzi, A. A. (1981). Defining and counting the chronically mentally ill. *Hospital and Community Psychiatry, 32*, 21–27.

Goldstein, M. J. (1985). Family factors that antedate the onset of schizophrenia and related disorders: The results of a fifteen year prospective longitudinal study. *Acta Psychiatrica Scandinavica, 71*, 7–18.

Goldstein, M. J. (1987). Family interaction patterns that antedate the onset of schizophrenia and related disorders: A further analysis of data from a longitudinal prospective study. In K. Hahlweg & M. J. Goldstein (Eds.), *The impact of family research on our understanding of family psychopathology*. New York: Family Process Press.

Goldstein, M. J., & Kopeikin, H. S. (1981). Short- and long-term effects of combining drug and family therapy. In M. J. Goldstein (Ed.), *New developments in interventions with families of schizophrenics*. London: Jossey-Bass.

Goldstein, M. J., Rodnick, E. H., Evans, J. R., May, P. R. A., & Steinberg, M. R. (1978). Drug and family therapy in the aftercare treatment of acute schizophrenia. *Archives of General Psychiatry, 35*, 169–177.

Goldstein, M. J., & Strachan, A. M. (1986). The impact of family intervention programs on family communication and the short-term course of schizophrenia. In M. J. Goldstein, I. Hand, & K. Hahlweg (Eds.), *Treatment of schizophrenia: Family assessment and intervention*. Heidelberg: Springer-Verlag.

Gunderson, J. G., Frank, A. F., & Katz, H. M. (1977). Effects of psychotherapy in schizophrenia: II. Comparative outcome of two forms of treatment. *Schizophrenia Bulletin, 10*, 564–598.

Gurman, A. S., & Razin, A. M. (1977). *Effective psychotherapy: A handbook of research*. Elmsford, NY: Pergamon Press.

Hatfield, A. B. (1978). Psychological costs of schizophrenia to the family. *Social Casework, 23*, 355–359.

Hatfield, A. B. (1981). Coping effectiveness in families of the mentally ill: An exploratory study. *Journal of Psychiatric Treatment and Evaluation, 3*, 11–19.

Herz, M. (1985). Prodromal symptoms and prevention of relapse in schizophrenia. *Journal of Clinical Psychiatry, 46*, 22–25.

Hogarty, G. E., Anderson, C. M., Reiss, D. J., Kornblith, S. J., Greenwald, D. P., Javna, C. D., Madonia, M. J., & the EPICS Schizophrenia Research Group. (1986). Family psycho-education, social skills training and maintenance chemotherapy in the aftercare treatment of schizophrenia: I. One year effects of a controlled study on relapse and expressed emotion. *Archives of General Psychiatry, 43*, 633–642.

Hogarty, G. E., Goldberg, S. C., & Schooler, N. R. (1974). Drug and sociotherapy in the aftercare of schizophrenic patients. III. Adjustment of non-relapsed patients. *Archives of General Psychiatry, 31*, 609–618.

Hogarty, G. E., Schooler, N. R., Ulrich, R., Mussare, F., Ferro, P., & Herron, E. (1979). Fluphenazine and social therapy in the aftercare of schizophrenic patients. *Archives of General Psychiatry, 36*, 1283–1294.

Holden, D. F., & Lewine, R. R. J. (1982). How families evaluate mental health professionals, resources, and effects of illness. *Schizophrenia Bulletin, 8*, 626–633.

Hooley, J. M., Orley, J., & Teasdale, J. D. (1986). Levels of expressed emotion and relapse in depressed patients. *British Journal of Psychiatry, 148*, 642–647.

Imber-Mintz, L., Liberman, R. P., Miklowitz, D. J., & Mintz, J. (1987). Expressed emotion: A call for partnership among relatives, patients, and professionals. *Schizophrenia Bulletin, 13*(2), 227–235.

Jenkins, J. H., Karno, M., De La Selva, A., Santana, F., Telles, C., Lopez, S., & Mintz, J. (1986). Expressed emotion, maintenance psychotherapy, and schizophrenic relapse among Mexican-Americans. *Psychopharmacology Bulletin, 22*(3), 621–627.

Kessler, S. (1980). The genetics of schizophrenia: A review. *Schizophrenia Bulletin, 6*, 404–416.

Kottgen, C., Sonnichsen, I., Mollenhauer, K., & Jurth, R. (1984a). The family relations of young schizophrenic patients: Results of the Hamburg Camberwell family interview study I. *International Journal of Family Psychiatry, 5*, 61–70.

Kottgen, C., Sonnichsen, I., Mollenhauer, K., & Jurth, R. (1984b). Group therapy with the families of schizophrenic patients: Results of the Hamburg Camberwell family interview study III. *International Journal of Family Psychiatry, 5*, 83–94.

Kuipers, L., Sturgeon, D., Berkowitz, R., & Leff, J. (1983). Characteristics of expressed emotion: Its relationship to speech and looking in schizophrenic patients and their relatives. *British Journal of Clinical Psychology, 22*, 257–264.

Laing, R. D., & Esterson, A. (1964). *Sanity, madness in the family*. London: Tavistock.

Leff, J., Berkowitz, R., Shavit, N., Strachan, A., Glass, I., & Vaughn, C. (1989). A trial of family therapy vs. a relatives group for schizophrenia. *British Journal of Psychiatry, 154*, 58–66.

Leff, J., Berkowitz, R., Shavit, N., Strachan, A., Glass, I., & Vaughn, C. (1990). A trial of family therapy versus a relatives' group for schizophrenia: Two-year follow-up. *British Journal of Psychiatry, 157*, 571–577.

Leff, J. P., Kuipers, L., Berkowitz, R., Eberlein-Fries, R., & Sturgeon, D. (1982). A controlled trial of social intervention in the families of schizophrenic patients. *British Journal of Psychiatry, 141*, 121–134.

Leff, J. P., Kuipers, L., Berkowitz, R., Eberlein-Fries, R., & Sturgeon, D. (1983). Social intervention in the families of schizophrenics: Addendum. *British Journal of Psychiatry, 142*, 313.

Leff, J. P., Kuipers, L., Berkowitz, R., & Sturgeon, D. (1985). A controlled trial of social intervention in the families of schizophrenic patients: Two year follow-up. *British Journal of Psychiatry, 146*, 594–600.

Leff, J. P., Kuipers, L., Berkowitz, R., Vaughn, C. E., & Sturgeon, D. (1983). Life events, relatives' expressed emotion and maintenance neuroleptics in schizophrenic relapse. *Psychological Medicine, 13*, 799–806.

Leff, J. P., & Vaughn, C. E. (1980). The interaction of life events and relatives' expressed emotion in schizophrenia and depressive neurosis. *British Journal of Psychiatry, 136*, 146–153.

Leff, J. P., & Vaughn, C. E. (1981). The role of maintenance therapy in relatives' expressed emotion in relapse of schizophrenia: A two year follow-up. *British Journal of Psychiatry, 139*, 102–104.

Leff, J. P., & Vaughn, C. E. (1985). *Expressed emotion in families*. New York: Guilford Press.

Leff, J. P., & Wing, J. K. (1971). Trial of maintenance therapy in schizophrenia. *British Medical Journal, 3*, 599–604.

Liberman, R. P. (1970). Behavioral approaches to couple and family therapy. *American Journal of Orthopsychiatry, 40*, 106–118.

Liberman, R. P. (1972). Behavioral methods in group and family therapy. *Seminars in Psychiatry, 4*, 145–156.

Liberman, R. P., DeRisi, W. J., & King, L. W. (1973). Behavioral interventions with families. In J. Masserman (Ed.), *Current psychiatric therapies*. New York: Grune & Stratton.

Liberman, R. P., Falloon, I. R. H., & Aitchison, R. A. (1984). Multiple family therapy for schizophrenics: A behavioral approach. *Psychosocial Rehabilitation Journal, 4*, 60–77.

Liberman, R. P., Massel, H. K., Mosk, M., & Wong, S. E. (1985). Social skills training for chronic mental patients. *Hospital and Community Psychiatry, 36*, 396–403.

Lukoff, D., Snyder, K., Ventura, J., & Nuechterlein, K. H. (1984). Life events, familial stress, and coping in the developmental course of schizophrenia. *Schizophrenia Bulletin, 10*, 258–292.

MacMillan, J. F., Gold, A., Crow, T. J., Johnson, A. L., & Johnstone, E. C. (1986). The Northwick Park study of first episodes of schizophrenia: IV. Expressed emotion and relapse. *British Journal of Psychiatry, 148,* 133–143.

May, P. R. A., & Tuma, A. H. (1976). The Paul H. Hoch Award Lecture: A follow-up study of the results of treatment of schizophrenia. In R. L. Spitzer, & D. F. Klein (Eds.), *Evaluation of psychological therapies.* Baltimore and London: Johns Hopkins University Press.

Miklowitz, D. J., Goldstein, M. J., Falloon, I. R. H., & Doane, J. A. (1965). Interactional correlates of expressed emotion in the families of schizophrenics. *British Journal of Psychiatry, 144,* 482–487.

Miklowitz, D. J., Goldstein, M. J., Nuechterlein, K. H., Snyder, K. S., & Mintz, J. (1988). Family factors and the course of bipolar affective disorder. *Archives of General Psychiatry, 45,* 225–231.

Miklowitz, D. J., Strachan, A. M., Goldstein, M. J., Doane, J. A., & Burtt, C. (1986). Expressed emotion and communication deviance in the families of schizophrenics. *Journal of Abnormal Psychology, 95,* 60–66.

Mintz, J., Mintz, L., & Goldstein, M. G. (1987). Expressed emotion and relapse in first episodes of schizophrenia: A rejoinder to MacMillan et al. (1986). *British Journal of Psychiatry, 151,* 314–320.

Moline, R. A., Singh, S., Morris, A., & Meltzer, H. Y. (1986). Family expressed emotion and relapse in schizophrenia in 24 urban American patients. *American Journal of Psychiatry, 142,* 1078–1081.

Nuechterlein, K. H., & Dawson, M. E. (1984). A heuristic vulnerability/stress model of schizophrenic episodes. *Schizophrenia Bulletin, 10,* 300–312.

Nuechterlein, K. H., Snyder, K. S., Dawson, M. E., Rappe, S., Gitlin, M., & Fogelson, D. (1986). Expressed emotion, fixed-dose fluphenazine decanoate maintenance and relapse in recent-onset schizophrenia. *Psychopharmacology Bulletin, 22,* 633–639.

Overall, J. E., & Gorham, D. R. (1962). The Brief Psychiatric Rating Scale. *Psychological Reports, 10,* 799–812.

Palazzoli, M. S., Boscolo, L., Cecchin, G., & Prata, G. (1978). Paradox and counterparadox. New York: Jason Aronson.

Parker, G., Johnson, P., & Hayward, L. (1988). Parental "expressed emotion" as a predictor of schizophrenic relapse. *Archives of General Psychiatry, 45,* 806–813.

Parloff, M. B., Wolfe, B., Hadley, S., & Waskow, E. E. (1978). *Assessment of psychosocial treatment of mental disorders: Current status and prospects.* Report to the Presidential Commission on Mental Illness. Washington, DC: National Institute of Mental Health.

Pederson-Hardesty, J., Falloon, I. R. H., & Shirin, K. (1985). The impact of life events, stress, and coping on the morbidity of schizophrenia. In I. R. H. Falloon (Ed.), *Family management of schizophrenia: A study of clinical, social, family, and economic benefits.* Baltimore, MD: Johns Hopkins University Press.

Peters, T., & Austin, N. (1985). *A passion for excellence.* New York: Random House.

Platman, S. R. (1983). Family caretaking and expressed emotion: An evaluation. *Hospital and Community Psychiatry, 34,* 921–925.

Platt, S., Weyman, A., Hirsch, S., & Hewett, S. (1980). The Social Behaviour Assessment Schedule (SBAS): Rationale, contents, scoring, and reliability of a new interview schedule. *Social Psychiatry, 15,* 43–55.

Snyder, K. S., & Liberman, R. P. (1981). Family assessment and intervention with schizophrenics at risk for relapse. In M. J. Goldstein (Ed.), *New developments in intervention with families of schizophrenics.* San Francisco: Jossey-Bass.

Spaniol, L., Jung, H., Zipple, A. M. & Fitzgerald, S. (1987). The needs and coping strengths of families of the mentally ill: Report of a national survey. In A. B. Hatfield, & H. P. Lefley (Eds.), *Families of the mentally ill.* New York: Guilford Press.

Stanton, A. H., Gunderson, J. G., Knapp, P. H., Frank, A. F., Vannicelli, M. L., Schnitzer, R., & Rosenthal, R. (1984). Effects of psychotherapy in schizophrenia: I. Design and implementation of a controlled study. *Schizophrenia Bulletin, 10,* 520–563.

Strachan, A. M., & Dunkel-Schetter, C. (1985). *Coping and expressed emotion in the relatives of schizophrenics.* Unpublished manuscript. Los Angeles: Psychology Department, University of California.

Strachan, A. M., Feingold, D., Goldstein, M. J., Miklowitz, D. J., & Nuechterlein, K. H. (1989). Is expressed emotion an index of a transactional process? II. Patient's coping style. *Family Process, 28,* 169–181.

Strachan, A. M., Goldstein, M. J., & Miklowitz, D. J. (1986). Do relatives express expressed emotion? In M. J. Goldstein, I. Hand, & K. Hahlweg (Eds.), *Treatment of schizophrenia: Family assessment and intervention* (pp. 51–58). Heidelberg: Springer-Verlag.

Strachan, A. M., Leff, J. P., Goldstein, M. J., Doane, J. A., & Burtt, C. (1986). Emotional attitudes and direct communication in the families of schizophrenics: A cross-national replication. *British Journal of Psychiatry, 149*, 279–287.

Tarrier, N., Barrowclough, C., Vaughn, C., Bamrah, J. S., Porceddu, K., Watts, S., & Freeman, H. (1988). The community management of schizophrenia: A controlled trial of a behavioural intervention with families to reduce relapse. *British Journal of Psychiatry, 153*, 532–542.

Tarrier, N., Barrowclough, C., Vaughn, C., Bamrah, J. S., Porceddu, K., Watts, S., & Freeman, H. (1989). Community management of schizophrenia: A two-year follow-up of a behavioral intervention with families. *British Journal of Psychiatry, 154*, 625–628.

Terkelson, K. G. (1983). Schizophrenia and the family: II. Adverse effects of family therapy. *Family Process, 22*, 191–200.

Valone, K., Norton, J. P., Goldstein, M. J., & Doane, J. A. (1983). Parental expressed emotion and affective style in an adolescent sample at risk for schizophrenia spectrum disorders. *Journal of Abnormal Psychology, 92*, 399–407.

Vaughn, C. E., & Leff, J. P. (1976). The influence of family and social factors on the course of psychiatric illness: A comparison of schizophrenic and depressed neurotic patients. *British Journal of Psychiatry, 129*, 125–137.

Vaughn, C. E., Snyder, K. S., Jones, S., Freeman, W., & Falloon, I. R. H. (1984). Family factors in schizophrenic relapse: A California replication of the British research on expressed emotion. *Archives of General Psychiatry, 41*, 1169–1177.

Ventura, J., Nuechterlein, K. H., & Lukoff, D. (1986). *Stressful life events and schizophrenic relapse*. Paper presented at 139th annual meeting of the American Psychiatric Association meeting, Washington, DC.

Wallace, C. J., & Liberman, R. P. (1985). Social skills training for patients with schizophrenia: A controlled clinical trial. *Psychiatry Research, 15*, 239–247, 1985.

Wallace, C. J., Nelson, C. J., Liberman, R. P., Aitchison, R. A., Lukoff, D., Elder, J. P., & Ferris, C. (1980). A review and critique of social skills training with schizophrenic patients. *Schizophrenia Bulletin, 6*, 62–63, 1980.

Weakland, J. H., Fisch, R., Watzlawick, P., & Bodin, A. M. (1974). Brief therapy: Focused problem resolution. *Family Process, 13*, 141–168.

Wing, J. K., & Brown, G. W. (1970). Institutionalism and schizophrenia. Cambridge: Cambridge University Press.

CHAPTER 10

CASE MANAGEMENT

Frank Baker
James Intagliata

About a decade ago, the authors began a collaboration that produced a number of papers focused on research and evaluation dealing with case management and community support systems (Baker, 1988; Baker, Burns, Libby, & Intagliata, 1985; Baker & Intagliata, 1982, 1984a, 1984b; Baker, Intagliata, & Kirshstein, 1980; Baker & Weiss, 1984; Intagliata, 1982; Intagliata & Baker, 1983, 1984; Intagliata, Willer, & Egri, 1986). The general purposes of this paper are to synthesize some of the products of this collaborative work and to update an earlier review of the growing case management literature (Intagliata, 1982). Although case management is not a new idea, it has recently gained popularity as a mechanism for improving services delivery to chronically mentally disabled persons. To appreciate the case management concept, it is useful to examine briefly some of the factors underlying its current popularity.

Case management has emerged in response to two trends that radically changed the environment for human services during the 1960s and 1970s: first, the rapid expansion of human service programs in general, and second, the deinstitutionalization of the mentally ill. As a result of both of these trends, the need for and availability of community services increased significantly. However, because funding for these programs has been provided through many different public and private sources, the resulting set of services is highly complex, fragmented, duplicative, and uncoordinated. Many separate programs provide specialized services to narrowly defined target groups. While this fragmentation of services interferes with accessibility for all potential users, it is particularly burdensome for those who require help from multiple programs.

SERVICES INTEGRATION

This situation was recognized by many professionals, even during the early 1960s.

For example, the President's Panel on Mental Retardation (1962) expressed concern about the ease with which consumers could secure needed services. According to this panel, the concept of a *continuum of care* was critical for service system planners. It involved

> the selection, blending and use in proper sequence and relationship of the medical, educational and social services required by a retarded person to minimize his disability at every point in his life span. . . . A continuum of care permits fluidity of movement of the individual from one type of service to another while maintaining a sharp focus on his unique requirements. The ongoing process of assuring that an individual receives the services he needs when he needs them and in the amount and variety he requires is the essence of planning and coordination. (p. 15)

Unfortunately, services in most areas were not developed with the planning or coordination needed to ensure continuity of quality care for consumers. For example, Test (1979) noted that most professionals' familiarity with continuity of care consisted of a variety of clichés that describe its absence. It became commonplace to hear them use such terms as "the fragmented system," or to refer to patients who "fall through the cracks" or "become lost in the system."

In response to these problems, increasing attention was given to the concept of services integration, especially by federal, state and local governments. In the early 1970s, the Department of Health, Education, and Welfare recognized the need for improved coordination of its own programs at state and local levels and proposed a legislative initiative, the Allied Services Act, to facilitate integration of services. The Department also began a series of demonstration projects—the Services Integration Targets of Opportunity (SITO) grants—to test various services integration techniques in states and localities.

Under SITO grants, numerous service integration techniques were developed and demonstrated, including client-tracking systems, information and referral mechanisms, one-stop service centers, specialized management information systems, interagency planning and service delivery agreements, computerized resource inventories, and management reorganization projects (Mittenthal, 1976). The one additional feature that was common to most of the SITO projects was creation of the role of systems agent, operationally a case manager, who was expected to coordinate system resources for individual clients and to be accountable for successful client transit through the system. Thus, the use of case managers in SITO programs directed attention to the case management concept.

DEINSTITUTIONALIZATION

Before the movement toward deinstitutionalization began, more than 500,000 mentally disabled persons resided in large public institutions. Although the institutions themselves were frequently characterized by overcrowding and dehumanizing conditions, the institutional model nevertheless offered the potential to meet all the needs of all the residents under one roof, and thus provide reasonable continuity of and clear accountability for care (Kirk & Therrien, 1975).

When mentally disabled persons were released from institutions, however, responsibility for their care and support generally became diffused among a variety of agencies and levels of government. The roles and responsibilities of these agencies and the specific actions that needed to be taken to meet the special needs of deinstitutionalized persons were not clearly defined, understood, or accepted (Government Accounting Office [GAO], 1976). As a result, deinstitutionalized persons were forced to depend for their support on a complex, uncoordinated network of community service agencies.

Although some people can manage such a situation through sufficient persistence and patience, persons with chronic mental illness, whose abilities to cope are significantly impaired, were generally incapacitated by it.

Thus, most did not receive the services they needed, either because the services did not exist or because they were unable to obtain and coordinate them on their own (Test, 1979). The negative consequences of failing to provide adequate and appropriate community care to deinstitutionalized persons received widespread attention (GAO, 1976; Bachrach, 1976; Bassuk & Gerson, 1978; Lamb & Goertzel, 1977; Segal & Aviram, 1978; Willer, Scheerenberger, & Intagliata, 1978).

In response, the National Institute of Mental Health (NIMH) developed the conceptual framework for a comprehensive network of required services—the community support system (CSS)—and provided funds to operationalize this concept through demonstration projects in 19 states and the District of Columbia (Mosher & Keith, 1980; Turner, 1977; Turner & Shiffren, 1979; Turner & TenHoor, 1978). The positive aspects of this comprehensive support approach for dealing with schizophrenic populations have been highlighted by Mosher and Keith (1980) in their review of psychosocial treatment strategies. At least 10 different potential elements of community support programs have been identified as part of the CSS concept. However, case management is considered to be the key element, since it is the mechanism for coordinating all system efforts.

More recently, the Medicaid law was amended to allow states, as an option, to include in their state medical assistance plans, coverage for defined case management services. In addition, PL 99-660, the Comprehensive Mental Health Services Act, requires that states develop and implement case management services as part of their required state mental health plans for community services for chronically mentally ill persons. These changes in federal law are too recent to permit an assessment of their impact, but it is clear that they provide incentives and requirements for the further use of case management for persons with severe mental illness.

THE CONCEPT OF CASE MANAGEMENT SERVICES

Numerous definitions of case management have appeared in the human services literature. Although they vary somewhat, they all suggest that case management is a process or method for ensuring that consumers are provided needed services in a coordinated, effective, and efficient manner. The specific meaning of case management in a particular situation, however, can vary widely and will depend upon the system that is developed to provide it. In turn, a system will be affected by four major sets of characteristics that can be defined for it. These are objectives, ideology, functions, and structural elements.

Objectives

A variety of objectives have been associated with case management systems. Perhaps the most fundamental is *continuity of care*. Test (1979) suggested that continuity of care has two kinds of dimensions and goals: (a) cross-sectional, so that the services provided to an individual at any given time are comprehensive and coordinated; and (b) longitudinal, so that the system provides comprehensive, integrated services over time, and is responsive to changes in the person's needs. This longitudinal dimension is particularly critical when case management systems serve populations whose disabilities are both significant and lifelong.

Other objectives frequently associated with case management systems are *accessibility* and *accountability*. Because the set of human services includes multiple programs, with differing and complex eligibility criteria, regulations, policies, and procedures, clients are likely to experience difficulties in gaining access to many of the services they need. Case management systems can help clients negotiate the system and make services more accessible. A case management system can enhance accountability as well, by designating a single person or agency as responsible for the overall effect of the service system (Baker & Northman, 1981).

A fourth objective of a case management system is *efficiency*. In the absence of case management, clients often fail to receive the services they need or, if they do receive services, often receive them in an improper sequence or untimely fashion. Thus, the potential positive effects of available services are greatly diminished. By fixing responsibility for developing and implementing a coordinated service plan on a single person or agency, a case management can improve the efficiency of the service system.

The objective of efficiency is sometimes equated with cost control. While a case management system may at times reduce costs, it is likely often to result in the identification of more client needs and the delivery of more services (Mittenthal, 1976; Morrill, 1976). Thus, while the specific services delivered to clients may be more cost-effective, total service costs per client may not be reduced by case management. Indeed, a conflict may be emerging between the goals of cost control and continuity of care, and it is important that mental health practitioners be alert to the possible negative effects of such a conflict and seek to reduce them (Baker & Vischi, 1989).

Ideology

Numerous studies have shown the importance of ideology in sustaining and rationalizing new approaches to providing caregiving services (Baker, 1982). Research evidence is also available that case management has an associated ideology. In an evaluation of the effects of an inservice training as case managers, 298 trainees were administered two measures of ideological orientation (Baker, Jodrey, & Morell, 1979). These measures were a brief version of the Community Mental Health Ideology (CMHI) Scale (Baker & Schulberg, 1967) and the Human Services Ideology (HSI) Scale (Baker & Baker, 1979). These new case managers, both at the beginning and on completion of 3 months of on-the-job training, showed little commitment to community mental health ideology, but strong endorsement of human service ideology. When the thematic content of the two scales is examined, it becomes clearer what beliefs appear to be important and which are less relevant to case managers.

The shortened version of the CMHI Scale consists of the 10 highest loading items on the first factor of the unifactorially derived scale as reported in the original scale development report (Baker & Schulberg, 1967). It emphasizes the public health themes of "population focus" and "primary prevention." As these case managers were focusing their efforts to help persons with severe and persistent mental illness get needed community-based services, it is not surprising that they were not strongly oriented to "preventing illness before it occurs" and "taking responsibility for a whole population including not only the sick but those who might become ill for the first time." On the other hand, they did embrace the initial version of the HSI that included items concerned with "systemic integration of services" and focusing on "problems-in-living of the whole client," beliefs quite consistent with the work that case managers do in attempting to pull together a system of services focused on individual client needs.

In trying to understand the case management concept, one should be aware of the ideology or belief system that accompanies it. This ideology typically includes the following principles:

1. The planning and implementation of service plans must be responsive to the fact that individual clients are unique, and that they have their own particular set of strengths and needs.
2. The services and supports provided to clients must vary over time in their type and intensity if they are to continue to fit the changing configuration of each client's strengths and needs.
3. The level of support provided to clients should match the degree of their indivi-

dual deficit. Clients should be encouraged to function as independently as they can.

4. The commitment of case management services to clients must be open ended. It is support that must be made available around the clock and throughout the lifespan according to clients' needs.

In developing a case management system, care must be taken to scrutinize and plan all aspects of the system if these principles are to be taken fully into account (Jessing & Dean, 1976). The following discussion of the functions and structures of case management systems will illustrate how these aspects of case management ideology can, in fact, be operationalized.

Functions

A case management system is frequently described as a process with multiple functions, but without the specification of the persons or structures responsible for carrying them out. According to Agranoff (1977), the five basic functions of a case management system include the following:

- assessing—assessing clients' needs
- planning—developing a comprehensive service plan
- linking—arranging for services to be delivered
- monitoring—monitoring and assessing the services delivered
- evaluating—evaluating and following up

These five functions appear in almost every description of a case management system, regardless of its context.

There are additional functions, however, that are considered to be important components of some case management systems. While some of these functions might be subsumed under Agranoff's five basic functions, a number of them clearly expand the role to be played by a case management system. The additional functions that appear most frequently in case management systems are *reaching out*, *advocating*, and *serving directly*.

The appropriate range of functions for a case management system varies with the context. Acknowledging this, Ross (1980) offers three different models for case management programs designed to serve elderly persons in need. Table 10.1 presents the set of functional components associated with each of the three models. According to Ross (1980), the major difference among them is the increasing amount of control over provider agencies that is exercised in the coordination model and the comprehensive model. This multimodel conceptualization is offered not to suggest that the more comprehensive models are necessarily more effective, but rather to illustrate that there is a range of options to consider when designing or implementing a case management system.

Structural Elements

There are two basic structural elements in a case management system: the case manager and the core agency. Though the functions that define a case management system do not necessarily require that one create a role for a person termed *case manager*, this is by far the most common structural characteristic of case management systems and it will be discussed first and at some length.

Case Manager

The need for a human services generalist whose function is to coordinate services for the individual client has been recognized since the early 1960s (Intagliata, 1978). The concept of an expeditor was adapted by Reiff and Reissman (1965). Since that time, various labels have been used for this role, including case manager, integrator, expeditor, broker, ombudsman, advocate, primary therapist, patient representative, personal program coordinator, systems agent, and continuity agent.

Case managers are the most critical components in the case management system.

Table 10.1. Three Models for Case Management Programs

COMPONENTS OF MINIMAL MODEL	COMPONENTS OF COORDINATION MODEL	COMPONENTS OF COMPREHENSIVE MODEL
Outreach	Outreach	Outreach
Client assessment	Client assessment	Client assessment
Case planning	Case planning	Case planning
Referral to service providers	Referral to service providers	Referral to service providers
	Advocacy for client	Advocacy for client
	Direct casework	Direct casework
	Developing natural support systems	Developing natural support systems
	Reassessment	Reassessment
		Advocacy for resource development
		Monitoring quality
		Public education
		Crisis intervention

They serve as the human link between the clients and the system. in collaboration with other providers, case managers seek to ensure continuity of care for clients by determining the services, environments, providers, and duration of service that will be of greatest advantage to each consumer. In addition, case managers are responsible for ensuring the achievement of high levels of social, economic, and physical functioning of consumers.

Although great care is often taken to define the scope of activities of case managers, substantial differences typically exist between officially mandated and actual patterns of case manager activity (Caragonne, 1979). The major reason for this is that case managers must confront and try to resolve a wide range of problems, many of which are unpredictable and/or even uncontrollable. Case managers have the unenviable task of assuring that clients receive appropriate, coordinated, and continuous care from service systems that were not designed to provide these. As a result, a person acting as a case manager must be ready to play whatever role the situation may require—outreach worker, broker, advocate, counselor, teacher, community organizer, planner, or administrator (McPheeters, 1974; Turner & Shiffren, 1979).

The comprehensiveness and intensity of the role that case managers assume should be tailored to fit the particular needs of the client populations being served. Functions judged to be essential when serving one type of client may be elective or even inappropriate for another. However, three functions must be viewed as essential for case managers regardless of their clientele.

The first and perhaps most basic function of case managers in any system is to *remain aware of the comprehensive needs of their clients*. Case managers must be aware of, though not necessarily directly involved in, the initial intake and assessment of their clients. If these functions are assigned to other workers in the system, case managers should be in close contact with them so that there is no slippage in the communication of crucial information. The assessment of client needs must be continued even after initial formal intake sessions. Thus, regardless of the role that case managers play during intake, they must stay in regular contact with their clients, remaining sensitive to and observant of changes in their clients' needs. This is crucial because the case manager is the only provider in the system whose responsibility is to be aware of the "whole" client.

A second basic function is to *link clients to services* that will meet their needs. To do this, case managers must be aware of the resources that are available to their clients. These resources include both services and entitlements (e.g., food stamps, Medicaid). To be effective linkers, it is also important that case managers function as advocates for clients. Though individual service plans may call for referral of clients to certain services, there may be barriers that inhibit clients from actually receiving those services. Potential barriers include restrictive regulations and policies or the reluctance of many generic providers to serve clients with particular disabilities (e.g., mental illness, mental retardation). In addition, the clients themselves sometimes resist being served or "drop out" of service. While respecting a client's right to refuse treatment, case managers should actively encourage clients to help maintain their motivation for treatment. This is especially true for adults with severe and chronic mental or emotional disorders (Turner & Shiffren, 1979).

The responsibility to link clients to services does not require that case managers also be responsible for clinical decisions about which services are appropriate. If, however, the development of an individual service plan is conducted by another professional or team of professionals, the case manager, as well as the client, should be actively involved in the process. Involvement of the case manager has several important benefits: (a) it acquaints the case manager with the rationale and expectations for the treatment prescribed; (b) it allows the case manager to inform clinical staff about the availability and adequacy of services being considered; and (c) it allows the case manager to serve as the client's advocate, raising questions about decisions or suggesting alternatives.

The third essential function of case managers is to *monitor the services being provided to clients*. The most basic aspect of the monitoring process is to ensure that the agreed upon services are being received. Case managers must maintain contact with clients and their service providers to ensure that appointments are kept. Case managers must also assess the appropriateness and effectiveness of services provided. To do this, a case manager must maintain contact with the client and service provider and, if feasible, visit the client while the service or program is being provided. This kind of firsthand contact often provides valuable information otherwise missed. If case managers are not allowed to change clients' treatment plans, then they should be allowed to communicate their observations and judgment to those persons who do make these decisions.

While the three activities of assessing, linking, and monitoring are the essential elements of the case manager's role, the "process" of carrying out these activities also requires consideration. Perhaps the most influential aspect of the case management process is the *quality of the personal commitment* that case managers develop for their clients. The case manager is the human link between the client and the system—the only service provider concerned with and responsible for the whole client. Individual case managers thus provide a mechanism for personalizing the service delivery system. The human relationships that develop between case managers and clients should be considered a fundamental strength of the case management model, and case management programs should be structured to facilitate and capitalize on this process.

While the essential aspects of the generic case manager role have been described, case managers who are expected to meet the needs of special populations, such as the mentally disabled, must assume more intensive and comprehensive client responsibilities. The special needs of mentally disabled persons necessitate that effective case management systems provide clients with such additional supportive services as

- assistance with managing problems of daily living
- crisis intervention
- individual level advocacy
- systems level advocacy

However, while case managers ought to have some role in providing these types of special support, the extensiveness of each of these additional case management functions necessitates that certain aspects be delegated to other direct care staff, supervisory or administrative level staff of the agency providing case management, other specialized service agencies, and even consumer groups. A brief discussion of each of the additional supportive services will illustrate the considerations involved.

Case managers for persons with severe and persistent mental illness are commonly expected to *assist their clients with the management of simple life activities and practical daily problems*. In New York state, for example, research showed that case managers of CSS clients often provided their clients with the assistance or encouragement they needed for the proper maintenance of their personal hygiene or individual households. Other supporting activities included helping clients prepare a grocery list, accompanying them on a shopping trip, or transporting clients to a needed service if no other arrangements could be made (Baker & Intagliata, 1984b; Baker & Weiss, 1984). Although case managers can be expected to provide some of the support that clients may need in managing daily activities, they clearly cannot meet all of their clients' direct service needs in this area. If system developers are not sensitive to this issue, there is a risk that case managers hired to coordinate and monitor the efforts of multiple direct service providers may themselves become specialized direct care staff. Thus, systems planners should consider assigning the responsibility of teaching clients community living skills to direct care staff who have special expertise in doing so. For clients who need continuous and intensive support in negotiating the community, other types of special service providers can be used.

Weinman and Kleiner (1978), for example, employed lay persons to act as enablers for chronic mental patients living in the community. These persons spent several hours each day with their individual clients teaching them basic community living skills, escorting and introducing them to services and resources in the community, and acting as a liaison to gain the understanding and support of neighbors and local merchants. This program was highly successful in facilitating clients' adjustment to the community and is an example of the way case manager functions can be extended and provided more intensely through the use of specialized ancillary staff.

Another important case management function is *crisis intervention*. The need for this type of support is particularly critical for those clients whose abilities to cope with living stresses are impaired or deficient. For example, the adjustment to community living made by many formerly institutionalized psychiatric patients is quite tenuous. Significant crises may be precipitated by unexpected changes in the environment, even events that seem trivial to persons with a "normal" level of coping ability. If such crises are not managed in a timely fashion, they can easily lead to significant deterioration in clients' levels of functioning and perhaps to their rehospitalization.

Because of their frequent contacts with clients, case managers are likely to encounter such crisis situations. At the minimum, they must be prepared to provide clients with personal support. However, case managers need not be expected to function as therapists or to assist their clients directly in resolving the crisis. Instead, it may be more appropriate for them to refer or accompany a client to a crisis intervention team or agency.

Another important case management function is *individual client advocacy* as some agencies may be resistant to providing entitlements or services to chronically disabled persons. In many situations such barriers can be overcome by the case manager through informal interpersonal negotiation (Riffer & Freedman, 1980). However, in more difficult cases it may be necessary for case managers to enlist the support of supervisory or administrative level staff within their own agency or even to make use of more formal channels to act as advocates for clients. This may involve seeking the assistance of legal aid services or of agencies that traditionally provide advocacy services for clients in need (e.g., mental health associations, associations for retarded citizens). In fact, because of administrative barriers and conflicts of interest, citizen groups and legal advocates rather than formal service providers are often in the best position to provide certain types of advocacy (Governor's Interagency Task Force, 1979).

Thus, while individual client advocacy is an important case management function, it cannot be delegated solely to case managers. As with other functions, other levels of agency personnel or specialized providers of services may have to provide clients with the support required.

A final case management function to be considered here is *systems level advocacy*. While trying to assure continuity of care for clients, case managers will often identify gaps in the service system. Needed services may simply not be available. Case managers should document such gaps and inform their supervisors. However, if the situation is to be alleviated, more direct action may be needed. Interventions required to develop new service resources, however, must take place on a systems level.

To facilitate such systems level change, case managers could band together to document the unmet need and to stimulate action from others (Horejsi, 1978), including clients and the agencies responsible for planning, funding, and implementing the needed services. If continuity of care is to be a reality, case management activities must take place at many levels within the system.

This discussion of case management structures has focused so far on the case manager. The individual in this role has responsibility for the coordination of services at the individual client level. The effectiveness of the case manager's efforts is constrained, however, by the support provided to case management by higher levels within the system. Thus, for a case management system to be effective, other formal structures must assure the coordination and linkage of services on a systems level.

Core Agencies

Almost all efforts to integrate services involve the allocation of special coordinating power and authority to a local agency. The President's Commission on Mental Health (Vol. II, Appendix, 1978), for example, recommended that "state mental health authorities, in consultation with local authorities, designate an agency in each geographic area to assume responsibility for assisting the chronically mentally ill from that area" (p. 367). Consistent with this suggestion, NIMH, in its contracting for the development of community support systems, expects state mental health agencies to specify a "core CSS agency" in each planning area to act as a convener and catalyst to assure that the comprehensive needs of the CSS population are met. More specifically, this core agency must assess the needs of the CSS population, negotiate interagency linkages and agreements necessary to provide needed support services including case management, and develop new service components to remedy any gaps in the existing service network (Turner & Shiffren, 1979).

The importance of establishing this type of structure cannot be overemphasized. Compliance with the efforts of case managers to coordinate services requires a formal set of contracts that bind providers to deliver specified services to case-managed clients (Mittenthal, 1976; Ross, 1980). The core agency for a given locale is the most appropriate negotiator of such contracts. However, it can effectively negotiate and implement such agreements only if it has enforcement power. Such power can result from the control of funds to purchase services, from legislation or guidelines that require providers to respond to case manager requests, or designation of the core agency as the single entry point into the local provider system.

A core agency can also develop new service components. While a major function of case managers is to link clients to services, they cannot perform effectively if needed services do not exist. Thus, one of the constraints that case managers face is the inadequacy of the service systems in which they often operate. If the system needs to be moved, a core agency is likely to be a far more effective change agent than is the case manager. Nevertheless, even a core agency is unlikely to function effectively in this role unless it is explicitly empowered with the authority or responsibility for local system development.

SYSTEMS DESIGN AND IMPLEMENTATION

In order for case management systems to function effectively, they need the support of all levels of government that affect the service system. Federal, state, and local governments all have important roles in fostering and maintaining case management systems.

The Role of Different Levels of Government

Federal

The federal government supports the development of case management services for chronically mentally ill individuals. Federal financial assistance has been provided through the NIMH Community Support Program, which has case management as a key service component. In addition, Medicaid has been amended to allow states to cover case management services, as an option, in their state medical assistance plans. Most recently, PL 99-660, the Comprehensive Community Mental Health Services Act, requires that states provide case management services as a part of statewide plans for comprehensive community mental health services for the chronically mentally ill. Ultimately, the states have the major responsibility for designing and implementing case management systems.

State

Within a state, the first step that should be taken to build a case management system is to fix responsibility for the program in a single state agency. Ideally, organizational structures for case management systems would be statewide, to ensure uniformity and equality in the services delivered (Lippman, 1976). However, the decision about which agency should be given authority for case management services for the mentally disabled will vary from state to state.

In states that have separate departments serving the mentally disabled, it is preferable for case management to be provided by the department most familiar with the population. Since case management systems, if they are to be effective, require the cooperation of almost all providers of human services, such a lead agency must coordinate its efforts with other departments in the state government. In New York state in the late 1970s, for example, the Office of Mental Health played the lead role in developing and managing CSS services for chronic psychiatric patients in the community. However, the Governor's Interagency Task Force was formed to bring together the various human service departments that relate to CSS clients to enable them to serve those clients better.

A subcommittee of that task force dealt specifically with case management services since they were such an essential component of the system. This subcommittee had representatives from the Office of Mental Health, Department of Social Services, Office of Vocational Rehabilitation, Office for Aging, and Office of Mental Retardation/Developmental Disabilities. Its purpose was to improve the practice of case management, determining which agencies were fulfilling the functions, and recommending how to reduce duplication and enhance the efficient and effective delivery of case management services to CSS clients (Governor's Interagency Task Force, 1979).

Such an interagency coordinating body is essential when responsibility for case management services is delegated to an agency that serves only a particular population, or provides only specific service functions. However, the need for such a mechanism may be less in states where the responsibility for human services is assigned to a single, generic agency. Clearly, the nature of the state human services structure will determine how case management efforts may best be organized and administered.

Nevertheless, it is also possible to alter the organizational structures for the purpose of strengthening case management. For example, a state could create a new agency whose sole responsibility is case management for human services clients. This model avoids potential conflicts of interest by separating case management from the provision of services. However, it may result in case management that is not as individualized to clients as that which could be provided by agencies more intimately familiar with the specific needs of their specialized target groups. In addition, the fiscal expenditures required for the creation of an entirely new department may be substantial. Given the current climate in which resources for human services are constrained, it is probably more realistic to build case management systems into the structures that already exist.

Local

Once a state agency has been given responsibility for case management for individuals who are severely mentally ill, that agency must develop a plan for fixing the responsibility of case management in selected local agencies. Each geographic subarea of the state should have a single agency responsible for it. Since these core agencies will be the primary responsible mechanisms for service integration within their regions, they must have a demonstrated ability to lead.

Most case management programs have encouraged flexibility in selecting the types of agencies that should provide local leadership. The core agencies designated for the NIMH Community Support Program have included public hospitals, community mental health centers, and county social service agencies (Turner & Shiffren, 1979). Core service agencies in New York state have included county departments of mental health, general county hospitals, family services agencies, and even state psychiatric centers. The regional centers that provided case management services to mentally retarded persons in California included hospitals, service or advocacy organizations, and nonprofit corporations developed specifically to assume the coordination role played by a regional center (Lippman, 1976). Openness to use of different models for the core agency is important for the development of effective case management systems, as the factors that contribute to effective leadership vary greatly among localities.

It is usually a good idea to establish formal mechanisms to facilitate the coordinating efforts of core agencies. The most essential of these is the "purchase of service" power, so that they can directly bring at least some services from other local agencies (Washington, Karmen, & Friedlob, 1974).

In addition, a local counterpart to the state interagency task force may be helpful. For example, local interagency cooperation could be facilitated if the core agency formed a local interagency committee (New York State Office of Mental Health, 1978). Such a committee could facilitate negotiations about which roles would be performed by which agencies and could help identify gaps in the service system. The core agency could use this committee to strengthen its ability to coordinate services for clients and to ensure that the entire range of needed services is available.

Another way to strengthen a core agency is to designate it as the single entry point to the service system in its geographic area. This approach has been used for the mentally retarded in California (i.e., Regional Centers) and was recommended for use in serving the developmentally disabled in New Jersey (New York State Office of Mental Health, 1978). A single-entry-point core agency has much greater control over clients than does a core agency that must rely on multiple outside agencies to refer clients for case management.

Since case management is primarily a service linking and coordinating function, its impact will be diluted if needed services are not available. For example, if a client must live in a supervised residence to be able to adjust to community living and no such residence is available, a case manager will not solve the problem. Case management can help clients improve the continuity of care they receive from a given service system, but case management cannot wholly succeed in a system that is missing major components. The development of needed services must precede, or at least be contemporaneous with, the development of a case management system if that system is to succeed. In most cases, a case manager should be a part of the core agency. Then, if the core agency has been given adequate authority and power, the case manager will be better able to gain the cooperation of other service providers in the area. However, a core agency may choose to contract with another local agency for case manager services. This approach may help avoid potential conflicts of interest, as when the core agency is a major provider of direct services to clients.

Regardless of where case managers are located, they are the key to the quality and effectiveness of any case management system because it is they who must interact with providers to improve services coordination for clients. Given the centrality of the role of the case manager in case management systems, it is important to consider how various aspects of the job and context can affect the effectiveness of case managers.

Case Manager Status

Perhaps the most essential aspect of the case manager's role is its status. One question frequently raised is whether the case manager should be a professional or paraprofessional. Since the demarcation between these two categories may vary from one human services discipline to another, however, it is probably more useful to discuss preparation for the role, including educational background and previous job experience.

Important aspects of educational background are the type and level of academic degree obtained. Case managers have typically been individuals trained in human services. However, it has been suggested that some human service disciplines are more relevant to the case manager role than are others. For example, individuals trained to use various providers of services to meet client needs (e.g., social workers, human service generalist workers) are likely to be better prepared as case managers than persons whose training has been focused primarily in a given discipline (e.g., psychology). Regarding level of education, the human services literature reports a wide range, from high school diploma (McPheeters, 1974) to doctoral degree (Altshuler & Forward, 1978). Depending on what is expected, individuals who fall anywhere in this range can function effectively.

The specific job experiences of individuals can also be relevant. Case managers for chronic psychiatric patients in New York state in the late 1970s included persons who did not have college degrees, but who had extensive experience with these patients in state psychiatric facilities; others had master's degrees in social work or counseling, but no prior contact with chronic psychiatric clients (Baker, Jodrey, & Morell, 1979). Each type of worker brought different strengths to the case manager's role. It is not clear which strength was more important, as level of education and number of years' experience in the specific problem field both seem to strengthen case manager effectiveness (Berkeley Planning Associates, 1977).

Most systems do not require case managers to have more than a B.A. level degree, which affords them a paraprofessional status. Such a status limits the range of activities that case managers can perform without supervision. It may also make it more difficult for case managers to establish credibility with the professionals to whom they must relate in coordinating client care. While case managers may be able gradually to resolve this problem (Baker, Intagliata, & Kirshstein, 1980), they may also need extra support from their core agency.

Some administrators feel that it is better to use professionals in the case manager role. However, while professionals may be able to function more independently, they are likely to be unwilling to devote time to many of the important but "less professional" services that paraprofessional case managers frequently provide to clients (e.g., transportation to an appointment, assistance in filling out forms to secure entitlements, visiting a day program to observe client activity). Caragonne (1981) found that many professional case managers in mental health settings spent much time directly serving clients (e.g., counseling, assessing) but neglected such key case management functions as linking, referring, following up, and evaluating. Further, since professionals are "overqualified" for many important case manager duties, they may burn out more quickly than paraprofessionals (Dormady, 1980). Finally, the use of professional case managers greatly increases the cost of any sizable case management effort.

The most cost-effective approach may be to use paraprofessionals for the essential case manager functions of linking and monitoring. The other important functions—assessing and planning—could be performed by these same individuals if they are capable, but could ultimately be the responsibility of professional clinician supervisors. Before making final decisions on the degree of discretion and authority that paraprofessional case managers should have in their jobs, however, it should be noted that case managers attach great importance to autonomy (Caragonne, 1980). Their job satisfaction reportedly increases when they have greater freedom and discretion to carry out their roles and responsibilities (Graham, 1980). There is no evidence that a particular level of autonomy is ideal, but the autonomy given to case managers should be matched to the expectations established when they were recruited and should be adjusted over time to reflect increasing competence.

Training/Preparation

A case manager training program should be viewed as essential in the building of an effective case management system. Regardless of the professional level, case managers should approach their role with a clear understanding of functions and responsibilities. Further, in order to insure a consistent and equitable statewide case management program, all case managers should be similarly oriented and prepared for the job.

The people who will become case managers will undoubtedly vary widely in the knowledge, skills, and competencies they bring to the job. To assure flexibility, a training program could be designed as a series of self-contained learning modules (Baker, Jodrey, & Morell, 1979). In this way, trainees who can demonstrate competency in a specific area need not take that module.

The statewide training program should focus on the basics of the case manager role. For example, it could include a module on the rationale for case management, making explicit the values that guide case managers. Such modules should be required for all trainees regardless of prior job experience. Additional modules could provide basic information in such content areas as the nature of mental illness or mental retardation (e.g., causes, definitions, associated consequences, limitations), common medications and side effects, local services, client entitlements (e.g., SSI, food stamps), clients' legal rights, and recordkeeping by case managers. Modules could also deal with the process of case management, focusing on teaching case managers skills for relating to clients, setting goals, solving practical problems, knowing how and when to intervene in crisis situations, and acting effectively as advocates for clients.

It is important that trainees understand that severely mentally disabled clients may be quite limited in their ability to achieve progress. Lamb (1979b) has noted that unless staff have a realistic conception of what they can expect to accomplish, frustration and burnout are inevitable. Case managers must realize that enhancing the quality of their clients' lives, rather than achieving totally independent functioning, is a reasonable and appropriate treatment goal for many in this population.

Several authors who have evaluated case manager training programs suggest that care should be taken to avoid assigning complete caseloads to case managers until they have completed their training (Amadio, 1976). It is useful for trainees to be responsible for some clients during training so that they can apply what they learn, but too much responsibility can interfere with learning. To avoid this, intensive, short-term training may be preferable to less intensive, prolonged training.

Plans should also be made to provide continuing education to case managers. An initial time-limited, intensive training program simply cannot be expected to meet all the needs of case managers for training. As with most positions, case managers will not know what they need to know until they have been on the job for a while. Thus, either at the state or local level, continuing education sessions should be planned. In addition, case managers should be assessed periodically to determine areas of need so that continuing education remains relevant and useful.

Supervision

If experienced professional case managers are hired, they will not require the extent of supervision that paraprofessional or less experienced individuals will require. However, since most programs are likely to use at least some paraprofessional persons, adequate support and supervision should be provided.

Case manager supervisors should perform several functions. For example, they should thoroughly and continually monitor the performance of case managers. They should meet regularly with individual case managers to discuss their caseload activities, and they should, at times, observe or even assist case managers in working with certain clients. While one might assume that supervisors would routinely do such things, Caragonne (1981) reported that many of the supervisors and program administrators at the 22 case management sites studied did not have accurate perceptions of the scope, extent, and pattern of their own case managers' activities. Further, it was exactly in those sites in which supervisors were most out of touch with their case managers' activities that the case managers departed most drastically from their defined roles.

A second important aspect of the supervisory role is staff development. Supervisors should be committed to the continuing education of case managers. Part of this education might be informal and as simple as encouraging case managers to develop a habit of generating alternative strategies for dealing with clients' problems before taking action. However, it is also appropriate for supervisors to consider more formal continuing education sessions for case managers. Such sessions could be didactic or experiential and should focus on specific areas in which the case managers themselves feel a need for more background.

A third and perhaps most important function of the supervisor is to support case managers. Graham (1980) found that the provision of consistent supervisory feedback and support was associated with greater case manager motivation on the job. Case managers seem to need such support to maintain a sense of the value of their work and the extent to which it is appreciated. Baker, Intagliata, and Kirshstein (1980) have reported that case managers identified regular supervision as essential to the prevention of burnout. They said that good supervision allowed them to "vent their frustrations with their clients and the system" and to receive support for their efforts. Caragonne (1979) found that case management sites in which supervision was more supportive and enabling, rather than monitoring and controlling, were also the sites in which case managers exhibited less antagonism toward management, lower levels of absenteeism and stereotyping of clients, and, in general, fewer overall symptoms associated with case manager burnout.

Clearly, the role of the case manager supervisor is very important. Establishing such a position allows case managers to receive support and backup, and offers them the possibility of upward job mobility. While such a position would provide just part of a case management career ladder, efforts along these lines enhance the likelihood that case managers will remain with a system after they have increased their expertise.

Individual Versus Team Case Management

Experienced observers have indicated that responsibility for clients might more appropriately be assigned to a case management team than to an individual (Altshuler & Forward, 1978; Gittelman, 1974; Kirk & Therrien, 1975; May, 1975; Test, 1979; Turner & TenHoor, 1978). Such a team consists of a group of individuals who are together responsible for the case management functions of assessing, linking, and monitoring to assure continuity of care for clients. The individuals on this team may all be case managers or may include professionals from different disciplines (e.g., psychiatrist, nurse, psychologist, social worker).

According to Test (1979), the advantages of a team are that it provides (a) more continuous coverage and coordination, as the unavailability of a single case manager does not incapacitate the client; (b) better planning, based on the availability of more points of view for managing difficult problems; and (c) a way to avoid isolation and burnout, which often afflicts individual case managers who must otherwise face seemingly endless and emotionally draining problems alone.

A report on case management efforts at one of the NIMH Community Support System demonstration sites in New York state provided support for Test's (1979) position. Reagles and Sheets (1979) reported that after a year of using the individual case management model to serve chronic psychiatric patients, two significant problems had surfaced: first, the overwhelming burden of responsibility that led to staff burnout, and second, the dysfunctional phenomenon of clients' becoming overly dependent on case managers. To address these problems, the program switched to a group case management model in which responsibility for a client's care rested with an interdisciplinary team rather than with one case manager.

While the team model may not be appropriate or feasible in all programs, those using an individual case manager model must pay serious attention to the need to provide case managers with adequate support. If case managers are not included as part of an interdisciplinary treatment team, then it is essential that the case managers themselves be organized either formally or informally for the purpose of mutual support. One possibility is to designate them as a distinct formal organizational entity, the "case management unit." Whether such a unit is formed, there is a need to provide mechanisms that facilitate regular interactions among case managers as a group. Examples would include daily morning meetings, weekly supervision sessions, and periodic training sessions.

Caseload Characteristics

A major factor influencing the style and effectiveness of services offered by case managers is the number of clients for whom they are responsible. As the number of clients assigned to a given case manager increases, the amount of time the case manager can potentially devote to each individual client decreases. Graham (1980) confirmed this relationship in his study of case managers who were serving varying sized caseloads of chronic psychiatric patients in New York state. He reported that as caseload size increased, case managers did not increase the number of clients seen each week. On the contrary, case managers saw individual clients less frequently as caseloads increased. This finding is extremely important, especially in view of the evidence that the quality of case management services increases as the intensity of contact between client and case manager increases (Berkeley Planning Associates, 1977).

Increasing caseload size can affect the nature and quality of client contacts as well. In a study of case management provided to chronic psychiatric patients in New York state, Baker, Intagliata, and Kirshstein (1980) found that increases in caseloads from about 15 clients to 30 to 50 clients had a significant impact on case managers' working styles. In addition to the inevitable consequence of having less time for each client, case managers reported the following:

1. Their efforts with clients had become primarily reactive rather than proactive, so that the majority of their time was consumed responding to crises rather than anticipating problems and helping clients plan ahead for them.
2. They were always "on the run" and no longer had the chance to get to know their clients and their needs.
3. To save time, they had begun to do things for clients instead of helping clients become more independent.
4. Their frequency of contact with clients was increasingly determined by clients' taking the initiative to contact them rather than vice versa (i.e., "the squeaky wheel gets the oil").
5. The amount of time they were required to spend simply documenting their efforts with clients was consuming an increasing portion of their time that otherwise might be spent with clients.

These are troublesome developments that threaten the quality and effectiveness of case managers' efforts.

Although caseload size can strongly influence case management, it is not at all easy to determine an ideal caseload size. The number of clients that a case manager can serve effectively will vary depending on the clients' levels of functioning (acute/chronic needs), the degree to which clients live close together or in scattered locations, and the competencies of individual case managers. Lannon (1979) reported that case managers serving chronic psychiatric patients tended to give more attention and service to those individuals who had poor community living skills or who exhibited behavior management problems. Graham (1980) reported that case managers serving only psychiatric clients living in family (foster) care homes spent significantly less time in direct client contact than did case managers assigned a mix of clients living in varied community residential settings.

Clearly, a variety of client characteristics affect case management activities, independent of caseload size. However, it is useful to discuss estimates of reasonable caseload levels based on program experience. For chronic psychiatric patients served in community support system programs in New York state, suggested reasonable caseloads for an individual case manager have ranged from 15 clients (Reagles & Sheets, 1979) to 30 clients (Baker, Intagliata, & Kirshstein, 1980). For case management teams serving a similar population, ratios of team members to clients ranged from 1 to 4 (Test, 1979) to 1 to 10 (Reagles & Sheets, 1979).

Recently, Harris and Bergman (1988) have underscored the need to determine caseload size on the basis of the scope of services to be delivered and the eventual outcomes the case management system is intended to achieve. They evaluated optimum caseload size for the patient population served by

Community Connections, a private case management agency in Washington, D.C. that provided clinical as well as coordinating services. They assert that their experience supports an optimum staff-to-patient ratio of about 1 to 15.

A low staff-to-client ratio of 1 to 10 is a key distinguishing characteristic of Intensive Case Management, the first major strategy for change implemented by Richard Surles as the new Commissioner of the Office of Mental Health in New York State (NYSOMH). This statewide program targets a relatively small number of people (5,000) with serious and persistent mental illness who have been identified as among the most severely mentally disabled community residents in the state (New York State Office of Mental Health, 1989).

Regardless of the client population served, reasonable caseload size ultimately depends on the type of case management program planners intend to offer. If, for example, case managers are expected to provide clients with support only when they are in crisis, they may be able to handle caseloads of 40 to 50 clients. However, if case managers are expected to assess clients' needs, develop treatment plans, link clients to services, monitor clients' progress, attend to the needs of clients' families, and continually update treatment plans, caseloads of 20 to 30 clients are likely to be more appropriate.

Reasonable or target caseload sizes should be determined separately for each program. As part of the planning for a case management program, caseload sizes should probably be set at low levels at first and then, if all goes well, gradually increased as the consequences are monitored. In this fashion, decisions on caseload sizes can be made more empirically and rationally.

Other Contextual Factors

Two other contextual factors can significantly influence how case managers perform their functions. The first is the degree to which the existing services meet client needs. A number of studies (Baker, Intagliata, & Kirshstein, 1980; Caragonne, 1979; Graham, 1980) have found that case managers' activities are significantly shaped by the service systems in which they operate. If, for example, there are relatively few services available, case managers spend relatively little time linking clients to services. Further, when certain important services are unavailable, case managers are likely to devote their own time to providing or creating the needed services. These findings indicate that the activities of case managers are shaped more by the environments in which they work than by their formal job descriptions.

The other contextual factor is that local agencies that provide case management are likely to develop unique case management programs. A state may try to impose structural and ideological uniformity on local programs, but the implementation of guidelines is usually shaped by unique local contexts.

Factors that result in variations among programs include the differences among regions in population, geography, services, interagency cooperation, and case management ideologies. Thus, a state's case management efforts typically comprise a variety of somewhat unique case management programs. While monitoring mechanisms may help ensure a certain amount of program uniformity and quality, local flexibility in program implementation should be both tolerated and encouraged. Flexibility enables programs to be tailored to meet both local and individual needs.

THE ROLE OF FAMILIES

The family can and does make significant contributions to the case management of their chronically mentally ill family members (Intagliata, Willer, & Egri, 1986). This is not to suggest that family members assume the primary case management responsibility for their relatives. There are aspects of case management for which effective performance requires special professional training or credentials. However, there is growing acknowledgement that many families already do play a crucial role in providing primary care and aftercare for mentally disabled individuals as a result of deinstitutionalization. Moreover, it is important that mental health professionals recognize the potential advantages of having the family involved in the basic functions of case management.

However, this does not mean that case managers should in any way neglect their responsibilities for those members of their case management caseloads who have families actively engaged in helping their sick relatives. Some families already are overburdened by the 24-hour-a-day responsibility for ongoing care that their family members require, while other families do not want and should not be encouraged to take a significant role in their relative's treatment.

Family members can make contributions to each of the six specific case management functions described earlier in this chapter including (a) assessing the needs of patients, (b) linking patients to services, (c) monitoring the quality of the services being provided, (d) assisting patients in daily living, (e) intervening in crisis, and (f) advocating for enhanced quality of the clients' services and lives (Intagliata, Willer, & Ergi, 1986). While the natural helping capabilities (Bachrach, 1983) of the family are highlighted, attention is also given to limitations in the involvement of family members in case management activities.

Assessment

With regard to the assessment function of case management, case managers should seek out information from all relevant sources regarding the patient's needs and functioning. This incudes the family which is in a unique position to provide information on the patient that may not be otherwise available to the mental health professional. Because of their knowledge of the patient over time, family members can provide information on the patient's history of illness and treatment and a longitudinal perspective on changes in the patient's needs, functioning, and symptoms. Through their close, ongoing, long-term contact with him or her, they may be the first to recognize the early signs of decompensation or relapse (Hansell, 1981; Herz & Melville, 1980; Leavitt, 1975; Miller, 1986). Also, because of their extensive daily contact with their relative, family members are in a better position to be sensitive to the many simple personal needs that may not be apparent to the mental health professionals who have less interaction with the patients and generally in more restricted settings (Sullivan, 1981).

Mental health professionals should invite and encourage the input of family members to the assessment and treatment planning process. Nevertheless, certain tasks related to assessment must continue to be the responsibility of the mental health system case manager. These include assessing the family unit itself regarding communication and affective styles and integrating information about a patient's needs into a systematic plan of treatment. While it would be inappropriate for family members to take primary responsibility for assessing their relative's treatment needs, they can still provide valuable assistance to the professional who has accepted formal case management responsibility.

Linking

Another major function of case management is linkage of clients to services that will meet their needs. Many mentally ill persons require assistance in accessing and coordinating the complex combinations of services that are required to meet their needs. They simply do not have the required information or capacity to deal with this by themselves. A knowledgeable case manager will be aware of the variety of programs and resources available to meet patient needs and will be able to help ensure that patients get the services and other supports (e.g., food stamps, SSI payments) that they need.

However, linking chronically mentally ill clients to needed services is not an easy task.

There are barriers to be overcome in the service system itself (e.g., eligibility criteria) and once mentally ill clients are referred to services, many of these persons will not get or stay linked (Anthony, Cohen, & Vitalo, 1978; Evans & Stellman, 1977; Krauss, 1980; Turner & Shiffren, 1979). One approach to this problem is to provide them with assertive case management (Beard, Malamud, & Rossman, 1978; Stein & Test, 1980); another method is to teach patients social skills, especially how to solve problems and locate needed services (Liberman, Wallace, & Falloon, 1981). It is important to seek a balance in approaches so that patients will be encouraged to function independently while still receiving any case management support they may need. For patients who do need assertive case management to be linked to services, less intense kinds of assistance can still be helpful, such as reminding patients about appointments, providing them with transportation, accompanying them to service appointments (to make sure they get there and to ensure that the providers understand and are responsive to their needs), and discussing with them any fears or misgivings they may have about treatment, so that they may maintain their motivation for treatment.

Some linkage activities are probably best handled by a professional case manager, including developing awareness of the range of services and supports that are available and assisting patients in getting through bureaucratic red tape. However, other types of assistance and encouragement that do not require complex or technical knowledge about the service system may make the difference between a patient's continuing with or dropping out of a needed treatment. The family's help may be particularly relevant since only someone who is concerned about the patient, has the time and motivation to take action, and can maintain a trusting and supportive relationship with the patient can provide this assistance effectively.

Case managers should encourage family members to take an active role in linking their relatives to services. Family members can provide encouragement and support that their patient-relative may need in using treatment as prescribed (e.g., providing reminders about taking medication). They can also support the patient in taking as much responsibility as possible for complying with the treatment plan (Schwartz & Schwartz, 1964).

Monitoring

The third essential case management function is to monitor the services provided to patients. Such monitoring requires that the case manager regularly assess whether the services provided seem to be appropriate and effective. The case manager must be familiar with the goals that the treatment team has set for a patient and must take into account the patient's satisfaction with the services provided. The case manager needs to maintain regular contact with the patient and family to monitor progress. Occasional visits to agencies providing services to the patient may be useful for the case manager in maintaining the regular contact with agencies that is necessary for effective monitoring. Monitoring can provide the system with feedback about whether the prescribed interventions are producing intended changes and meeting patient needs and can thus lead to important needed changes in treatment plans.

The monitoring activities of family members and professional staff are generally similar; they differ only in that each brings a different perspective to the monitoring responsibility. While treatment staff are trained to observe and understand how patients respond to treatment in clinical settings, family members are good observers of the behavioral adjustments of their patient-relatives in community settings. They can be particularly helpful in keeping a historical perspective on what does or does not seem to help the patient. Family members can provide clinical staff, including the case manager, important information about medication side effects and behaviors at home and in other community settings. Family members can also encourage behaviors that are the focus of treatment. Finally, because they are not a part of the service system itself, family members can be a source of information regarding the value of services that is not biased by consideration of the costs to the system of these services—although they may have to consider the implications of additional costs to themselves.

Assistance in Daily Living

In some mental health systems, case managers are expected to assist their chronic mentally ill patients with simple life activities that the patients may be unable to handle on their own. The case managers provide the personal support that many patients need if they are to succeed. Assistance with practical daily problems need not be provided by professional case managers alone but can be provided by other helpers as well. For example, Weinman and Kleiner (1978) used lay persons as enablers for chronic mental patients living in the community. These enablers spent several hours each day with their clients. They taught them basic community living skills, escorted and introduced them to community services and resources, and acted as liaisons with neighbors and local merchants. The program was quite successful in helping patients adjust to the community.

Family members are already experienced in helping their patient-relatives to manage practical, everyday problems. In fact, in many mental health service systems the family are the only ones available to assume these responsibilities, whether the patients live with their families or not.

Although it can be convenient to the service system for family members to assist patients with problems in daily living, this assistance can easily become overinvolvement; it can lead to higher relapse rates for the patient (Anderson, Hogarty, & Reiss, 1981) and to the physical and emotional exhaustion of family members (Doll, 1976; Hatfield, 1978). Mental health professionals should acknowledge the contributions that family members can make in meeting the daily needs of their patient-relatives, but they should also help family members avoid the problems of overinvolvement. This can be done by providing family members with advice on how to set limits on their involvement and by ensuring that there are trained support staff (e.g., case managers, enablers) available to help patient-relatives with at least some of their daily problems. Family members may have no alternative to becoming "overinvolved" because they often are the only ones available or willing to assist their relatives. The needs of family members for assistance in caring for their relatives must be recognized by case managers.

Crisis Intervention

Another important case management function is crisis intervention. Significant crises may be precipitated by unexpected changes in a patient's environment, even by events that seem trivial to persons with a "normal" level of coping ability. The adjustment to community living made by many formerly institutionalized psychiatric patients is often quite tenuous, and if such crises are not managed reasonably quickly, they can easily lead to deterioration in functioning and often to rehospitalization. The case manager, by being available to patients and their families in times of crisis, can play a crucial role in providing or linking them to crisis intervention supports.

One of the most important aspects of crisis intervention is timing. It is important that a developing crisis be identified quickly and that appropriate action be taken assertively to prevent further patient deterioration. Because of their ongoing contact, family members can be the first to recognize the early stages of decompensation and can call this to the attention of their relative's case manager or other treatment staff (Herz & Melville, 1980; Leavitt, 1975). With other types of crises, they may be able to alleviate their relative's stress by providing food, money, or housing. Such resources may simply not be available through the mental health system.

Advocacy

A final case management function is advocacy—for the individual and for the system. The need for individual-level advocacy can arise when a patient is having difficulty getting into a service program, or when a patient is dropped from a program. When such situations can be managed through informal negotiations between the case manager and the service provider, this activity can be considered a part of the linking function described earlier. When informal negotiations are ineffective, however, the case manager may have to become involved in more formal advocacy. This may involve enlisting the support of supervisory or administrative staff within his or her own agency, or using more formal channels, such as legal aid services or mental health associations.

Systems-level advocacy is somewhat different since it generally requires that someone call attention to a deficiency in a service system that adversely affects a large number or class of patients. Systems-level advocacy often entails political action and is especially appropriate for citizen groups. In the mental retardation field, for example, parents established in the 1950s the Association for Retarded Citizens for advocacy purposes. Since then, they have been able to focus national attention on the needs of the mentally retarded. Similar advocacy groups for the mentally ill have also emerged—such as the National Alliance for the Mentally Ill. In addition to providing families with information and emotional support, they are increasing public awareness about mental illness, and are advocating improved services for the mentally ill and a greater commitment to research into the causes and treatments of mental illness.

Because of their considerable personal commitment and concern about mental illness, parents and other family members of the mentally ill can be extremely effective advocates for systems-level change. Their voices may be as powerful as those of mental health professionals, if not more so. The mental health establishment has thus gained a strong and influential ally in the family. What professionals must understand, however, is that the objectives of such advocacy groups may not always be consistent with their own. Family members are beginning to demand changes from both the system and the professionals. For example, relatives of the mentally ill are demanding larger service and research budgets as well as more responsiveness and respect for the family from mental health professionals.

EVALUATION AND RESEARCH

Ongoing case management evaluation and research are clearly needed to enhance the quality of case management services. Both formative and summative efforts are important.

Formative Evaluation

In the early phases of developing a case management program, it is vital to assess program implementation. All too often, the label of "case management" is attached to professional activities without sufficient careful examination of whether these services relate in any meaningful way to the goals and assumptions of case management. Offering old wine in bottles with new labels has a strong survival value in the human services for people who want to maintain their jobs, doing what they have done before, although funding is shifting to "new" program initiatives. Goal statements are not enough to ensure real case management; resources have to be invested in appropriate service system structures and processes to achieve dependent outcomes (Schulberg & Baker, 1968). Information that is produced from this type of formative evaluation can provide system planners with feedback that can be used to keep program development on track or to modify or reshape a program if necessary. Such process evaluation activities should help to pinpoint how case management services are provided and the factors that seem to affect their delivery. This descriptive information is important if providers or administrators are to understand or replicate the results of any case management program.

Several recent reviews summarize the growing descriptive literature dealing with case management. These include a small book by Levine and Fleming (1985), a set of case management action guidelines based on a synthesis of research (Rothman, 1987), and two journal article reviews (Anthony, Cohen, Farkas, et al., 1988; Intagliata & Baker, 1983). However, additional implementation studies are necessary to help define different types of case management, and formative evaluations are needed to serve as a basis for further program planning and development.

Summative Evaluation

Once a case management program has developed to the point of functioning as intended, the focus of evaluation should shift to summative evaluation, with controlled experimental designs used to measure the outcomes the program produces. The various objectives of case management services should be studied, including those described earlier, such as enhancing the continuity and comprehensiveness of care, improving the accessibility of services to clients, and increasing the efficiency and cost effectiveness with which services are provided.

Recently a few controlled outcome studies of case management have been published. These experiments have produced inconsistent results in terms of effects of case management on patients, with some indicating positive outcomes and some indicating little or no impact. It is difficult to compare the studies because of inadequate descriptions of the services being compared and because of differences in outcome measures employed.

One of the strongest studies from an experimental design point of view was conducted in Texas by Franklin and colleagues (Franklin & Solovitz, 1986; Franklin, Solovitz, Mason, et al., 1987). This study employed a randomized pretest/posttest control group experimental design. A group of 417 individuals, who had been discharged at least twice from a mental hospital, were randomly assigned to an experimental group who received case management services or to a control group who received the usual aftercare services available to chronic mentally ill individuals in the community. At the end of 1 year, the experimental group had received more services than the control group and incurred more costs. However, they had not improved more in their quality of life than the control group and they had experienced more mental hospital readmissions.

Franklin et al. (1987) acknowledge that the follow-up period they used in their study may be too brief to measure the impact of case management adequately. However, there are also several other problems with this study related to not giving adequate attention to the implementation analysis issues described above. The independent variable, case management, was apparently not carefully distinguished from the "usual and customary aftercare services" provided to the "control" group. Further, some of the services that the experimental group had received would usually be considered case management services, such as assessments, evaluations, and referrals, and therefore should not be counted as additional services or costs because one would expect them to be part of the independent variable, that is, the provision of case management services.

Case management was more carefully defined in a study in Kansas by Modrcin, Rapp, and Poertner (1988) who used an experimental design to compare two types of case management services in a large mental health center. All 89 individuals referred for community support service during a 4-month period were randomly assigned to an experimental group that received case management using a "developmental-acquisition model" or a control group that received the "normal" case management services. The developmental-acquisition model focused on the strengths of the client and the community environment, rather than on individual pathology or environmental obstacles. Experimental group case managers were found to have more contact with clients and more interaction with clients outside the office than did control group case managers. When compared to the control group, the experimental subjects showed changes in the hypothesized direction on five of the six measures used. Experimental subjects were more likely to be rated by significant others as better in community living skills and the appropriateness of community behaviors. As contrasted with the control subjects, experimental subjects were also more likely to take vocational training, tolerate stress better, and perceive their use of leisure time as more meaningful. However, there was also a significant finding that the experimental group did not socialize as well as the control group. This result may reflect a problem in the reliability of the socialization ratings made by control group case managers who were less involved with their subjects and thus might have attributed to them a higher than accurate level of performance because of a lack of information.

Goering et al. (1988) compared 82 patients in a rehabilitation-oriented case management program with 82 matched control patients who had been discharged from the same Toronto inpatient settings before the case management program was implemented. At 6-month follow-up, only occupational functioning was better for the case managed group as compared to the control group. At the 2-year follow-up, the patients in the case management program not only had better occupational functioning, but also lived in more independent living situations and were less socially isolated. However, this study is flawed by the use of historical controls and lack of randomization.

Bond et al. (1988) randomly assigned 167 clients at risk of rehospitalization at three community mental health centers in Indiana to experimental groups receiving assertive case management or to control groups eligible for other available aftercare services at the centers. Outcomes assessed 6 months later showed that clients receiving assertive case management had significantly lower rehospitalization rates and shorter stays than controls at two of the centers. No differences were found between the experimental and control groups on quality of life, medication compliance, involvement in center programs, or contacts with the legal system. The most cost-effective center showed an average cost per client of $5,490 less than for the control group.

Problems in Current Evaluation of Outcome

This brief discussion of available outcome evaluations of case management points to a number of problems still to be dealt with in the current evaluation practice in this area. Advances in measuring the effectiveness of case management depend on clear definition of the following terms: (a) specification of the case management intervention, (b) characterization of the client population, (c) adequacy of outcome measures, (d) consideration of time in program, and (e) specification of community context (Baker, 1988).

Specification of Case Management Interventions

Published reports are often unclear as to the type(s) of case management interventions offered. In some comparisons across groups, it is difficult to know what was offered to the experimental group that was not offered to the control group. Sometimes it seems that the control group of patients receiving services from aftercare workers are receiving services as much or more in line with the spirit and substance of case management than those receiving services from people designated as case managers. Evaluations of case management outcomes need to be explicit in their operational definition of the kinds of services offered patients in the case management programs being studied. Without such information, effectiveness comparisons across programs are meaningless because of lack of clarity about what is being compared. Some attempts have been made to develop standardized operational definitions of case management, such as the efforts by Hargreaves et al. (1984), but more is needed. A further complicating factor is that family members, as described earlier in this paper, also must become actively involved in providing case management support to their patient-relative. When experimental and control groups are being compared, researchers must take care to control for any differential levels of such family involvement.

Characterization of the Client Population

A salient issue in the evaluation of case management is the match or mismatch between the target populations and the type of case management offered. The chronic mentally ill differ in important ways that should be taken into account in analyzing the impact of the services provided to them. Among the key variables that need to be considered in sampling are diagnosis; severity and refractoriness of symptoms; and risk of relapse, as indexed by the family emotional climate and recency of last relapse. Despite efforts to specify the characteristics of the target patient population for the program, most definitions allow for considerable variability in the characteristics of those who meet given eligibility criteria.

The clientele of most case management programs have demonstrated impairments in functioning because of psychiatric illness and are at some risk of hospitalization, but they differ considerably on a number of important variables. One of these variable is age, and client age can be a factor in differences in previous hospitalization history, chronicity, and level of functioning (Goldstrom & Manderscheid, 1983; Intagliata & Baker, 1983, 1984; Schulberg & Baker, 1968; Tessler, Bernstein, Rosen, et al., 1982). In recent years, increasing attention has been given to at least one age group, "young adult chronic patients" (Bachrach, 1982; Lamb, 1979a; Pepper, Kirshner, & Ryglewicz, 1981; Prevost, 1982; Sheets, Prevost, & Reihman, 1982). One way to handle issues of client heterogeneity is to collect information on various client variables, divide the sample into subgroups based on those variables, and then, in data analysis, examine the range of patient outcomes for each of the subgroups.

Collecting Adequate Outcome Measures

There are several relevant outcome goals for case management programs: (a) minimizing the number and length of rehospitalizations of patients, thereby increasing their tenure in community settings; (b) improving their psychiatric status by reducing or controlling the level of psychiatric symptomatology; (c) improving their functional capacities so that they can function in a more independent fashion, both socially and vocationally; (d) helping them to lead more personally satisfying and less oppressive lives.

Because case management programs have multiple goals, evaluations of such programs require the use of multiple outcome measures. It is advisable that various vantage points or perspectives be taken into consideration (Ellsworth, 1975; Fontana & Dowds, 1975). Moreover, good outcome studies must be founded on the theoretical principles that guided the program being evaluated (Schulberg & Bromet, 1981). These theoretical principles must stipulate not only the intended outcomes of the program but also the process by which program inputs are expected to result in such outcomes.

It is important to realize that not all outcomes are goals for, or achievable by, all patients. One might not expect to see changes in vocational performance either among patients for whom improved vocational functioning was not a goal or among patients who were not involved in a program designed to enhance vocational functioning.

Another factor that must be considered, and which becomes apparent when reading the relevant literature, is that the various outcomes of interest are not unidirectional. Positive outcome on one measure does not necessarily imply positive outcomes on others. Measures of client vocational changes are often uncorrelated with measures of change in psychosocial functioning (Anthony & Farkas, 1982). Even more striking are the findings illustrating that positive effects on one client outcome may be associated with negative effects on others. Some research findings have indicated that clients in an intensive skills training program may improve their interpersonal skills but at the same time become more anxious. Similarly, clients in high-expectation environments demonstrate greater levels of social functioning and report greater life satisfaction even though they have higher rates of rehospitalization than clients in low-expectation settings (Carpenter & Bourestom, 1976).

Current relevant literature gives some important cues that can be used to generate hypotheses and guide the analysis and interpretation of data linking case management program inputs and client outcomes. For example, evidence indicates that rehospitalization can be influenced both by clients' compliance with prescribed neuroleptic medication (Hogarty & Goldberg, 1973; Hogarty, Goldberg, & Schooler, 1974) and by their participation in aftercare programs (Anthony, Cohen, & Vitalo, 1978; Paul, 1969; Test & Stein, 1978; Weinman, Sanders, Kleiner, et al., 1970). While there is clear indication of the impact of psychotropic medication in controlling psychiatric symptomatology (Hansell, 1981), such medication does not teach clients life and coping skills. Only those programs that have worked intensively with chronic patients on specific skills (especially when training has taken place in actual community settings) have been able to effect changes. Even then, however, the changes have been maintained only so long as treatment was provided (Test & Stein, 1978).

These case management programs have not used behavioral training methods, and there is evidence that when programs employ behaviorally based learning principles (modeling, behavioral rehearsal, reinforcement, etc.) in skills training in an intensive, comprehensive, and lengthy (at least 3 months) fashion, substantial improvement in functional skill levels can accrue that are both durable and generalizable (Austin et al., 1976; Falloon, 1985; Wallace & Liberman, 1985). Case management programs attempting to induce durable and generalized improvements in social and living skills will have to employ training methods that adhere closely to behavioral learning principles, including the "programming" for generalization that requires systematic techniques such as fading, multiple exemplars, involvement of natural caregivers in reinforcing skills, and the like. Corrigan, Schade and Liberman, in Chapter 5 on skills training in this book, document at length the importance of linking social skills training to case management in community settings.

Consideration of Time in Program

A significant factor in evaluating outcome of service programs is the amount of time that clients have been receiving service. Several of the case management outcome studies described earlier recognized the importance of allowing enough time for program impact between entry and follow-up assessments. While this is difficult to accomplish within the limitations of small contrived experiments, time in program can make a difference. Hogarty et al. (1974) have shown that some benefits from a particular treatment emerge relatively quickly while the effects of other interventions may not emerge for some time. Hogarty and colleagues (Hogarty & Goldberg, 1973; Hogarty, Goldberg, & Schooler, 1974, 1975; Hogarty, Schooler, Ulrich, Mussare, Ferro, & Herron, 1979) found that, for newly discharged outpatient schizophrenics, the beneficial effects of adding sociotherapy to drug therapy did not emerge until follow-up had reached the 18- to 24-month point.

Other studies, using a variety of outcome criteria, have shown that the cessation of community treatment results in gradual deterioration until no significant differences exist between research groups. This has been particularly true for measures of recidivism (Davis, Dinitz, & Pasamanick, 1974; Langsley, Mochotka, & Flomenhalft, 1971; Mosher & Menn, 1978; Weinman, Sanders, Kleiner, & Wilson, 1970) and psychosocial functioning (Test & Stein, 1978). Clearly, time in treatment is an important variable in determining the impact of case management interventions on clients.

Specification of Community Context

Difficulties in deciphering underlying contextual circumstances of programs further complicate evaluation of effectiveness data. Few published studies provide information regarding community context, mental health system policies, rural vs. urban settings, historical changes, and the nature of the existing service network. It is relevant to know the extent of interagency cooperation and the type, if any, of core agency functioning within the locale. Important research questions in this area involve assessment of how the extent of cooperation and connectedness between key agencies influences the case management process and what types of core agency models work best to enhance case management effectiveness.

Need for Further Evaluation and Research

Obviously, more research and evaluation are called for, to strengthen and refine the case management process further. Weak intervention cannot be expected to produce measurable differences, and future evaluators of case management must define clearly the independent variables they are examining and develop more sensitive measures of the dependent variables.

Case management cannot be accomplished by case managers working alone. Supportive organizational arrangements must be developed to assure the availability of services to which case managers can link clients. Organizational structures, such as a core service agency, are also needed for interagency affiliation and cooperation agreements, resource development, and other organizational structures that support a coordinated community service system.

To enhance the quality of case management services, greater attention must be given to systematic research and evaluation of case management systems. The importance of such research and evaluation to case management should not be minimized. Given the present economic and political climate, in which funding for human services programs is shrinking, case management programs will be particularly vulnerable because they provide indirect services to clients. If a choice has to be made between funds for case managers or for work-skills training programs for clients, it is likely that the more direct client services will be funded. If case management programs are to continue to grow in the 1990s, program administrators should have information to demonstrate their value and effectiveness.

Evaluations of service integration projects have reported that case manager teams and case managers can increase the accessibility, comprehensiveness, and volume of services to clients (Baker & Northman, 1981). Caragonne (1979) came to similar conclusions and, in addition, reported that the use of case managers led to more effective packaging of client service plans, documented gaps and duplications in service networks, and generally promoted organizational responsiveness to consumer needs. Although this evidence is encouraging, many questions remain unanswered. As with many human service activities, case management is more art than science. Thus, as we implement case management systems for the chronically mentally disabled, we must continue to learn and change.

REFERENCES

Agranoff, R. (1977). Services integration. In W. F. Anderson, B. J. Frieden, & M. J. Murphy (Eds.), *Managing human services*. Washington, DC: International City Management Association.

Altshuler, S. C., & Forward, J. (1978). The inverted hierarchy: A case manager approach to mental health services. *Administration in Mental Health, 6*, 57–58.

Amadio, S. B. (Ed.). (1976). *An evaluation of the Jackson County integrated human services delivery project*. Murphysboro, IL: Jackson County Mental Health Department.

Anderson, C. M., Hogarty, G., & Reiss, D. J. (1981). The psychoeducational family treatment of schizophrenia. In M. Goldstein (Ed.), *New directions for mental health services: New developments in interventions with families of schizophrenics* (No. 12, pp. 70–94). San Francisco: Jossey-Bass.

Anthony, W. A., Cohen, M. R., Farkas, M., & Cohen, F. (1988). Case management—More than a response to a dysfunctional system. *Community Mental Health Journal, 24*, 219–228.

Anthony, W. A., Cohen, R. M., & Vitalo, R. (1978). The measurement of rehabilitation outcome. *Schizophrenia Bulletin, 4*, 365–383.

Anthony, W. A., & Farkas, J. M. (1982). A client outcome planning model for assessing psychiatric rehabilitation interventions. *Schizophrenia Bulletin, 8*, 13–38.

Austin, N. K., Liberman, R. P., King, L. W., & DeRisi, W. J. (1976). A comparative evaluation of two day hospitals: Behavior therapy vs. milieu therapy. *Journal of Nervous & Mental Disease, 163*, 253–261.

Bachrach, L. (1976). *Deinstitutionalization: An analytical review and sociological perspective*. Publication No. (ADM) 76-351. Washington, DC: Department of Health, Education and Welfare, Government Printing Office.

Bachrach, L. L. (1982). Assessment of outcomes in community support systems: Results, problems, and limitations. *Schizophrenia Bulletin, 8*, 39–62.

Bachrach, L. L. (1983). New directions in deinstitutionalization planning. In L. L. Bachrach (Ed.), *New directions in mental health services: Deinstitutionalization* (No. 17, pp. 93–106). San Francisco: Jossey-Bass.

Baker, F. (1982). Effects of value systems on service delivery. In H. C. Schulberg & M. Killilea (Eds.), *The modern practice of community mental health* (pp. 246–264). San Francisco: Jossey-Bass.

Baker, F. (1988). Case study: An approach to evaluating state-funded community support services for the chronically mentally ill. In L. Blackwell & L. K. Cartwright (Eds.), *Program consultation with human service programs: A clinical perspective* (pp. 155–163). Oakland, CA: Third Party Publishing Company.

Baker, F., & Baker, A. P. (1979). *The construction and validation of the human service ideology scale*. Buffalo: Division of Community Psychiatry, State University of New York.

Baker, F., Burns, T. F., Libby, M., & Intagliata, J. (1985). The impact of life events on chronic mental patients. *Hospital & Community Psychiatry, 36*, 299–301.

Baker, F., & Intagliata, J. (1982). Quality of life in the evaluation of community support systems. *Evaluation and Program Planning, 5*, 69–79.

Baker, F., & Intagliata, J. (1984a). The New York state community support system. *Hospital & Community Psychiatry, 35*, 39–44.

Baker, F., & Intagliata, J. (1984b). Rural community support services for the chronically mentally ill. *Journal of Rural Community Psychology, 5*, 13–14.

Baker, F., Intagliata, J., & Kirshstein, R. (1980). *Case management evaluation: Second interim report*. Buffalo, NY: TEFCO Services.

Baker, F., Jodrey, D., & Morell, M. (1979). *Evaluation of a case management training program: Final report*. New York: New York School of Psychiatry.

Baker, F., & Northman, J. E. (1981). *Helping: Human services for the 80s*. St. Louis: C V Mosby.

Baker, F., & Schulberg, H. C. (1967). Development of a community mental health ideology scale. *Community Mental Health Journal, 3*, 216–225.

Baker, F., & Vischi, T. (1989). Continuity of care and control of costs: Can case management assure both? *Journal of Public Health Policy, 10*(2), 204–213.

Baker, F., & Weiss, R. S. (1984). The nature of case manager support. *Hospital & Community Psychiatry, 35*, 925–928.

Bassuk, E. L., & Gerson, S. (1978). Deinstitutionalization and mental health services. *Scientific American, 238*, 46–53.

Beard, J. H., Malamud, T. J., & Rossman, E. (1978). Psychiatric rehabilitation and long-term rehospitalization rates: The findings of two research studies. *Schizophrenia Bulletin, 4*, 622–635.

Berkeley Planning Associates. (1977). *The quality of case management process: Final report*, Vol. III. In *The evaluation of child abuse and neglect projects 1974–1977*, Washington, DC: U.S. Department of Commerce, National Technical Information Service.

Bond, G. R., Miller, C. D., Krumwied, R. D., & Wand, R. S. (1988). Assertive case management in three CMHCs: A controlled study. *Hospital & Community Psychiatry, 39*, 411–418.

Caragonne, P. (1979, April 6). *Implications of case management: A report on research*. Presented at the Case Management Conference, Buffalo, NY.

Caragonne, P. (1980). *An analysis of the function of the case manager in four mental health social services settings*. Austin, TX: Report of the Case Management Research Project.

Caragonne, P. (1981). *A comparative analysis of twenty-two settings using case management components*. Austin, TX: Report of the Case Management Research Project.

Carpenter, J. O., & Bourestom, N. C. (1976). Performance of psychiatric hospital discharges in strict and tolerant environments. *Community Mental Health Journal, 12*, 45–51.

Corrigan, P., Schade, M., & Liberman, R. P. (In press). Social skills training. In R. P. Liberman (Ed.), *Case management of the seriously mentally ill*. Elmsford, NY: Pergamon Press.

Davis, A. E., Dinitz, S., & Pasamanick, B. (1974). *Schizophrenics in the new custodial community: Five years after the experiment*. Columbus: Ohio State University Press.

Doll, W. (1976). Family coping with the mentally ill: An unanticipated problem of deinstitutionalization. *Hospital & Community Psychiatry, 24*, 183–185.

Dormady, J. M. (1980). *New York State Board of Social Welfare case management concept paper* (Draft). Albany, NY.

Ellsworth, R. (1975). Consumer feedback in measuring the effectiveness of mental health programs. In M. Guttentag & E. Streuning (Eds.), *Handbook of evaluation research*, Vol. 2. Beverly Hills, CA: Sage Publications.

Evans, D. A., & Stellman, V. P. (1977). Community leaders assess quality of life. *Journal of Existentialism, 4*, 7–12.

Falloon, I. R. H. (1985). *Family management of schizophrenia*. Baltimore, MD: Johns Hopkins University Press.

Fontana, F., & Dowds, B. (1975). Assessing treatment outcome, I: Adjustment in the community. *Journal of Nervous & Mental Disease, 161*, 221–230.

Franklin, J. L., & Solovitz, B. (1986, October). *Evaluation of case management*. Paper presented at the annual convention of the American Public Health Association, Las Vegas.

Franklin, J. L., Solovitz, B., Mason, M., Clemons, J. R., & Miller, G. E. (1987). An evaluation of case management. *American Journal of Public Health, 77*, 675–678.

Gittelman, M. (1974). Coordinating mental health systems: A national and international perspective. *American Journal of Public Health, 64*, 496–500.

Goering, P. N., Wasylenki, D. A., Farkas, M., Lancee, W. J., & Ballantyne, R. (1988). What difference does case management make? *Hospital & Community Psychiatry, 39*, 272–276.

Goldberg, S. C., Schooler, N. R., & Hogarty, G. E. (1977). Prediction of relapse in schizophrenic outpatients treated by drug and sociotherapy. *Archives of General Psychiatry, 34*, 171–184.

Goldstrom, I. D., & Manderscheid, R. W. (1983). A descriptive analysis of community support program case managers serving the chronically mentally ill. *Community Mental Health Journal, 19*(1), 17–26.

Government Accounting Office. (1976). *Return-*

ing the mentally disabled to the community: Government needs to do more. Washington, DC: Comptroller General's Report to the Congress.

Governor's Interagency Task Force on Mental Health Community Support Systems. (1979, December 1). Subcommittee on Case Management: Final Report. Albany, NY.

Graham, K. (1980). *The work activities and work-related attitudes of case management personnel in New York State Office of Mental Health Community Support Systems*. Unpublished doctoral dissertation, Union College, Albany, NY.

Hansell, N. (1981). Medication. In J. Talbott (Ed.), *The chronically mentally ill* (pp. 29–46). New York: Human Sciences Press.

Hargreaves, W. A., Shaw, R. E., Shadoan, R., Walker, E., Surber, R., & Gaynor, J. (1984). Measuring case management activity. *Journal of Nervous & Mental Disease, 172*, 296–300.

Harris, M., & Bergman, H. C. (1988). Misconceptions about use of case management services by the chronic mentally ill: A utilization analysis. *Hospital & Community Psychiatry, 39*, 1276–1280.

Hatfield, A. B. (1978). Psychological costs of schizophrenia to the family. *Social Work, 34*, 355–359.

Herz, M. I., & Melville, C. (1980). Relapse in schizophrenia. *American Journal of Psychiatry, 137*, 801–805.

Hogarty, G. E., & Goldberg, S. C. (1973). Drug and sociotherapy in the aftercare of schizophrenic patients: One year relapse rates. *Archives of General Psychiatry, 28*, 54–64.

Hogarty, G. E., Goldberg, S. C., & Schooler, N. R. (1974). Drug and sociotherapy in the aftercare of schizophrenic patients: Adjustment of nonrelapsed patients. *Archives of General Psychiatry, 31*, 609–618.

Hogarty, G. E., Goldberg, S. C., & Schooler, N. R. (1975). Drug and sociotherapy in the aftercare of schizophrenic patients: A review. In M. Greenblatt (Ed.), *Drugs in combination with other therapies*. New York: Grune & Stratton.

Hogarty, G. E., Schooler, N. R., Ulrich, R., Mussare, F., Ferro, P., & Herron, E. (1979). Fluphenazine and social therapy in the aftercare of schizophrenic patients. *Archives of General Psychiatry, 36*, 1283–1295.

Horejsi, C. (1978). What is case management? *Foster family care: A handbook for social workers*. Missoula, MT: University of Montana.

Intagliata, J. (1978). The history and future of associate degree workers in the human services. In K. Nash, M. Lifton, & S. Smith (Eds.), *The paraprofessional: Selected readings* (pp. 206–215). New Haven, CT: Center for Paraprofessional Evaluation and Continuing Education.

Intagliata, J. (1982). Improving the quality of community care for the clinically mentally disabled: The role of case management. *Schizophrenia Bulletin, 8*, 655–674.

Intagliata, J., & Baker, F. (1983). Factors affecting case management services for the chronically mentally ill. *Administration in Mental Health, 11*, 75–91.

Intagliata, J., & Baker, F. (1984). A comparative analysis of the young adult chronic patients in New York State's community support system. *Hospital & Community Psychiatry, 35*, 45–50.

Intagliata, J., Willer, B., & Egri, G. (1986). Role of the family in case management of the mentally ill. *Schizophrenia Bulletin, 12*, 699–708.

Jessing, B., & Dean, S. (1976). Case advocacy: Ideology and operation. In L. Baucom & G. Bensberg (Eds.), *Advocacy systems for persons with developmental disabilities*. Lubbock, TX: Research and Training Center for Mental Retardation.

Kirk, S. A., & Therrien, M. E. (1975). Community mental health myths and the fate of former hospitalized patients. *Psychiatry, 38*, 209–217.

Krauss, J. B. (1980). The chronic psychiatric patient in the community: A model of care. *Nursing Outlook, 5*, 308–314.

Lamb, H. R. (1979a). Roots of neglect of the long-term mentally ill. *Psychiatry, 42*, 201–297.

Lamb, H. R. (1979b). Staff burnout in work with long-term patients. *Hospital & Community Psychiatry, 30*, 396–398.

Lamb, H. R., & Goertzel, V. (1977). The long-term patient in the era of community treatment. *Archives of General Psychiatry, 34*, 679–682.

Langsley, D. G., Mochotka, P., & Flomenhalft, K. (1971). Avoiding mental hospital admission: A follow-up study. *American Journal of Psychiatry, 127*, 127–130.

Lannon, P. B. (1979, November). *Functional assessments and service utilization patterns of clients within New York state community sup-*

port systems. Paper presented at the Pennsylvania Evaluation Network Conference, Philadelphia.

Leavitt, M. (1975). The discharge crisis: The experience of families of psychiatric patients. *Nursing Research, 24*, 33–40.

Leff, J., Kuipers, L., Berkowitz, R., Eberlein-Vries, R., & Sturgeon, D. (1982). A controlled trial of social intervention in families of schizophrenic patients. *British Journal of Psychiatry, 141*, 121–134.

Levine, I. S., & Fleming, M. (1985). *Human resource development: Issues in case management*. College Park, Center of Rehabilitation and Manpower Services, University of Maryland.

Liberman, R. P., Wallace, C. J., & Falloon, I. R. H. (1981). Interpersonal problem-solving therapy for schizophrenics and their families. *Comprehensive Psychiatry, 22*, 627–630.

Lippman, L. (1976). Three examples of case management advocacy. In L. Baucom & G. Bensberg (Eds.), *Advocacy systems for persons with developmental disabilities* (pp. 167–176). Lubbock, TX: Research and Training Center in Mental Retardation.

May, P. (1975). Adopting new models for continuity of care: What are the needs? *Hospital & Community Psychiatry, 26*, 599–601.

McPheeters, H. L. (1974, March). Theme II: Optimal continuity of care—second faculty presentation. *Proceedings of the Conference on Creating the Community Alternative: Options and Innovations*. Philadelphia, PA: Horizon House Institute.

Miller, G. (1986). The future of the chronically mentally ill. *Proceedings of the Sixteenth Annual Texas Research Institute of Mental Sciences Symposium*. New York: SP Medical & Scientific Books.

Mittenthal, S. D. (1976). Systems approach to human services integration. *Evaluation, 3*, 142–148.

Modrcin, M., Rapp, C. A., & Poertner, J. (1988). The evaluation of case management services with the chronically mentally ill. *Evaluation & Program Planning, 11*, 307–314.

Morrill, W. (1976). Services integration and the Department of Health, Education, and Welfare. *Evaluation, 3*, 52–55.

Mosher, L. R., & Keith, S. J. (1980). Psychosocial treatment: Individual, group, family, and community support approaches. *Schizophrenia Bulletin, 6*, 10–41.

Mosher, L. R., & Menn, A. Z. (1978). Community residential treatment for schizophrenia: Two year follow-up. *Hospital & Community Psychiatry, 29*, 715–723.

New York State Office of Mental Health. (1978). *Request for Proposal: Community support system services*. Albany: Author.

New York State Office of Mental Health. (1989). *Intensive case management: Executive summary*. Albany: Author.

Paul, G. L. (1969). Chronic mental patients: Current status—future directions. *Psychological Bulletin, 71*, 81–94.

Pepper, B., Kirshner, M. C., & Ryglewicz, R. (1981). The young adult chronic patient: Overview of a population. *Hospital & Community Psychiatry, 32*, 463–469.

President's Commission on Mental Health. (1978). *Report to the President from the President's Commission on Mental Health* (Vol. 1). Washington, DC: Superintendent of Documents, U.S. Government Printing Office.

President's Panel on Mental Retardation. (1962). *A proposed program for national action to combat mental retardation*. Washington, DC: Superintendent of Documents, U.S. Government Printing Office.

Prevost, J. A. (1982). Youthful chronicity: Paradox of the 80s. *Hospital & Community Psychiatry, 33*, 173.

Reagles, S., & Sheets, J. (1979, October). Hutchings Psychiatric Center second year CSP project report. In S. Steindorf (Ed.), *Second year community support program progress report*. Albany, NY: New York State Office of Mental Health.

Reiff, R., & Reissman, F. (1965). The indigenous nonprofessional. *Community Mental Health Journal Monograph, 1* (Suppl. No. 1).

Riffer, N., & Freedman, J. (1980). *Case management in community based services: A training manual*. Albany: New York Office of Mental Health.

Ross, H. (1980). Volunteers for services to older persons. *Proceedings of the Conference on the Evaluation of Case Management Programs*. Los Angeles.

Rothman, J. (1987). *Case management action guidelines: A synthesis of social research*. Los Angeles: UCLA School of Social Welfare.

Schulberg, H., & Baker, F. (1968). Program evaluation models and the implementation of research findings. *American Journal of Public Health, 58*, 1248–1255.

Schulberg, H. C., & Bromet, E. (1981). Strategies for evaluating the outcome of community services for the chronically mentally ill. *American Journal of Psychiatry, 138*, 930–935.

Schwartz, M., & Schwartz, C. G. (1964). *Social approach to mental patient care*. New York: Columbia University Press.

Segal, S., & Aviram, V. (1978). *The mentally ill in community-based sheltered care*. New York: John Wiley.

Sheets, J. L., Prevost, J. A., & Reiham, J. (1982). Young adult chronic patients: Three hypothesized subgroups. *Hospital & Community Psychiatry, 33*, 197–203.

Stein, L. I., & Test, M. A. (1980). Alternative to mental hospital treatment: I. Conceptual model, treatment program, and clinical evaluation. *Archives of General Psychiatry, 37*, 392–397.

Stevens, B. C. (1972). Dependence of schizophrenic patients on elderly relatives. *Psychological Medicine, 2*, 17–32.

Sullivan, J. P. (1981). Case management. In J. Talbott (Ed.), *The chronically mentally ill* (pp. 119–131). New York: Human Sciences Press.

Tessler, R. C., Bernstein, A. G., Rosen, B. M., & Goldman, H. H. (1982). The chronically mentally ill in community support systems. *Hospital & Community Psychiatry, 33*, 208–211.

Test, M. A. (1979). Continuity of care in community treatment. *New Directions in Mental Health Services, 2*, 15–23.

Test, M. A., & Stein, L. I. (1978). Community treatment of the chronic patient: Research review. *Schizophrenia Bulletin, 4*, 350–364.

Turner, J. C. (1977). Comprehensive community support systems for severely disabled adults. *Psychosocial Rehabilitation Journal, 1*, 39–47.

Turner, J., & Shiffren, I. (1979). Community support system: How comprehensive? In L. Stein (Ed.), *Community support systems for the long-term patient* (pp. 1–13). San Francisco, CA: Jossey-Bass.

Turner, J. C., & TenHoor, W. J. (1978). The NIMH community support program: Pilot approach to a needed social reform. *Schizophrenia Bulletin, 4*, 319–349.

Wallace, C. G., & Liberman, R. P. (1985). Social skills training for schizophrenics. *Psychiatry Research, 15*, 239–247.

Washington, R. O., Karmen, M., & Friedlob, A. (1974, February). *Second year evaluation report (SITO) of the East Cleveland Community Human Services Center*. Cleveland, OH: Case Western Reserve University.

Weinman, B., Sanders, R., Kleiner, R., & Wilson, S. (1970). Community based treatment of the chronic psychotic. *Community Mental Health Journal, 6*, 13–21.

Weinman, B., & Kleiner, R. J. (1978). The impact of community living and community member intervention on the adjustment of the chronic psychiatric patient. In L. Stein & M. A. Test (Eds.), *Alternatives to mental hospital treatment* (pp. 139–162). New York: Plenum Press.

Willer, B., Scheerenberger, R. C., & Intagliata, J. (1978). Deinstitutionalization and mentally retarded persons. *Community Mental Health Review, 3*, 1–12.

CHAPTER 11

VOCATIONAL REHABILITATION

Gary R. Bond

This chapter provides a glimpse of the past, present, and possible future of vocational programming for persons with severe mental illness. To use a historical metaphor, the post-deinstitutionalization period can be divided into three eras: the rule of imperial institutions, the dark ages, and a renaissance. The first era started in the 1950s and extended into the 1960s. Vocational programs were implemented in hospitals, sheltered workshops, and halfway houses (Black, 1988). However, the optimism that prompted these facility-based efforts was soon overtaken by a deeply felt pessimism about the employment potential for psychiatric patients.

The 1970s and early 1980s were the "dark ages," in which vocational rehabilitation for persons with severe mental illness was not considered the mission of either community mental health centers (CMHCs) or comprehensive rehabilitation centers. During this time, psychosocial rehabilitation (PSR) centers, such as Fountain House (New York) (Malamud & McCrory, 1988; Vorspan, 1988), Thresholds (Chicago) (Dincin, 1975), Horizon House (Philadelphia) (Cnaan, Blankertz, Messinger, & Gardner, 1988), and the Club (Piscataway, NJ) (Lehrer & Lanoil, 1977) developed transitional employment (TE) programs. These programs were seen either as "maverick" or as "model" programs, depending on one's ideology. They existed as isolated fiefdoms within pervasively nonvocational mental health systems. Adaptations of TE are only now becoming part of the services within community support programs (CSPs) in CMHCs.

Now we may be on the verge of a renaissance in the form of the supported employment (SE) movement (Wehman & Moon, 1988). SE represents a paradigm shift in vocational thinking. By advocating the placement of clients with minimal prevocational training in community employment and the provision of time-unlimited support, SE has led to explorations of employment possibilities for persons with severe disabilities. Whether these explorations shall result in enduring social inventions remains to be seen.

Vocational approaches for persons with severe psychiatric disabilities will be examined against this historical backdrop. Three general questions guide this chapter: (a) What vocational approaches are effective? To be deemed effective, a program must result in paid employment outcomes for its clients. (b) What exactly do these programs do? We urgently need clear, operational descriptions of program services. (c) For whom are different vocational approaches successful? An appreciation of the potential of vocational programs has been muddled by vague sample descriptions. We need to develop more precise and appropriate taxonomies to describe clients successfully served by various programs.

A LOOK AT THE PAST: PRIOR RESEARCH

The research literature on the effectiveness of vocational approaches in psychiatric programs was examined, including the rare occasions in which researchers reported client-treatment interactions. Researchers have not built a cumulative knowledge base, and it was therefore necessary to impose an external structure on a scattered literature.

Method

Inclusion Criteria

Evaluation studies were included if they met five criteria: (a) The study was conducted after 1955, the approximate date for the inception of deinstitutionalization. (b) The program evaluated had an explicit vocational component. Several studies have shown that nonvocational approaches with emphases on insight and improved social functioning do not generalize to better work functioning (Gunderson et al., 1984; Vitale & Steinbach, 1965; Wilder, Levin, & Zwerling, 1966). (c) The sample studied consisted solely of clients with psychiatric disabilities. Or, if a mixed disability sample was used, statistics were reported on a psychiatric subgroup. (d) Random assignment, or a close approximation, was used. Subject as own control, ex post facto matched group, and single-subject designs were excluded. (e) Employment outcomes were reported. Twenty-four studies were located that met the requirements, as listed in Table 11.1.

Typology

Vocational programs were grouped into the seven categories briefly described below. The last three approaches (the job club, assertive community treatment, and psychosocial rehabilitation) are discussed further in the section, A Look at the Present: Current Popular Approaches, p. 251.

1. *Hospital programs* included those in which the participants were inpatients, regardless of whether the vocational programming occurred in the community or in-hospital.

2. *Halfway houses* included programs in which the primary site of rehabilitation was conceptualized as a community residence. The best-known model was the Fairweather Lodge, which provides a structured setting for living, employment, and peer support (Fairweather, Sanders, Maynard, Cressler, & Bleck, 1969).

3. *Sheltered workshops* included programs in which training and employment were provided by securing subcontract work from industry (Black & Kase, 1986). The vocational activity generally occurred in segregated facilities. Programs included comprehensive rehabilitation centers offering training to a range of disability populations (Weinberg & Lustig, 1968) and workshops specifically designed for clients with psychiatric disabilities (Meltzoff & Blumenthal, 1966).

4. *Vocational counseling* included programs in which the primary activity evaluated

Table 11.1. Controlled Studies of Vocational Programs for Persons with Severe Psychiatric Disabilities

PROGRAM TYPE	STUDY	SAMPLE SIZE		FOLLOW-UP PERIOD (MONTHS)	EXPERIMENTAL COMPARISON
		EXPERIMENTAL	CONTROL		
Hospital programs	Paquette & Lafave (1964)	140	140	Not stated	Halfway house and vocational training vs. custodial
	Becker (1967)	25	25	8	Intensive social/vocational program vs. custodial
	Walker et al. (1969)	14	14	6	Community transitional employment (TE) vs. hospital job placement
	Marx et al. (1973)[a]	19	20	5	Progressive inpatient vs. regular ward
	Kuldau & Dirks (1977)	41	48	18	Day hospital and workshop vs. rapid discharge
	Ryan & Bell (1985)	31	26	6	Hospital and community job placements vs. traditional inpatient
Halfway house	Fairweather et al. (1969)	57	48	12	Lodge vs. aftercare
	Lamb & Goertzel (1972)	28	20	24	High expectation halfway house vs. low expectation family care
	Velasquez & McCubbin (1980)	36	36	6	Community residence vs. waiting list
Sheltered workshop	Meltzoff & Blumenthal (1966)	33	36	18	Day treatment with workshop vs. psychotherapy
	Soloff (1967)	55	91	12	Sheltered workshop vs. state hospital or recreation therapy

	Weinberg & Lustig (1968)	20	18	24	Sheltered workshop vs. vocational counseling
	Griffiths (1974)	14	14	18 (mean)	Sheltered workshop vs. aftercare
Vocational counseling	Briggs & Yater (1966)	74	60	13 (mean)	Vocational counseling vs. no treatment
	Purvis & Miskimins (1970)	99	50	not stated	Group and individual counseling vs. no follow-up
	Kline & Hoisington (1981)	10	10	6	Career exploration at a psychosocial rehabilitation (PSR) center vs. PSR only
Job club	Azrin & Philip (1980)	19	6	4	Job club vs. vocational lecture
Assertive community treatment	Marx et al. (1973)[a]	21	20	5	Assertive community treatment (ACT) vs. hospital
	Field et al. (n.d.)	18	18	18	Job developer + ACT vs. sheltered work + ACT
	Stein & Test (1980)	57	59	12	ACT vs. short-term hospital and aftercare
Psychosocial rehabilitation centers	Beard et al. (1963)	163	69	12	PSR with TE vs. waiting list
	Wolkon et al. (1971)	106	185	12	PSR vs. aftercare
	Dincin & Swift (1969)	160	76	24	PSR + TE vs. PSR day program only or no services
	Dincin & Witheridge (1982)	46	44	9	PSR + TE vs. social club
	Bond & Dincin (1986)	56	54	15	PSR + rapid placement vs. PSR + gradual placement

[a]This study is listed twice. It had two hospital control groups, which have been treated as separate experiments in the ensuing analyses.

was verbal interaction, in either a one-to-one or group format. Vocational counseling typically involved identification of client needs, development of a rehabilitation plan, and career selection (Farley, Schriner, & Roessler, 1988; Rubin & Roessler, 1978).

5. *Job club* included programs in which a behavioral approach was used to help any unemployed group acquire and use the skills needed to obtain jobs (Azrin & Besalel, 1979).

6. *Assertive community treatment (ACT)* was an approach consisting of helping clients in their natural environment with frequent home and community visits, and assisting clients to obtain funding, housing, and jobs on a time-unlimited basis (Stein & Test, 1980).

7. *Psychosocial rehabilitation (PSR) centers* included programs that evolved from the clubhouse model developed by Fountain House in New York (Beard, Propst, & Malamud, 1982; Dincin, 1975). They provided an accepting peer-oriented clubhouse. They also offered a continuum of vocational opportunities, ranging from prevocational work crews, usually unpaid work opportunities within the center, to TE, which consists of temporary community jobs employing clients under an arrangement between the PSR agency and a community employer.

Outcome Measures

Six variables measuring paid employment were examined: employment status at the end of the follow-up period (either *paid* or *competitive* employment), *duration* (number of weeks worked), *earnings, job starts* (i.e., any community employment at any time during study period), and *intensity* (i.e., full-time competitive employment status). Paid employment included competitive, transitional, and sheltered employment.

Findings from 24 Controlled Studies

Study Characteristics

The classification of studies is shown in Table 11.1. The median publication dates for the studies reviewed in each of the seven vocational program categories showed an approximate temporal progression from institutional to industry-integrated approaches: sheltered workshop (1967), hospital programs (1971), halfway houses (1972), vocational counseling (1970), PSR (1971), ACT (1980), job club (1980). The mean study sample size was 104 subjects and the mean study follow-up period was 12.5 months. The studies had various methodological problems, including vague descriptions of both experimental and control treatment conditions, low statistical power, brief follow-up periods, ambiguities about when vocational programming was terminated, and high dropout and refusal rates (Bond, 1988).

Vocational Outcomes

Vocational programs have been consistently, although modestly, successful in helping clients obtain and hold jobs, as shown in Table 11.2. When meta-analytic techniques (Rosenthal, 1984) were used to evaluate the findings for this group of studies, the experimental condition showed greater vocational gains than controls on all six of the vocational outcome variables, as shown in Table 11.3. However, it is also true that none of the 13 studies reporting competitive employment outcomes found an experimental effect when examined individually.

Hospital Outcomes

Clients assigned to the experimental conditions had significantly less hospitalization than controls in over half the studies examining this outcome. However, in addition to vocational programming, these experimental groups received other services not provided to the control group. The studies were designed this way because they were not intended to evaluate the vocational intervention in isolation from all other services. Thus, this set of comparisons does not directly test the efficacy of vocational programs in preventing rehospitalizations.

Table 11.2. Frequency of Significant Findings on 7 Outcome Measures Favoring Experimental Conditions Among Studies Reported in Table 11.1[a]

	OUTCOME VARIABLE						
PROGRAM TYPE	PAID EMPLOYMENT	COMPETITIVE EMPLOYMENT	FULL-TIME EMPLOYMENT	JOB STARTS	DURATION	EARNINGS	HOSPITAL ADMISSIONS
Hospital-based	2/3	0/3	2/4	2/3	2/3	2/3	2/5
Halfway house	1/2	–	0/1	–	2/2	–	2/3
Sheltered workshop	–	0/4	–	1/2	0/2	–	1/1
Vocational counseling	0/1	0/1	–	–	0/1	–	–
Job club	–	–	–	1/1	–	–	–
Assertive community treatment	2/2	0/3	1/2	–	1/2	1/2	2/3
Psychosocial rehabilitation	0/4	0/2	1/1	1/2	1/2[b]	0/2	2/5
Total	5/12	0/13	4/8	5/8	6/12[b]	3/7	9/17

[a]The first number in each pair is the frequency of studies significantly favoring experimental condition. The second number is the total number of studies examining a particular outcome variable.
[b]Control group in one study had worked significantly more weeks than the experimental group.

Table 11.3. Meta-Analytic Results for 24 Controlled Studies Reported in Table 11.1

VARIABLE	OVERALL Z-SCORE	NUMBER OF STUDIES
Paid employment	6.0**	12
Competitive employment	2.9*	13
Full-time employment	4.1**	8
Job starts	5.7**	8
Duration	4.3**	12
Earnings	2.8*	5
Rehospitalization	6.2**	14

Note: All z-scores favor the experimental conditions; $^{*}p < .01$; $^{**}p < .001$.

Client Factors

Three studies used prior work experience to classify clients (Bond & Dincin, 1986; Kuldau & Dirks, 1977; Ryan & Bell, 1985) and one study stratified clients on their general psychosocial adjustment (Meltzoff & Blumenthal, 1966). A simple dichotomy was used in each case; for example, Bond and Dincin (1986) classified clients as *work-experienced* if they had been employed continuously for at least 1 year before admission, and classified the remainder as *work-inexperienced.* All four studies found that clients with more work experience (or better adjustment) benefited significantly more from the enriched vocational programs than did controls. Clients with little or no work experience did poorly regardless of the vocational training provided.

Discussion of the Literature Review

Early reviews by Anthony and his colleagues (Anthony, Buell, Sharratt, & Althoff, 1972; Anthony, Cohen, & Vitalo, 1978) documented a lack of differences in employment rates for clients attending vocational programs compared with baseline rates for this population. The current review qualifies this conclusion. It shows that these programs *have* succeeded in placing clients in jobs and in helping clients retain these jobs. The consistent deficiency of these programs has been their failure to prepare clients for future competitive employment outside the support provided by the rehabilitation program. Thus, the success of vocational programs has been in helping clients adjust to a specific vocational environment, which has sometimes been sheltered or transitional employment. Given what is known about the psychiatric population, it is not surprising that these skills have not generalized to new environments. Extrapolating from these data, one hypothesis is that clients have a decent likelihood of retaining community employment positions as long as they continue to receive intensive support.

Research on the effectiveness of sheltered workshops for persons with severe mental illness stopped in the United States after 1968. This was in contrast to the half-dozen active research programs in the 1960s (Black, 1988; Criswell, 1970). The reason that this line of research was abandoned is quite simple: Sheltered workshops have been ineffective in helping clients with psychiatric disabilities achieve competitive employment.

Among disability populations, clients with psychiatric disabilities do especially poorly in sheltered workshops (Ciardiello, 1981). The larger issue, however, is the poor track record these facilities have for placing in competitive employment clients with *any* disability. A national survey found that only 10% of workshop clients were placed in competitive employment annually (Greenleigh Associates, 1975). Bellamy, Rhodes, Bourbeau, and Mank (1986) have estimated that clients with mental retardation (MR) who are placed in day activity and work activity centers require an average of 47 years to "graduate" to competitive employment.

This points to the need to "triage" the vocational needs of the psychiatric population in a more meaningful way than has been done in the past. For example, the generally positive results from controlled studies of hospital-based programs illustrate the capacity for institutionalized patients for work, and to a greater extent than is sometimes acknowledged. Industry-integrated programs for long-term patients are possible, and should be encouraged when discharge is not a current option (Forman, 1988). At the other end of the continuum, the evidence is compelling that many clients with prior work experience can benefit from high expectation programs. Another subgroup not adequately served by existing programs consists of well-educated clients who aspire to more than entry-level jobs (Collignon, Noble, & Toms-Barker, 1987).

Finally, the subgroup that is perhaps least understood and who may benefit the least from existing programs are clients with little prior work experience. The current experimentation with "supported education" may prove to be an optimal pathway to employment for clients not suited for traditional programs (Unger, Danley, Kohn, & Hutchinson, 1987).

Overall, experimental clients had a *lower* hospital rate than controls in the studies reviewed. The inference, therefore, is that most clients who receive vocational programming within a comprehensive rehabilitation program have no greater risk of rehospitalization than those who are not involved in a vocational program. This conclusion is somewhat at odds with that reached by Test (1984) and Hogarty et al. (1986) for high expectancy programs in general. There are, in fact, examples in the literature (Goldberg, Schooler, Hogarty, & Roper, 1977; Lamb & Goertzel, 1972) in which some clients had poorer outcomes in high expectancy programs. Further research is needed to delineate client and treatment combinations in which high expectancy vocational programs are contraindicated. One characteristic of successful programs may be that they attend to the warning signs of relapse (Herz, 1984) and provide additional support or crisis intervention at those times. Successful programs may also assist clients in a graded, incremental trajectory of rehabilitation as well as in avoiding too many major life changes at the same time.

Comparison between different vocational approaches is difficult, because of the different populations each typically serves (Black, 1988). Research is needed to determine, for example, whether clients served by sheltered workshops differ systematically from those attending PSR programs, as has been sometimes argued. Such research would clarify whether different success rates are a result of sampling differences. Only a few of the studies reviewed used "grand prix" designs (Gottman & Markman, 1978) that pitted one approach against another. This research strategy has the unfortunate side effect of heightening competitiveness in a field in which cooperation is an essential ingredient of success. Perhaps quasi-experimental designs (e.g., Lam, 1986) are a partial answer.

A LOOK AT THE PRESENT: CURRENT POPULAR APPROACHES

Table 11.4 lists five vocational rehabilitation strategies currently being used in the United States. Although a few controlled studies have been conducted on these models, as described in the last section, many gaps remain in our knowledge. The following summaries are impressionistic, and the conclusions may well change as more data accumulate.

Table 11.4. Current Vocational Approaches in Psychiatric Rehabilitation

PROGRAM APPROACH	EXAMPLES	STRENGTHS	WEAKNESSES
Boston University psychiatric rehabilitation model	Transitional Employment Enterprises, Boston	Well articulated Emphasis on client choice	Lengthy prevocational preparation Not empirically validated
Job club	Brentwood Job Club, Los Angeles	Stresses client responsibility Most direct strategy for higher functioning clients Positive empirical findings	Not suitable for lower functioning clients Job retention unclear
Assertive community treatment	Program for Assertive Community Treatment, Madison, Wis, Harbinger, Grand Rapids, Mich	Closest to Wehman's Individual Placement Promising controlled research Adaptable to small programs Wide range of clients served	Cost effectiveness not clear
Psychosocial rehabilitation/ transitional employment	Fountain House	Clear model National network Long track record	Null findings from controlled studies Step to competitive employment hard
"Job bank" extensions of transitional employment	Thresholds Rise, Minneapolis, Minn, Incentive Community Enterprises, Mass	Menu of job options Eclectic – both Place-Train & Train-Place Wide range of clients served	Takes years to establish More suitable for urban areas No published evaluations

Boston University's Psychiatric Rehabilitation Model

At the Boston (BU) Center for Psychiatric Rehabilitation, Anthony and his colleagues have been developing a conceptually grounded rehabilitation approach that has roots in both client-centered therapy and skills training (Anthony, 1980; Farkas & Anthony, 1989). Unlike the other four current approaches described in this section, the Boston University (BU) psychiatric rehabilitation model has developed in an academic setting.

In a quasi-experimental evaluation of the BU psychiatric rehabilitation model, Goering, Wasylenki, Farkas, Lancee, and Ballantyne (1988) examined 2-year outcomes for 82 clients, comparing experimental subjects to historically matched controls. The experimental treatment was a case management program, using case managers trained according to the Boston model. The rate of paid employment was 20% for the experimental group, compared with 13% for controls, a nonsignificant difference. However, using a measure of "instrumental role," defined as ability to function as worker, student, volunteer, or homemaker, significantly more of the experimental subjects than controls were rated as successful.

Danley and Rogers (1989) have further articulated the vocational aspect of the BU model as entailing a *Choose-Get-Keep* sequence. Transitional Employment Enterprises (TEE), an agency experienced in providing vocational training to a range of vocationally disadvantaged clients, adopted the Choose-Get-Keep model in a new project designed for persons with severe mental illness (Trotter, Minkoff, Harrison, & Hoops, 1988). The BU model emphasizes extended exploration of career options before community placement. Accordingly, TEE's program included two phases of preemployment training, averaging 2 to 6 months, before clients graduated to the job-seeking phase. An evaluation of their program showed that 35% of program participants obtained competitive employment. Role functioning in nonvocational life domains did not predict successful placement.

The strength of the BU model is its focus on client choice, an emphasis that has been overlooked in many vocational programs. One effect of this counseling focus has been to enable clients to feel more satisfied with their vocational choices (Goering et al., 1988). Other studies suggest that a focus on career development increases client involvement in the rehabilitation process (Farley et al., 1988; Kline & Hoisington, 1981). Career exploration seems especially appropriate for addressing "career immaturity" that characterizes a significant subset of clients with severe mental illness (Ciardiello & Bingham, 1982). Poor job retention rates occur partly because clients are placed in jobs they do not choose. Often these are dead-end jobs that they find demeaning.

One indication that client preferences have been neglected is their absence in the empirical literature. The next generation of evaluations will undoubtedly examine quality of life, quality of the work place, and client satisfaction (Schalock, 1988).

A drawback to the BU model is its untested assumption that extended prevocational career exploration will lead to better outcomes. What has been shown to date is that career exploration leads to greater satisfaction with choices. However, satisfaction with choices is different from success in employment, as noted by Bolton (1988): "Vocational interests are relatively independent of the abilities that determine occupational success" (p. 180). More research is needed to determine how success and satisfaction can be jointly maximized.

Job Club

The job club is an intensive behavioral counseling program based on Skinnerian principles. The focus is on job finding with clients taking ultimate responsibility for obtaining jobs. Job finding is viewed as involving interpersonal skills, a social information network, and motivational factors (Azrin & Philip, 1980).

The emergence of the job club in the 1980s as a major VR activity is consistent with the mounting evidence that the only counselor activities associated with successful VR closures are services in close proximity to the job search itself (Vandergoot, 1986). According to past surveys, rehabilitation professionals typically spend less than 10% of their time on placement-related activities, thus partially explaining low competitive employment rates for clients with severe disabilities (Vandergoot, 1986).

Azrin and Philip's (1980) initial study with a heterogeneous sample of unemployed persons reported extraordinary success rates for job club participants. For job club clients who had been in a mental institution, the employment rate was 90%, compared to 33% for controls. Job club clients "with mental problems" achieved a 94% employment rate. A replication reported that 42% of the job club members were placed in employment, compared with 13% of controls (Keith, Engelkes, & Winborn, 1977). Unfortunately, this study did not report separate statistics for different disability groups. Eisenberg and Cole (1986) compared veterans with mental illness participating in a job club with a demographically matched control group. During a 5-month follow-up period, 61% of the 26 experimental subjects had found employment, compared with only 10% of the controls, a significant difference.

A series of uncontrolled studies on the Brentwood Job Finding Club by Jacobs and his colleagues (Jacobs, Kardashian, Kreinbring, Ponder, & Simpson, 1984; Jacobs et al., 1988) provides the most extensive information on the application of the job club to the psychiatric population. A study with a Veterans Administration (VA) psychiatric population found that 56% of those entering the program obtained a job; 68% of those employed who were located after 6 months were still employed (Jacobs et al., 1984). In a subsequent study, 51% of all participants found vocationally productive placements (Jacobs et al., 1988). However, a third study obtained a more heterogeneous sample than the preceding two studies. In this last study, which included referrals from community-based treatment and residential care programs, the success rate dropped to 29% (Jacobs et al., 1988). VA referrals had a 37% success rate, compared to a 17% success rate for non-VA referrals. Moreover, only 12% of clients diagnosed with schizophrenia or bipolar disorder achieved employment, compared to 45% of the remainder, who had diagnoses of substance abuse, anxiety disorder, or depression. Recipients of Supplemental Security Income (SSI) had significantly poorer outcomes. Poor work history and poor interviewing also were negatively associated with employment. Thus, the job club is an excellent option for clients who are not overly disabled, but it is apparently an inadequate response for clients with severe psychiatric disabilities.

One drawback to the job club model is that it does not address job retention. Similarly, the job club literature has generally not reported job retention statistics beyond a short follow-up period. Moreover, documentation of program dropouts has been weak.

A logical extension of the job club model is use of behavioral strategies to improve job retention. Mueser and Liberman (1988) report a successful case study of a behavioral approach to helping a client acquire the social skills necessary to retain a job. A large sample controlled study of this individualized approach applied to vocational issues would be a major contribution to the literature.

Assertive Community Treatment

ACT includes programs in which assertive outreach and service coordination is used to help clients in their natural environment.

The prototype is the Program for Assertive Community Treatment (PACT) in Madison, Wisconsin, developed by Stein and Test (1980). Unlike facility-based models, PACT provides in vivo training in the activities of daily living.

ACT is widely regarded as a promising, commonsense approach. Its demonstrated efficacy in increasing community tenure is substantial. It is flexible, in that it can be adapted to both small and large programs. It is also well suited to rural communities (Rutkowski & Howick, 1986). Because the approach is individualized, clients with a wide variety of characteristics are appropriate for referral. ACT programs provide time-unlimited support, which is believed to be important for job retention. The ACT philosophy of defining client services as the responsibility of a single core team avoids the fragmentation that has hampered vocational initiatives.

Harbinger, a Michigan ACT program, was evaluated in a controlled study of 91 clients (Mulder, 1982). The study results are difficult to evaluate because of compromises made in the randomization procedure, the lack of a fixed follow-up period, and lack of details in the final report. However, it is the only controlled study outside of Madison of an ACT program with a vocational focus. Harbinger placed clients in volunteer positions in community businesses. Follow-up interviews were completed on 90% of Harbinger clients and only 56% of control clients. The difference in employment rates—26% for Harbinger clients and 18% for controls—was not significant. The mean annual earnings from employment was $537 higher for Harbinger clients than for controls.

Another controlled study of ACT found no differences in employment status between ACT clients and controls (Hoult, Reynolds, Charbonneau-Powis, Weekes, & Briggs, 1983). However, the description of the ACT program did not include any mention of a vocational emphasis.

Unfortunately, few ACT programs have developed their vocational capacity as extensively as the PACT program in Madison, so it remains unclear how easily the vocational aspect of the ACT model can be replicated. Finally, the cost effectiveness of the ACT model's individual placement approach to employment remains an open question.

Psychosocial Rehabilitation and Transitional Employment

PSR developed out of a self-help group for ex-psychiatric patients (Dincin, 1975). Accordingly, it deemphasizes the patient role and stresses the client's own responsibility for rehabilitation. Clients are referred to as *members*, and the rehabilitation process stresses principles of normalization. Status distinctions between staff workers and members are often blurred. PSR programs attempt to address basic needs of members for housing, recreation, social support, and employment. Most PSR programs emphasize the principle of gradualism (Dincin, 1975). According to this principle, clients may move through a continuum in each of several critical life domains (such as employment, independent living, and socializing) in the process of achieving full integration in the community.

A key element in the vocational continuum is TE. Beard et al. (1982) have listed 18 formal characteristics of TE, including the following: The positions are temporary, and they "belong" to the PSR agency, not the members. Members typically work half-time, in entry-level jobs in community settings. Job failures are accepted as part of the vocational process, and members may work many different TE positions.

PSR is a well-defined model with a strong national network. These are valuable characteristics for implementation and community acceptance. The long history of PSR suggests that it has survived a trial-and-error process during which its methods have been refined.

Several recent surveys suggest the extent

to which the PSR model has been disseminated. Stratoudakis (1986) has reported 178 clubhouses modeled after Fountain House. Rutman and Armstrong (1985) surveyed 114 TE programs and found that among clients completing TE, 35% were employed and 16% were on another TE placement. One of the key findings was a fair degree of fidelity in emulating the Fountain House model among those programs surveyed.

One drawback to PSR programs is that clients develop an institutional dependency on the prevocational work crews (Bond & Boyer, 1988). Some studies have suggested that PSR clubs have difficulty moving the majority of clients beyond prevocational activities. A Maryland survey of 28 PSR centers found that only 5% of their clients were placed in competitive employment in a 12-month period (Connors, Graham, & Pulso, 1987). A case study of one PSR program found that clients had alternating cycles of progress and regression, and that they returned more frequently to prevocational crews than to any other program component (Turkat & Buzzell, 1982). Clinical impressions suggest that the step from TE to competitive employment may simply be too large for some clients.

The nonexperimental evidence on the efficacy of the PSR and TE models is equivocal. Some reports suggest competitive employment rates exceeding 40% for graduates (Rehab Brief, 1986; Ruffner, 1986). To what degree these figures are affected by self-selection is hard to judge. Moreover, none of the controlled studies of PSR have shown positive results for employment.

Another criticism of Fountain House and other clubhouses following its paradigm is that they have traditionally taken a fairly rigid stance to the kinds of agency-employer relationships they will undertake. For example, the TE model stipulates that jobs belong to the PSR agency, not the member. Consistent with this principle, Rutman and Armstrong's (1985) survey reported that only 15% of TE participants converted their TE position into a permanent job. Thus, the disadvantage of a clearly defined model is a tendency to rule out other options.

Job Bank Extensions of Transitional Employment

A label for the final type of vocational approach is approximated, although inadequately, by the term *job bank*. This approach is characterized by expansion of vocational services into a wide array of options, partly as a function of community business opportunities. The job bank capitalizes on relationships with a variety of cooperating employers. Employment specialists therefore already have a list of available employment possibilities when they begin vocational planning with a new or returning client. The menu of job opportunities the job bank affords its members distinguishes it from all the other models described above. Clients have the advantage of a range of options in terms of types of jobs, work schedules, duration of employment, and hours worked per week. Moreover, such programs offer relatively easy entry, exit, and reentry to new jobs.

Three agencies that exemplify this eclectic approach are Thresholds (in Chicago), Rise (in Minneapolis) (Barrett & Lavin, 1987; Prieve & DePoint, 1987), and Incentive Community Enterprises (in Massachusetts) (Campbell, 1988). Unlike Fountain House, these agencies have experimented widely with different vocational options. These agencies are pragmatic, and they have avoided a rigid ideology regarding the single "best" agency-employer arrangement.

For example, over the past 30 years many innovations have transformed the Thresholds vocational program from a clubhouse approach based on Fountain House to a complex and eclectic set of vocational strategies. A partial list of strategies includes a factory enclave (Bond, 1987; Forman, 1988), arrangements with local food services industries to supply them with trainees, supported employment opportunities, a mobile job support team, and special arrangements with community employers in which Thresholds, in essence, functions as an employment agency. In the realm of supported employment, Thresholds staff have been examining supportive roles for coworkers. A recent program development has been the Community Scholars Program, a "supported education" approach in which clients are assisted in the completion of university and technical school coursework. Thirty-six clients had enrolled in the Community Scholars Program by the end of 1988 (Thresholds Community Scholars, 1990). Thresholds also continues to have a strong TE program. In a 1986 survey of 135 agencies offering TE to persons with severe mental illness in the United States, Thresholds ranked first in the number of members on job placement, first in the total annual wages paid to members, and fourth in the total number of employers (Thresholds Newsletter, 1987).

The Rise program provides a similar range of options: enclaves, typically for lower functioning clients with multiple disabilities; training programs for data entry and for nursing assistant certification; and conventional TE (Barrett & Lavin, 1987; Prieve & DePoint, 1987).

Discussion of Current Approaches

These five vocational approaches vary on a number of critical dimensions. None emphasizes traditional psychometric assessment. The BU model employs a functional assessment approach that explores the skills necessary for a client to be successful and satisfied in the environment of choice (Anthony, Cohen, & Danley, 1988). The job club uses behavioral assessment to identify specific skill deficits in job acquisition. ACT stresses community-based assessments and job tryouts (Bond, 1987). PSR programs have used prevocational work crews as a context for situational assessments (Bond & Friedmeyer, 1987). The job bank agencies use a combination of strategies. Among the five approaches discussed, ACT is most similar to the individual placement SE approach, to be described in the next section.

With regard to prevocational training, the approaches vary from the BU model, which stresses extensive prevocational exploration, to the job club, which consists of only 20 hours of training prior to the job search. Empirically, PSR programs appear to have extended prevocational preparation for most clients. ACT and job bank programs are individualized and in theory are flexible about preparatory time.

As we look toward the future, Wehman's (1986) *place-train* paradigm may affect both the conceptualization and implementation of psychiatric vocational programs. Of the five current approaches presented, only the BU approach explicitly stresses the desirability of extended preparation in protected environments. Accordingly, programs adopting BU principles have not encouraged rapid entry of clients into community employment (Bond, 1990a).

Important comparative issues remain unanswered. What are the self-selection biases to the respective approaches? Clients with prior work history appear to do better, regardless of vocational approach, but are some approaches more adaptable? How easily can each approach be implemented in new areas? The clubhouse has had the widest dissemination. Is it incompatible with medically oriented CMHCs? How has the clubhouse been adapted? Aspects of the ACT approach have similarly been widely adopted, but the inclusion of a vocational counselor on the ACT team, as found in some Wisconsin CSPs, is rare. With regard to ongoing support, which approaches actually provide the necessary intensity of intervention? Only the job club approach explicitly excludes ongoing support from its program description. How cost-effective is each approach? Which approaches do clients prefer? This is only a sampling of questions that merit attention.

A LOOK AT A POSSIBLE FUTURE: SUPPORTED EMPLOYMENT

Definition of Supported Employment

Supported employment as defined by 1987 federal guidelines consists of three elements: (a) competitive employment (defined as employment paid at commensurate wages with an average of 20 hours of work per week), (b) an integrated work setting, and (c) the provision of ongoing support services (Wehman, 1988). The guidelines stipulate three types of integrated work settings, which have become known as (a) the individual placement approach, (b) the enclave, and (c) the mobile work crew (Moon & Griffin, 1988). These guidelines also state that SE is intended for "individuals who, because of the severity of their handicaps, would not traditionally be eligible for VR services" (Wehman, 1988, p. 5).

In the federal guidelines, TE is listed explicitly as a type of SE. Its inclusion in the SE guidelines was *political*, and not a conceptually elegant decision. The prospects for VR funding to SE programs explains the lobbying activity on behalf of the TE language.

Historically, TE has evolved quite differently from SE, although the motivations for the development of each are related. As previously described, TE was originally developed by Fountain House for persons with severe mental illness. By contrast, SE developed out of the normalization movement for persons with MR.

Definitionally, the chief distinction between SE and TE is that TE is *time-limited* whereas SE is not. Edelstein (1988) has noted three assumptions of TE not shared by SE: (a) prevocational training should precede placement, (b) clients should be able to function at the competitive production levels at the time of placement, and (c) follow-up supports are not permanent and ongoing.

Philosophically, there are points of convergence and divergence (Anthony & Blanch, 1987; Bond, 1987). Both SE and TE stress the importance of placing clients in real work settings, and both deemphasize traditional assessment approaches. TE, however, minimizes the importance of the job match for a TE client, because the TE work experience is valued as an opportunity to work and to earn money in an integrated setting. Because the job is temporary, the specific content of the job is less important.

The SE Movement

Wehman, Kregal, and Shafer (1989) have documented the growth of SE services in 27 states that received federal SE funding. According to their survey, these states reported serving 9,633 SE clients in 1986. By 1988 this number had grown to 24,817. The vast majority (72%) of 1988 SE clients had a primary disability of MR. However, 14.6% had long-term mental illness. Individual placements accounted for 65% of the 1988 placements, followed by the enclave (20%), the work crew (6%), and small businesses (4%). The most popular SE occupations have been custodial (35%), food service (23%), manufacturing (12%), and clerical (3%). The majority of clients (73%) met the federal guidelines by working at least 20 hours per week, although 40% of the individual placement clients did not. Hill's (1988) surveys suggest that SE programs have not fulfilled the intent of federal guidelines in that most SE recipients are only mildly or moderately disabled. Wehman (1988) has acknowledged this discrepancy.

To summarize, SE is a popular movement at present, probably fostered in part by economic conditions that brought a demand for new workers in the service sector. Campbell (1988) notes that supported employment involves a reconceptualization of the problem from a client to a societal focus. The problem is defined in terms of unemployment, not disability. Following this logic, the solution lies with local industries, *not* with human service organizations.

Although SE can be conceptualized as a program model, the existing literature has focused largely on the systems aspects implied by its introduction. This emphasis is not accidental because adoption of SE requires a radical shift in thinking in both the VR and MH systems. Moreover, the proponents of SE have been politically astute and sensitive to the problems of assimilation of new models into the existing VR system. Despite Wehman's assertions that SE is a movement for all disabilities, in most states it has remained focused mainly on the MR population. We now turn to efforts directed specifically at the psychiatric population.

SE for Persons with Severe Mental Illness

In 1978 a cooperative agreement was made between the Rehabilitation Services Administration and the National Institute of Mental Health to improve vocational services for the chronically mentally ill. This agreement led many state vocational rehabilitation (VR) and mental health (MH) departments to follow suit (Stratoudakis, 1986). Additionally, supported employment legislation provided funding for SE demonstration projects. In some states this funding resulted in projects targeting the psychiatric population (Rehab Brief, 1987).

Statewide SE projects aimed at the psychiatric population are a recent phenomenon, and virtually no statistical data on them are available. The early results from these demonstration projects have been mixed.

In 1983 Pennsylvania funded 33 "industry-integrated" projects at a cost of $2.5 million. During the first year of operation, 920 clients were served and 174 were placed. However, only 47 clients were rehabilitated, using VR criteria for successful closure. The second year brought a large increase in successful closures (Forbrich, 1986).

In 1983, the Ohio DMH initiated a study of vocational services for persons with severe mental illness (Saveanu & Roth, 1986). Over a 4-year period, 2,323 clients were rehabilitated, at an average per-client cost of $2601. Of the 7,164 clients referred, 71% were accepted for rehabilitation services. This is an encouraging rate because of the history throughout the United States of screening out clients believed to be too severely disabled. The fact that only 20% of the referrals came directly from the CMHCs suggested a major gap in the full implementation of the interagency agreement. In a survey of VR and MH practitioners, each tended to blame the *other's* system for implementation problems (Saveanu & Roth, 1986).

Indiana provided $1.2 million targeted for 10 vocational projects during 1986–1987. The guidelines for these projects included the requirements that they be "industry integrated, complement existing services, and lead to competitive employment" (Indiana, DMH, 1985, p. 1). The success in implementation of the 10 projects was mixed. Five were judged moderate successes, and five had major implementation problems.

Outcome Findings from an SE Demonstration Project

Nichols (1989) evaluated one of the 10 Indiana demonstration projects. It used an individual placement approach provided by Morgan County Rehabilitation Services (MCRS), a comprehensive rehabilitation center in central Indiana. The sample consisted of 25 clients who were followed for an average of 66 weeks after admission to the program. The clients were mostly referred from local CMHCs. Although the target population was intended to be clients with severe mental illness, the sample characteristics suggested that this population was less impaired than typical CSP clientele. For example, only 36% were SSI or Social Security Disability Income (SSDI) recipients and only 32% had a diagnosis of schizophrenia. Nevertheless, the majority of clients were severely disabled, as suggested by an average of three prior psychiatric hospitalizations and an average of only 1 month of employment in the preceding year.

During the study period, 80% of the clients were employed at least once, and 52% were employed at the end of the study period. Nineteen clients were employed at least once before the last month of the study period. They averaged 30.7 weeks of employment, earning an average of $2,616. They also averaged 28 hours of employment per week with an average hourly wage of $4.00. The average number of hours worked per week varied widely; 36% averaged fewer than the 20 hours per week stipulated by the federal definition of SE.

The 19 clients achieving competitive employment received an average of only 19.4 hours of job coaching, or approximately 40 minutes of job coaching per week of employment. Clients also averaged 75.9 hours of attendance in an employment support group. Number of hours of job coaching was negatively correlated with average number of hours worked per week. Thus, clients who worked full time had far less job coaching than those who worked only a few hours a week, as might be expected.

The "VR process" was a major interest in this study. MCRS conceptualized their program as consisting of two major phases, a *prevocational* phase and a *placement* phase. The prevocational phase was further sequenced into: *VR referral* (the time required for establishing the client's eligibility for VR services), *vocational evaluation*, and *work adjustment* (consisting of sheltered workshop and TE placements). Periods of time in which clients temporarily dropped out of the vocational program were classified as *hold* time. Hold status occurred for a wide range of reasons, including medication problems, attempts by clients to find jobs on their own outside the rehabilitation program, concerns about losing Social Security benefits, and requests by staff at the CMHC. Once in the placement phase, clients began the job search in collaboration with the job developer. The placement phase consisted of three types of activities: searching for jobs (*search*), working (*job*), and periods of inactivity (*hold*).

The average duration in each of the program phases for the sample of 25 clients is displayed in Figure 11.1. Time was apportioned as follows: prevocational phase (28%), searching for a job (19%), hold status (19%), and competitive employment (36%). The length of time spent in the various preparation phases was either unrelated, or negatively related, to vocational outcomes, after controlling for time in program. Thus, these data do not support the notion that an extended preparation time enhances one's job retention.

The obstacles to employment can be clarified by examining the apportionment of time across the various phases. Clients averaged 18.4 weeks in the prevocational phase before starting the job search. This delay is noteworthy, because the program was conceptualized as a rapid placement approach. Moreover, MCRS was the most committed of the 10 Indiana demonstration projects to reducing the administrative and other barriers to community employment. Specifically, MCRS streamlined the VR eligibility process and deemphasized both vocational evaluation and prevocational preparation. Thus the prevocational phase was *shorter* than in the other projects. Even so, the 4-month preparation period may be less than optimal.

After clients entered the placement phase, the process of vocational rehabilitation was not linear. Three factors influenced the stability of job tenure: hold status, job changes, and hospitalizations. Clients averaged 12.9 weeks in hold status, 91% of which occurred *after* they entered the placement phase. Twelve clients held two or more jobs. Three of the 25 clients were hospitalized during the study period.

Demographic and diagnostic variables had little bearing on either the rehabilitation process (as measured by length of time in the program components and amount of job

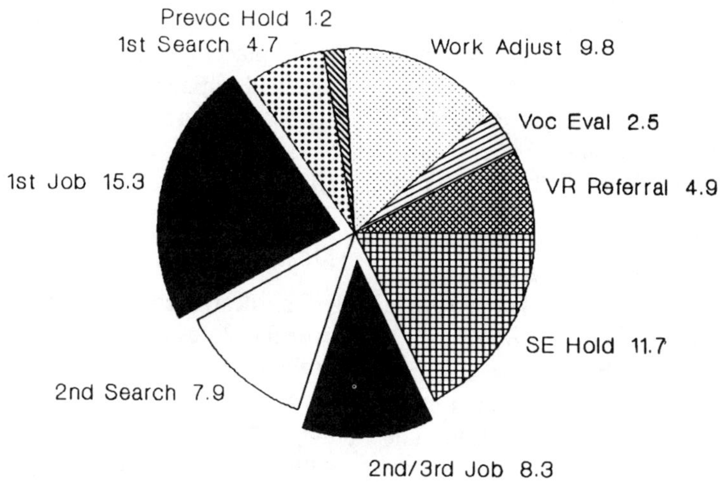

Figure 11.1. Average duration in SE phase. Average number of weeks spent in each vocational program phase for 19 clients with severe mental illness. *Note:* Values are weeks in each phase. SE = supported employment; VR = vocational rehabilitation; Voc Eval = vocational evaluation; Prevoc Hold = prevocational hold. (Adapted from Nichols, 1989.)

coaching and number of support groups attended), or on outcomes. SSI and SSDI recipients, however, had significantly poorer outcomes compared to nonrecipients.

Discussion of Supported Employment

The debate on the merits of SE for the psychiatric population has been obscured by a lack of hard data, conceptual confusion, and the confluence of *program* and *systems* issues. The Pennsylvania, Ohio, and Indiana projects suggest that systems change is slow. Others have also concluded that cooperation between VR and MH programs is problematic (Dellario, 1985; Noble & Collignon, 1988).

The Nichols study shows that achievement of competitive employment is difficult even when rapid placement is an objective. The barriers included both client resistance and administrative barriers. Client resistance became more salient when clients were closer to actual employment than when they were engaged in prevocational activities. As other studies have found, client resistance was also greater when clients were receiving Social Security benefits. Long-standing administrative barriers included those imposed by both the VR system, with its cumbersome eligibility process, and the MH system, with the lack of referrals.

Future research should differentiate SE approaches for clients with psychiatric disabilities from the approaches used with the MR population. One difference already widely reported is a different conception of job coaching with the psychiatric population than with MR clients. Quantitatively, clients with severe mental illness receive far less job coaching at the job site. For example, the average of 19.4 hours of job coaching in the Nichols study for an average 30-week employment period is far less than the 113-hour average during an initial 12-week training period for MR clients reported by Hill (1988), or the average of 233.2 hours reported more recently by Wehman et al. (1989). Supplementing the job coaching in the mental health system is case management. The empirical literature suggests that the consistency of follow-along support is instrumental in job retention (Bond, 1987), although this has not been shown directly for supported employment. Wehman (1986) has described SE as a *place-train* model. For the psychiatric population a more apt term may be *place/follow-along*, because the support does not typically involve job coaches training clients in job-specific skills.

The nonlinearity of the rehabilitation process observed in the Nichols study has also been noted by Strauss, Hafez, Lieberman, and Harding (1985). Insofar as SE provides time-unlimited support and allows for flexible arrangements in the number of hours clients work, it is well suited to the frequent and unpredictable variations in status characteristic of the psychiatric population. The finding that clients in the Nichols study were given a second and third opportunity for competitive employment is consistent with the Fountain House philosophy of tolerating job failures (Beard et al., 1982).

ONE FUTURE DIRECTION FOR RESEARCH: THE *TIMING* OF PLACEMENT

Wehman (1986) has hypothesized that a place-train sequence is more effective for persons with severe disabilities than the conventional train-place approach. This hypothesis should be tested directly, especially because it goes against the conventional VR wisdom. Not all experts agree that Wehman's hypothesis applies to the psychiatric population. In particular, the BU model represents a dissenting viewpoint (Anthony & Blanch, 1987).

One fact is apparent. If clients are to have rapid entry into integrated work experiences, employment specialists must take an assertive approach to both the VR and MH systems. To date, the main evidence that a place-train model is effective is based on demonstration projects showing reasonable placement and retention rates for MR clients who have had little prior competitive employment within the traditional sheltered workshop programs. The Thresholds accelerated placement study (Bond & Dincin, 1986), although conducted between 1980 and 1983 and therefore somewhat dated, offers the only direct experimental evidence on a rapid placement approach with any severely disabled population. For this reason it is described in some detail.

Method

Design

The design compared two vocational approaches designated as *accelerated* and *gradual*. Clients randomly assigned to the accelerated condition were placed in a TE position (typically an enclave) 1 month after admission to Thresholds. Clients in the gradual condition attended prevocational work crews for a minimum of 4 months before they were eligible for TE.

Sample Characteristics

The study eligibility criteria for clients were the following: (a) 18 years of age, (b) unemployed, (c) stated goal of employment, and (d) minimum attendance of 40 hours during the first 4 weeks at Thresholds.

In the sample of 131 clients accepted into the study, the mean age was 24.5. Modally, the clients were males (69%), whites (75%), and high school graduates (80%). Diagnoses, obtained by the client's case worker from the most recent hospital records, indicated 55% with schizophrenia, 19% with a major affective disorder, and 26% with a personality disorder. The sample averaged 3.2 prior psychiatric hospitalizations. At the time of admission, 61% were receiving government assistance (either SSI or SSDI), 31% were supported by their parents, and 8% stated they were self-supporting. The median number of years in prior competitive employment was 2 years. The median length of unemployment immediately prior to admission was 9 months.

Predictor Variables

Client background variables were obtained during an interview conducted 1 month after program admission. In addition to demographics, three employment variables were coded: work experience, months employed, and months unemployed. Work experience was a dichotomous variable distinguishing between clients who had worked 1 year continuously in competitive employment and those who had never done so. Months employed was defined as the time in paid employment before admission. Months unemployed was measured between the termination from the last job held and date of admission (with a value of 70 months assigned to those who had never worked).

Two types of staff ratings were obtained. At study admission, a research assistant made ratings on the Global Assessment Scale (GAS) (Endicott, Spitzer, Fleiss, & Cohen, 1976). A situational assessment, based on staff ratings of client work performance in prevocational work crews and TE placements, was obtained for 84 clients an average of 5 months after program admission (Bond & Friedmeyer, 1987). (Situational assessments were not obtained for early program dropouts.)

At study admission, clients made self-ratings of general capacity to cope with problems on a 7-point Coping-Mastery scale (Pearlin & Schooler, 1978). Clients also completed the Work Performance Inventory, a 22-item inventory of common obstacles to job retention (e.g., symptoms, lack of education, work conditions, work stress) adapted from Westermeyer and Harrow (1987).

Dropout status was coded as a 3-point scale, based on whether a client dropped out during the first 4 months in the program, dropped out between the fourth and ninth months, or was an active client of the program for the entire 15-month study period.

Vocational Outcome Variables

Three outcome variables were examined for 107 clients located for interviews 15 months after study admission. Employment status was based on the client's status at the time of the follow-up interview. A 5-point scale was used: (a) competitive employment, (b) individual TE placement, (c) group TE placement, (d) prevocational work crew, (e) unemployed. Weeks worked was defined as the total number of weeks of paid employment over the final 11-month period. Earnings referred to all wages earned during that time.

Findings from the Accelerated Placement Study

As shown in Table 11.5, the two most potent predictors of vocational success were dropout status and situational assessment ratings. The correlations for the dropout status variable are probably underestimates, in that employment information on many of the early program dropouts could not be obtained at follow-up. The third largest correlation in Table 11.5 was between assignment to experimental condition and weeks worked during follow-up.

Among the employment history variables, work experience was modestly correlated with vocational outcome, and length of unemployment was negatively correlated with earnings. Reception of government assistance was negatively correlated with outcome. Finally, education showed a marginal correlation with outcomes. Except for those variables already mentioned, client characteristics were not helpful in predicting vocational success. Hospitalization history, global functioning, and client's self-report were not correlated with outcomes.

Three Conditions Enhancing Vocational Success

The pattern of correlations suggested a post hoc representation of the findings based on the intuitive notion that the pathway to employment consists of a series of successive hurdles. The findings were organized around a division of the sample into five subsamples defined by an *approximate* chronological hierarchy, based on clients' progression through the program. This is diagrammed

Table 11.5. Predictors of Vocational Outcomes in Thresholds Study by Bond & Dincins, 1986

PREDICTOR VARIABLE	SAMPLE SIZE	15-MONTH EMPLOYMENT STATUS[a]	WEEKS WORKED	EARNINGS
Demographic Variables				
Age	107	.06	.10	.09
Sex[b]	107	.02	−.16	−.06
Race[c]	107	.10	.04	−.02
Education	107	.17	.19*	.15
Diagnosis, Disability, and Duration				
Schizophrenia/other	107	.15	.00	.03
Income assistance[d]	107	−.21*	−.21*	−.23*
No. of psychiatric hospitalizations	107	.04	−.07	−.11
Vocational Variables				
Work experience[a]	107	.21*	.23*	.20*
Months employed	107	.13	.09	.11
Months unemployed	107	−.18	−.10	−.20*
Staff Ratings				
Global assessment scale[a]	102	−.03	−.01	.08
Situational assessment[a]	77	.48**	.55**	.57**
Client Self-Ratings				
Coping mastery[a]	85	.03	−.02	.09
Work performance inventory[a]	103	−.08	.00	−.01
Vocational Program Variables				
Dropout status[e]	107	−.51**	−.46**	−.22*
Gradual/accelerated	107	.15	.38**	.21*

Note: Categorical variables were coded as follows for calculating Pearson correlations:
[a]Higher scores indicate better functioning.
[b]Sex: Male = 1, Female = 2.
[c]Race: White = 1, Black or Latino = 2.
[d]Income assistance: Self-support = 1, Parental support = 2, Government assistance = 3.
[e]Dropout status: Active for 15 months = 1, Terminated between 4 and 9 months = 2, Terminated within 4 months = 3.
*$p < .05$.
**$p < .001$.

in Figure 11.2. The first variable, labeled *persistence*, was defined by duration in the Thresholds program. Two subgroups of dropouts were defined: those who dropped out within 4 months and those who dropped out between 4 and 9 months. The second variable, labeled *performance*, was defined by staff ratings on the situational assessment. Among clients active for at least 9 months, those who scored below the median on the situational assessment rating were classified in this third group. The third variable, labeled *placement*, was defined by the experimental condition. Two groups were identified among clients who were active for at least 9 months and who scored above the median on the situational assessment: those who were randomly assigned to the standard gradual program with prevocational preparation, and those assigned to the accelerated TE program.

The three variables were not statistically independent. Although persistence and placement were uncorrelated, performance

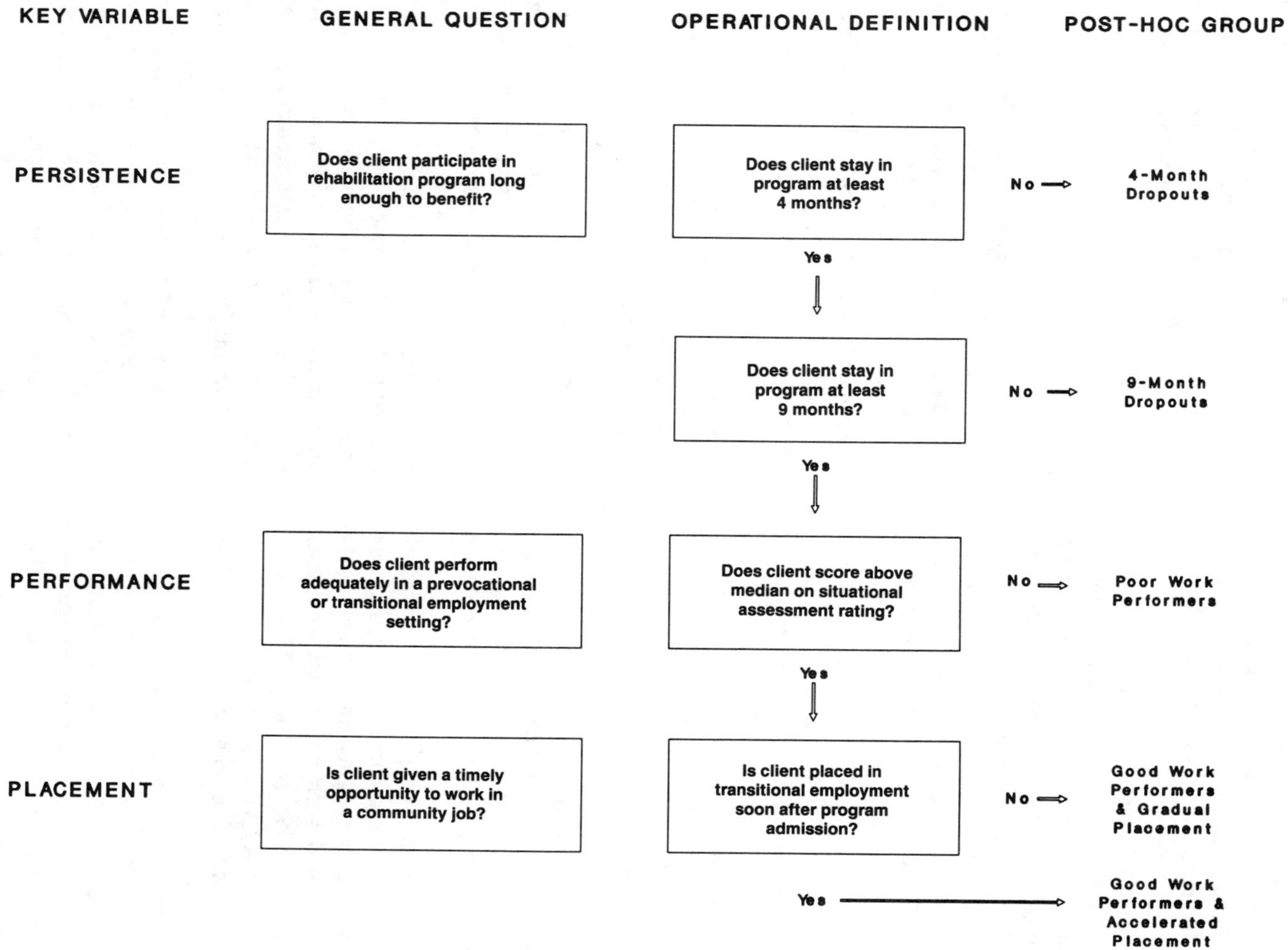

Figure 11.2. Three conditions for employment success among persons with serious mental illness.

was related to both persistence and placement. Dropout status was correlated with poorer performance on the situational assessment (r (82) = −.26, $p < .01$). More surprising was the finding that accelerated clients had higher assessment ratings than did gradual clients (t (75) = 2.00, $p < .05$).

Persistence appeared to be a critical precondition for successful rehabilitation. As seen in Table 11.6, dropout status identified two subgroups of unsuccessful clients. It is logical to ask further if any client characteristics predict dropout status. In the current study, however, the only predictor variable listed in Table 11.5 that was correlated with dropout status was educational level (r = −.27, $p < .001$). More educated clients were less likely to drop out.

Performance in the vocational domain (as measured by the situational assessment) is a second condition for employment success. In the current study, various global indicators of role functioning, including a rating of global functioning and client's self-assessments, were not predictive of outcomes. In contrast, those who received low ratings on the situational assessment had poor vocational outcomes regardless of their accelerated or gradual vocational programs assignment.

Months employed prior to study admission was the only client background variable among those listed in Table 11.5 that was correlated with situational assessment ratings (r = .19, $p < .05$). Thus, client background information yielded little predictive information on a client's actual work performance.

Placement was also important for enhancing employment outcomes. Among the subgroup of clients who demonstrated adequate work performance, those in the accelerated TE program were compared to clients in the standard (gradual) program. Accelerated clients had better vocational outcomes than gradual clients: over twice as many accelerated clients were competitively employed and had worked significantly more weeks.

Discussion of the Accelerated Placement Study

From the standpoint of program planning, the findings from the preceding analysis are cause for optimism. The identified factors are all within the control of rehabilitation programs, at least in principle, as discussed below.

Persistence

Several studies have shown that clients who persist, that is, clients who attend PSR programs for an extended period, have the best employment outcomes (Barry, 1982; Bond, 1984; Dincin & Kaberon, 1979; Malamud & McCrory, 1988; Rehab Brief, 1986). Persistence is typically a characteristic attributed to clients and not to programs. However, assertive outreach can increase client participation in rehabilitation (Stein & Test, 1980). No research has yet directly tested the viability of assertive outreach as a means to increase attendance in vocational programs.

Assuming that assertive outreach does increase persistence among clients who otherwise would drop out, a second question is whether reluctant clients so encouraged will benefit from vocational rehabilitation. SE proponents have advanced an idealistic "zero exclusion model," which states that all clients are assumed candidates for employment until proven otherwise (Wehman, 1988). Although this study was not designed to evaluate a zero reject model, its findings can be reexamined in terms of this perspective. Specifically, we examined the outcomes for the subgroup of 30 clients who persisted beyond 9 months but who performed poorly on the situational assessment (see Table 11.6). This subgroup would be viewed by the VR system as poor employment risks. Consistent with that view, they did not have any better vocational outcomes than did program dropouts. Thus, persistence alone provides no guarantee of success in competitive employment.

Table 11.6. Employment Outcomes for the Five Subgroups Identified in Figure 11.2

			EMPLOYMENT STATUS AT 15 MONTHS					
						CREWS		
CLIENT SUBGROUP	WEEKS WORKED[a]	EARNINGS[b]	COMPETITIVE EMPLOYMENT	INDIVIDUAL TRANSITIONAL EMPLOYMENT	GROUP TRANSITIONAL EMPLOYMENT	PREVOCATIONAL	UNEMPLOYED	UNKNOWN
A: 4-month dropouts (N = 19)	5.2	$559	0%	0%	0%	5%	53%	42%
B: 9-month dropouts (N = 35)	10.0	$913	3%	0%	0%	11%	60%	26%
C: Poor work performance (N = 30)	16.1	$731	3%	0%	13%	53%	23%	7%
D: Good performance and gradual preparation (N = 21)	23.1	$1625	14%	19%	19%	33%	5%	10%
E: Good performance and accelerated placement (N = 26)	39.7	$2140	39%	19%	15%	15%	12%	0%

[a]According to the Newman-Keuls test for post hoc comparisons, the following subgroups differ at $p < .05$: A,B < D,E; C,D < E.
[b]According to the Newman-Keuls test for post hoc comparisons, the following subgroups differ at $p < .05$: A,B,C < E.

Clients who do become engaged in rehabilitation but who have limited vocational skills represent a large and important segment of the total population of persons with serious mental illness. Finding appropriate vocational options for this subgroup remains a vexing problem. At a commonsense level, it appears that some form of systematic skills training may be necessary for these clients to achieve employment success.

Performance

The priority of current vocational performance over work history is an affirmation of the Fountain House principle that every consumer deserves a chance to work, regardless of past problems (Beard et al., 1982). The intent of prevocational and TE programs is to improve client work habits and attitudes. We have surprisingly little literature to show that a client's work performance and attitudes in psychosocial rehabilitation settings does improve over time (Growick, 1976). It would be relatively easy to determine whether situational assessment ratings in PSR programs typically show a steady progression, or whether, as is more likely, a nonlinear path to improvement is more common.

Clients working on the prevocational crews had lower situational assessment ratings than did those on TE. Possibly clients in the prevocational crews felt that little was expected of them, as suggested by frequent reference to poor attendance on their rating forms (Bond & Friedmeyer, 1987). The monetary incentive in TE also may have made a difference in performance (Lehrer & Lanoil, 1977).

A further speculation is that the TE job coaches gave higher ratings because they expected more of their clients in an integrated setting. This possible explanation is reminiscent of the finding from educational studies in which teachers' expectations have been experimentally demonstrated to affect student performance (Rosenthal & Jacobson, 1968). In a similar vein, Kiernan and Brinkman (1988) have also noted an interaction between work performance and the work site. One implication is that community-based assessments may be more ecologically valid indicators of a client's potential than are those obtained in artificial settings (Menchetti & Rusch, 1988).

From a programmatic standpoint, it would seem logical to provide skills training in order to improve client performance in prevocational and transitional work settings. The efficacy of skills training has been examined in over 50 studies (Anthony, Cohen, & Cohen, 1984; Liberman, 1988), yet most PSR proponents have adamantly maintained that an experiential learning approach is superior to more structured approaches. In any case, research has not yet closed the causal chain that hypothesizes that clients can be taught vocational skills and thereby achieve success in community employment.

Placement

The provision of job opportunities is a simplistic addition to the rehabilitation model, yet one that has not been fully appreciated. A study using a similar research paradigm but with individual supported employment placements as the accelerated condition is now in progress (Bond, 1990b). Early anecdotal evidence makes it clear that many clients clearly *prefer* early placement over gradual work preparation *including group TE programs* in CMHCs. This unexpected pattern suggests a strong client aversion to prevocational training programs that are considered progressive in many CMHCs. It is reminiscent of recent survey findings on supported and transitional housing: Most clients prefer to live in their own apartments with adequate support from professionals, despite the opinion of most professionals who think the majority of clients need structured group homes (Blanch, Carling, & Ridgway, 1988).

SUMMARY

Like Dickens' *Christmas Carol*, we have examined the past, present, and possible future of vocational programs for persons with severe mental illness.

The limitations of sheltered approaches for most clients with psychiatric disabilities have been widely documented. Although it is customary to note that sheltered alternatives are appropriate for some clients, to operationalize this assumption has proved difficult. Too often the belief that some clients are more suited to sheltered settings has been used to justify wholesale exclusion of clients from competitive employment. Clients themselves are often reluctant to enter vocational programs. Clients who have self-defeating attitudes perhaps are influenced by rehabilitation workers who believe that psychiatric disabilities are a barrier to employment (Bingham, 1988).

The opposite viewpoint, that clients simply need an opportunity in competitive employment, with supports, is also an insufficient formulation. In the accelerated placement study (Bond & Dincin, 1986), for example, there was a subgroup of clients who did not succeed in TE, even though they attended the rehabilitation program for over a year. Multiple vocational options are necessary to address the spectrum of clients who are admitted to CSP programs.

Although prognostication is a risky business, some observers are predicting expansion of SE services for persons with severe mental illness. A recent comprehensive national survey of SE practices in rehabilitation facilities (NARF, 1989) notes that "individuals with chronic mental illness are receiving more attention nationally" (p. 39), although the survey showed only 11% of the individuals served in surveyed SE programs had chronic mental illness. Another recent survey (Tashjian, Hayward, Stoddard, & Kraus, 1989) showed a large discrepancy between the percentage of clients believed by mental health workers to have access to SE and TE programs (70%) and the percentage of clients actually receiving these services (11%). How much and how fast expansion occurs will depend on many factors, including solving the problems of short-term and long-term funding. SE requires attention to systems issues and financing at the program level, whereas VR has historically funded most of its services on a case-by-case *client* basis. The funding problems are not insurmountable, but they require new thinking.

This chapter has argued that our future includes the incorporation of the *principles* of supported employment. It is already clear that Wehman's provocative model, developed for persons with mental retardation, must be modified considerably for persons with severe mental illness. That adaptation is already being attempted across the United States.

Because current programs with vastly different philosophies have adopted the label of *supported employment*, the term has lost its meaning. In place of labels and slogans, we need empirical benchmarks: Whom does your program admit? What is the dropout rate? What self-selection occurs? What is the average duration in each program phase? What do vocational staff do? What are your employment rates? How long do clients hold jobs? How satisfied are they with the jobs they have?

Supported employment has in no sense been "proven." It conforms with a number of working hypotheses, but has not been examined within a rigorous evaluation framework. Several scenarios for the future of SE for persons with severe mental illness are possible, including the following: (a) SE is implemented only under special conditions, such as in agencies that have charismatic administrators, or in communities where the local VR and MH politics are somehow bypassed. (b) Its evolution is heavily influenced by the characteristics of the local communities and economies. For example, the job bank model may become the dominant model in some large cities, whereas the individualized placement model may evolve in less populated areas. (c) Administrators conclude that SE is not cost effective or that the funding dilemmas are insoluble. In the short term, SE programs appear costly and inefficient. As Wehman (1989) notes, "It usually takes 2 to 3 years for the full benefit and placement outcomes of supported employment to accumulate" (p. 8). Questions about economic feasibility have already surfaced in the Pennsylvania and Indiana projects described above, in which the placement rates were low during the early stages of implementation. In fact, in both states, demonstration sites only first began to make genuine progress during the second year of implementation. In the case of Indiana, the projects were funded for only 2 years, thus severely hampering their development from the outset.

The intent of this chapter has been to generate hypotheses. We are still at an early stage of program description (Brekke, 1988), and better classification of vocational approaches will need to be developed in the future. Some process and outcome variables have been suggested in this chapter that may contribute to a consensus battery of measures that all investigators might use.

Time has been a motif of this chapter. In the past, extensive resources have been directed to prevocational activities, with little demonstrable impact. Conversely, few resources have been directed to the postplacement period (Tashjian et al., 1989), resulting in disappointing rates of job retention (Solberg & Raschmann, 1980). It is time to reverse these priorities.

REFERENCES

Anthony, W. A. (1980). *The principles of psychiatric rehabilitation*. Baltimore, MD: University Park Press.

Anthony, W. A., & Blanch, A. (1987). Supported employment for persons who are psychiatrically disabled: An historical and conceptual perspective. *Psychosocial Rehabilitation Journal, 11*(2), 5–23.

Anthony, W. A., Buell, G. J., Sharratt, S., & Althoff, M. E. (1972). The efficacy of psychiatric rehabilitation. *Psychological Bulletin, 78*, 447–456.

Anthony, W. A., Cohen, M. R., & Cohen, B. F. (1984). Psychiatric rehabilitation. In J. A. Talbott (Ed.), *The chronic mental patient: Five years later* (pp. 137–157). Orlando, FL: Grune & Stratton.

Anthony, W. A., Cohen, M. R., & Danley, K. S. (1988). The psychiatric rehabilitation model as applied to vocational rehabilitation. In J. A. Ciardiello & M. D. Bell (Eds.), *Vocational rehabilitation of persons with prolonged mental illness* (pp. 59–80). Baltimore, MD: Johns Hopkins Press.

Anthony, W. A., Cohen, M. R., & Vitalo, R. (1978). The measurement of rehabilitation outcome. *Schizophrenia Bulletin, 4*, 365–383.

Azrin, N. H., & Besalel, V. B. (1979). *Job club counselor's manual: A behavioral approach to vocational counseling*. Baltimore, MD: University Park Press.

Azrin, N. H., & Philip, R. A. (1980). The job club method for the job handicapped: A comparative outcome study. *Rehabilitation Counseling Bulletin, 23*, 144–155.

Barrett, J., & Lavin, D. (1987). *The industrial work model: A guide for developing transitional and supported employment*. Menomonie: Materials Development Center, University of Wisconsin-Stout.

Barry, P. (1982). Correlational study of a psychosocial rehabilitation program. *Vocational Evaluation and Work Adjustment Bulletin, 15*, 112–117.

Beard, J. H., Pitt, R. B., Fisher, S. H., & Goertzel, V. (1963). Evaluating the effectiveness of a psychiatric rehabilitation program. *American Journal of Orthopsychiatry, 33*, 701–712.

Beard, J. H., Propst, R. N., & Malamud, T. J. (1982). The Fountain House model of rehabilitation. *Psychosocial Rehabilitation Journal, 5*(1), 47–53.

Becker, R. E. (1967). An evaluation of a rehabilitation program for chronically hospitalized psychiatric patients. *Social Psychiatry, 2*, 32–38.

Bellamy, G. T., Rhodes, L. E., Bourbeau, P. E., & Mank, D. M. (1986). Mental retardation in sheltered workshops and day activity programs. In F. R. Rusch (Ed.), *Competitive employment: Issues and strategies* (pp. 257–281). Baltimore, MD: Brookes.

Bingham, W. C. (1988). A vocational psychology perspective on rehabilitation. In J. A. Ciardiello & M. D. Bell (Eds.), *Vocational rehabilitation of persons with prolonged mental illness* (pp. 137–149). Baltimore, MD: Johns Hopkins Press.

Black, B. J. (1988). *Work and mental illness: Transitions to employment*. Baltimore, MD: Johns Hopkins Press.

Black, B. J., & Kase, H. M. (1986). Changes in programs over two decades. In B. J. Black (Ed.), *Work as therapy and rehabilitation for the mentally ill* (pp. 3–37). New York: Altro Health and Rehabilitation Services, 40 East 30th Street.

Blanch, A. K., Carling, P. J., & Ridgway, P. (1988). Normal housing with specialized supports: A psychiatric rehabilitation approach to living in the community. *Rehabilitation Psychology, 33*, 47–55.

Bolton, B. (1988). Vocational assessment of persons with psychiatric disorders. In J. A. Ciardiello & M. D. Bell (Eds.), *Vocational rehabilitation of persons with prolonged mental illness* (pp. 165–180). Baltimore, MD: Johns Hopkins Press.

Bond, G. R. (1984). An economic analysis of psychosocial rehabilitation. *Hospital and Community Psychiatry, 35*, 356–362.

Bond, G. R. (1987). Supported work as a modification of the transitional employment model for clients with psychiatric disabilities. *Psychosocial Rehabilitation Journal, 11*(2), 55–75.

Bond, G. R. (1988, August). *Employment outcomes from psychiatric rehabilitation*. Paper presented at a poster session at the annual meeting of the American Psychological Association. Atlanta, GA.

Bond, G. R. (1990a). [Review of *Psychiatric rehabilitation programs: Putting theory into practice*]. *Hospital and Community Psychiatry, 41*, 682–684.

Bond, G. R. (1990b, May). *Controlled studies of transitional and supported employment*. Presentation at annual conference of the International Association of Psychosocial Rehabilitation Services, St. Louis, MO.

Bond, G. R., & Boyer, S. L. (1988). Rehabilitation programs and outcomes. In J. A. Ciardiello & M. D. Bell (Eds.), *Vocational rehabilitation of persons with prolonged mental illness* (pp. 231–263). Baltimore, MD: Johns Hopkins Press.

Bond, G. R., & Dincin, J. (1986). Accelerating entry into transitional employment in a psychosocial rehabilitation agency. *Rehabilitation Psychology, 31*, 143–155.

Bond, G. R., & Friedmeyer, M. H. (1987). Predictive validity of situational assessment at a psychiatric rehabilitation center. *Rehabilitation Psychology, 32*, 99–112.

Brekke, J. S. (1988). What do we really know about community support programs? Strategies for better monitoring. *Hospital and Community Psychiatry, 39*, 946–952.

Briggs, P. F., & Yater, A. C. (1966). Counseling and psychometric signs as determinants in the vocational success of discharged psychiatric patients. *Journal of Clinical Psychology, 22*, 100–104.

Campbell, J. F. (1988). Rehabilitation facilities and community-based employment services. In P. Wehman & M. S. Moon (Eds.), *Vocational rehabilitation and supported employment* (pp. 193–202). Baltimore, MD: Brookes.

Ciardiello, J. A. (1981). Job placement success of schizophrenic clients in sheltered workshop programs. *Vocational Evaluation and Work Adjustment Bulletin, 14*, 125–28, 140.

Ciardiello, J. A., & Bingham, W. C. (1982). The career maturity of schizophrenic clients. *Rehabilitation Counseling Bulletin, 26*, 3–9.

Cnaan, R. A., Blankertz, L., Messinger, K. W., & Gardner, J. R. (1988). Psychosocial rehabilitation: Toward a definition. *Psychosocial Rehabilitation Journal, 11*(4), 61–77.

Collignon, F. C., Noble, J. H., & Toms-Barker, L. (1987). Early lessons from the Marion County demonstration in integrating vocational and mental health services. *Psychosocial Rehabilitation Journal, 11*(2), 75–85.

Connors, K. A., Graham, R. S., & Pulso, R. (1987). Playing the store: Where is the vocational in psychiatric rehabilitation? *Psychosocial Rehabilitation Journal, 10*(3), 21–33.

Criswell, J. H. (1970). Community roles in psychiatric rehabilitation. *Welfare in Review, 8*, 8–15.

Danley, K. S., & Rogers, E. S. (1989). A psychiatric rehabilitation approach to vocational rehabilitation. In M. D. Farkas & W. A. Anthony (Eds.), *Psychiatric rehabilitation programs: Putting theory into practice* (pp. 81–131). Baltimore, MD: Johns Hopkins University Press.

Dellario, D. J. (1985). The relationship between mental health, vocational rehabilitation interagency functioning, and outcome of psychiatrically disabled persons. *Rehabilitation Counseling Bulletin, 28*, 167-170.

Dincin, J. (1975). Psychiatric rehabilitation. *Schizophrenia Bulletin, 1*, 131-148.

Dincin, J., & Kaberon, D. A. (1979). *Attendance as a predictor of success in rehabilitation of former psychiatric patients.* Final report to the Chicago Community Trust, Thresholds, Chicago, IL.

Dincin, J., & Swift, J. W. (1969). *The post-hospital schizophrenic patient.* Final report for SRS Project RD-1058-P. Thresholds, Chicago.

Dincin, J., & Witheridge, T. F. (1982). Psychiatric rehabilitation as a deterrent to recidivism. *Hospital and Community Psychiatry, 33*, 645-650.

Edelstein, T. B. (1988). Rehabilitation facilities and supported employment: Implementation issues. In P. Wehman & M. S. Moon (Eds.), *Vocational rehabilitation and supported employment* (pp. 213-218). Baltimore, MD: Brookes.

Eisenberg, M. G., & Cole, H. W. (1986). A behavioral approach to job seeking for psychiatrically impaired persons. *Journal of Rehabilitation*, April/May/June, pp. 46-49.

Endicott, J., Spitzer, R. L., Fleiss, J. L., & Cohen, J. (1976). The Global Assessment Scale: A procedure for measuring overall severity of psychiatric disturbance. *Archives of General Psychiatry, 33*, 766-771.

Fairweather, G. W., Sanders, D. H., Maynard, H., Cressler, D. L., & Bleck, D. S. (1969). *Community life for the mentally ill.* Chicago: Aldine.

Farkas, M. D., & Anthony, W. A. (1989). *Psychiatric rehabilitation programs: Putting theory into practice.* Baltimore, MD: Johns Hopkins University Press.

Farley, R. C., Schriner, K. F., & Roessler, R. T. (1988). The impact of the Occupational Choice Strategy on the career development of rehabilitation clients. *Rehabilitation Psychology, 33*, 121-125.

Field, G., Allness, D., Knoedler, W., & Test, M. A. (n.d.). *Employment training for chronic mental patients in the community.* Unpublished paper, Program for Assertive Community Treatment, Mendota Mental Health Institute, Madison, WI.

Forbrich, C. B. (1986). *OVR/OMH grant program review.* Rehabilitation in the Community, Bulletin #10. Division of Community Support Programs, Office of Mental Health, Harrisburg, Pennsylvania.

Forman, J. D. (1988). Sheltered work in a non-sheltered setting. *Psychosocial Rehabilitation Journal, 10*(3), 19-28.

Goering, P. N., Wasylenki, D. A., Farkas, M. D., Lancee, W. J., & Ballantyne, R. (1988). What difference does case management make? *Hospital and Community Psychiatry, 39*, 272-276.

Goldberg, S. C., Schooler, N. R., Hogarty, G. E., & Roper, M. (1977). Prediction of relapse in schizophrenic outpatients treated by drug and sociotherapy. *Archives of General Psychiatry, 34*, 171-184.

Gottman, J. M., & Markman, H. J. (1978). Experimental designs in psychotherapy research. In S. L. Garfield & A. E. Bergin (Eds.), *Handbook of psychotherapy and behavior change: An empirical analysis* (2nd ed.) (pp. 23-62). New York: Wiley.

Greenleigh Associates. (1975). *The role of sheltered workshops in the rehabilitation of the severely disabled.* New York: Department of Health, Education, and Welfare.

Griffiths, R. D. (1974). Rehabilitation of chronic psychotic patients. *Psychological Medicine, 4*, 316-325.

Growick, B. S. (1976). Effects of a work-adjustment program on emotionally handicapped individuals. *Journal of Applied Rehabilitation Counseling, 7*, 119-123.

Gunderson, J. G., Frank, A. F., Katz, H. M., Vannicelli, M. L., Frosch, J. P., & Knapp, P. H. (1984). Effects of psychotherapy in schizophrenia: II. Comparative outcome of two forms of treatment. *Schizophrenia Bulletin, 10*, 564-596.

Herz, M. I. (1984). Recognizing and preventing relapse in patients with schizophrenia. *Hospital and Community Psychiatry, 35*, 344-349.

Hill, M. L. (1988). Supported competitive employment: An interagency perspective, In P. Wehman & M. S. Moon (Eds.), *Vocational rehabilitation and supported employment* (pp. 31-49). Baltimore, MD: Brookes.

Hogarty, G. E., Anderson, C. M., Reiss, D. J., Kornblith, S. J., Greenwald, D. P., Javana, C. D., & Madonia, M. J. (1986). Family psychoeducation, social skills training, and maintenance chemotherapy in the aftercare treatment of schizophrenia. I. One-year effects on relapse and expressed emotion. *Archives of General Psychiatry, 43*, 633-642.

Hoult, J., Reynolds, I., Charbonneau-Powis, M., Weekes, P., & Briggs, J. (1983). Psychiatric hospital versus community treatment. The results of a randomized trial. *Australian and New Zealand Journal of Psychiatry, 17*, 160–167.

Indiana Department of Mental Health. (1985, September). *Request for proposals: Projects to improve and expand vocational services to chronically mentally ill persons*. Indianapolis: Author.

Jacobs, H. E., Kardashian, S., Kreinbring, R. K., Ponder, R., & Simpson, A. S. (1984). A skills-oriented model for facilitating employment among psychiatrically disabled persons. *Rehabilitation Counseling Bulletin, 28*, 87–96.

Jacobs, H. E., Wissusik, D., Collier, R., Stackman, D., Burkeman, D., Fitzpatrick, M., Dorrington, C., Lee, L., Liberman, R. P., Mintz, J., Simpson, A. P., & Rush, T. V. (1988). *The Brentwood job finding club: Predictors of vocational outcome for the psychiatrically ill*. Submitted for publication.

Keith, R. D., Engelkes, J. R., & Winborn, B. B. (1977). Employment-seeking preparation and activity: An experimental job-placement training model for rehabilitation clients. *Rehabilitation Counseling Bulletin, 21*, 159–165.

Kiernan, W. E., & Brinkman, L. (1988). Disincentives and barriers to employment. In P. Wehman & M. S. Moon (Eds.), *Vocational rehabilitation and supported employment* (pp. 221–233). Baltimore, MD: Brookes.

Kline, M. N., & Hoisington, V. (1981). Placing the psychiatrically disabled: A look at work values. *Rehabilitation Counseling Bulletin, 24*, 365–369.

Kuldau, J. M., & Dirks, S. J. (1977). Controlled evaluation of a hospital-originated community transitional system. *Archives of General Psychiatry, 34*, 1331–1340.

Lam, C. S. (1986). Comparison of sheltered and supported work programs: A pilot study. *Rehabilitation Counseling Bulletin, 30*, 66–81.

Lamb, H. R., & Goertzel, V. (1972). High expectations of long-term ex-state hospital patients. *American Journal of Psychiatry, 129*, 471–475.

Lehrer, P., & Lanoil, J. (1977). Natural reinforcement in a psychiatric rehabilitation program. *Schizophrenia Bulletin, 3*, 297–302.

Liberman, R. P. (1988). *Psychiatric rehabilitation of chronic mental patients*. Washington, DC: American Psychiatric Association Press.

Malamud, T. J., & McCrory, D. J. (1988). Transitional employment and psychosocial rehabilitation. In J. A. Ciardiello & M. D. Bell (Eds.), *Vocational rehabilitation of persons with prolonged mental illness* (pp. 150–162). Baltimore, MD: Johns Hopkins Press.

Marx, A. J., Test, M. A., & Stein, L. I. (1973). Extrohospital management of severe mental illness. *Archives of General Psychiatry, 29*, 505–511.

Meltzoff, J., & Blumenthal, R. L. (1966). *The day treatment center: Principles, application, and evaluation*. Springfield, IL: Charles C. Thomas.

Menchetti, B. M., & Rusch, F. R. (1988). Vocational evaluation and eligibility for rehabilitation services. In P. Wehman & M. S. Moon (Eds.), *Vocational rehabilitation and supported employment* (pp. 79–90). Baltimore, MD: Brookes.

Moon, M. S., & Griffin, S. L. (1988). Supported employment service delivery models. In P. Wehman & M. S. Moon (Eds.), *Vocational rehabilitation and supported employment* (pp. 17–30). Baltimore, MD: Brookes.

Mueser, K. T., & Liberman, R. P. (1988). Skill training in vocational rehabilitation. In J. A. Ciardiello & M. D. Bell (Eds.), *Vocational rehabilitation of persons with prolonged mental illness* (pp. 81–103). Baltimore, MD: Johns Hopkins University Press.

Mulder, R. (1982). *Final evaluation of the Harbinger program as a demonstration project*. Unpublished report. Grand Rapids, MI: Harbinger.

National Association of Rehabilitation Facilities. (1989). *Supported employment in context: NARF's national scope supported employment survey and policy implications*. Washington, DC: Author.

Nichols, M. (1989). *Demonstration study of a supported employment program for persons with severe mental illness: Benefits, costs, and outcomes*. Unpublished master's thesis, Indiana University-Purdue University at Indianapolis.

Noble, J. H., & Collignon, F. C. (1988). Systems barriers to supported employment for persons with chronic mental illness. In P. Wehman & M. S. Moon (Eds.), *Vocational rehabilitation and supported employment* (pp. 325–340). Baltimore, MD: Brookes.

Paquette, A., & Lafave, H. (1964). Halfway house. *American Journal of Nursing, 64*(3), 121–124.

Pearlin, L., & Schooler, C. (1978). The structure of coping. *Journal of Health and Social Behavior, 19*, 2–21.

Prieve, K., & DePoint, B. (1987). *Making it work: Supported employment for persons with severe and persistent mental illness*. Minneapolis, MN: Rise.

Purvis, S. A., & Miskimins, R. W. (1970). Effects of community follow-up on post-hospital adjustment of psychiatric patients. *Community Mental Health Journal, 6*, 374–382.

Rehab Brief. (1986). *Community adjustment: Evaluation of the clubhouse model for psychiatric rehabilitation* (Vol. 9, No. 2). Falls Church, VA: PSI International, 510 N. Washington.

Rehab Brief. (1987). *Supported employment* (Vol. 10, No. 1). Falls Church, VA: PSI International, 510 N. Washington.

Rosenthal, R. (1984). *Meta-analytic procedures for social research*. Beverly Hills, CA: Sage Publications.

Rosenthal, R., & Jacobson, L. (1968). *Pygmalion in the classroom*. New York: Holt, Rinehart.

Rubin, S. E., & Roessler, R. T. (1978). Guidelines for successful vocational rehabilitation of the psychiatrically disabled. *Rehabilitation Literature, 39*, 70–74.

Ruffner, R. H. (1986). The last frontier: Jobs and mentally ill persons. *Psychosocial Rehabilitation Journal, 9*(3), 35–42.

Rutkowski, P., & Howick, M. (1986). Creating opportunities for persons with serious mental illness in rural areas: The Green County Community Support Program. In L. V. Daniels (Ed.), *Community support programs in rural areas*. Hot Springs: Arkansas Department of Human Services.

Rutman, I. D., & Armstrong, K. (1985). *A comprehensive, national evaluation of transitional employment programs for the psychiatrically disabled*. Unpublished paper. Philadelphia, PA: Matrix Research Institute.

Ryan, E. R., & Bell, M. D. (1985, August). *Rehabilitation of chronic psychiatric patients: A randomized clinical study*. Paper presented at the American Psychological Association Convention, Los Angeles, CA.

Saveanu, T. I., & Roth, D. (1986). *Evaluation of the impact of a state-level interdepartmental agreement for the provision of rehabilitation services to severely mentally disabled persons in Ohio*. Unpublished report. Columbus, OH: Ohio Department of Mental Health.

Schalock, R. L. (1988). Critical performance evaluation indicators in supported employment. In P. Wehman & M. S. Moon (Eds.), *Vocational rehabilitation and supported employment* (pp. 163–174). Baltimore, MD: Brookes.

Solberg, A., & Raschmann, J. K. (1980). The effects of vocational services provided to the mentally disabled. *Community Mental Health Journal, 16*, 112–120.

Soloff, A. (1967). *A work therapy research center*. Monograph No. 7. Chicago, IL: Jewish Vocational Service.

Stein, L. I., & Test, M. A. (1980). An alternative to mental health treatment. I: Conceptual model, treatment program, and clinical evaluation. *Archives of General Psychiatry, 37*, 392–397.

Stratoudakis, J. P. (1986). Rehabilitation of the mentally ill: Psychosocial, vocational, and community support perspectives. *Annual Review of Rehabilitation, 5*, 255–284.

Strauss, J. S., Hafez, H., Lieberman, P., & Harding, C. M. (1985). The course of psychiatric disorder, III: Longitudinal principles. *American Journal of Psychiatry, 142*, 289–296.

Tashjian, M. D., Hayward, B. J., Stoddard, S., & Kraus, L. (1989). *Best practice study of vocational rehabilitation services to severely mentally ill persons*. Washington, DC: Policy Study Associates.

Test, M. A. (1984). Community support programs. In A. S. Bellack (Ed.), *Schizophrenia: Treatment, management, and rehabilitation* (pp. 347–373). Orlando, FL: Grune & Stratton.

Thresholds Community Scholar Program. (1990, February). *Community Support Network News, 6*(3), 5–6.

Thresholds Newsletter. (1987, Spring). Thresholds, 2700 N. Lakeview, Chicago, IL.

Trotter, S., Minkoff, K., Harrison, K., & Hoops, J. (1988). Supported work: An innovative approach to the vocational rehabilitation of persons who are psychiatrically disabled. *Rehabilitation Psychology, 33*, 27–36.

Turkat, D., & Buzzell, V. (1982). Psychosocial rehabilitation: A process evaluation. *Hospital and Community Psychiatry, 33*, 848–850.

Unger, K. V., Danley, K. S., Kohn, L., & Hutchinson, D. (1987). Rehabilitation through education: A university-based continuing education program for young adults with psychiatric disabilities on a university campus. *Psychosocial Rehabilitation Journal, 10*(3), 35–49.

Vandergoot, D. (1986). *Review of placement research literature: Implications for research and practice*. (Rehabilitation Research Review, NARIC). Washington, DC: DATA Institute.

Velasquez, J. S., & McCubbin, H. I. (1980). Towards establishing the effectiveness of community-based residential treatment: Program evaluation by experimental research. *Journal of Social Service Research, 3*, 337–359.

Vitale, J. H., & Steinbach, M. (1965). The prevention of relapse of chronic mental patients. *International Journal of Social Psychiatry, 11*, 85–95.

Vorspan, R. (1988). Activities of daily living in the clubhouse: You can't vacuum in a vacuum. *Psychosocial Rehabilitation Journal, 12*(2), 15–21.

Walker, R., Winick, W., & Frost, E. S. (1969). Social restoration of hospitalized psychiatric patients through a program of special employment in industry. *Rehabilitation Literature, 30*, 297–303.

Wehman, P. (1986). Supported competitive employment for persons with severe disabilities. *Journal of Applied Rehabilitation Counseling, 17*, 24–29.

Wehman, P. (1988). Supported employment: Toward zero exclusion of persons with severe disabilities. In P. Wehman & M. S. Moon (Eds.), *Vocational rehabilitation and supported employment* (pp. 3–14). Baltimore, MD: Brookes.

Wehman, P. (1989). Supported employment implementation in 27 states: An introduction. In P. Wehman, J. Kregel, & M. S. Shafer (Eds.), *Emerging trends in the national supported employment initiative: A preliminary analysis in twenty-seven states* (pp. 1–14). Richmond, VA: Virginia Commonwealth University.

Wehman, P., Kregel, J., & Shafer, M. S. (1989). *Emerging trends in the national supported employment initiative: A preliminary analysis of twenty-seven states*. Richmond, VA: Virginia Commonwealth University.

Wehman, P., & Moon, M. S. (1988). *Vocational rehabilitation and supported employment*. Baltimore, MD: Brookes.

Weinberg, J. L., & Lustig, P. (1968). A workshop experience for post-hospitalized schizophrenics. In G. N. Wright & A. B. Trotter (Eds.), *Rehabilitation research* (pp. 72–78). Madison: University of Wisconsin.

Westermeyer, J., & Harrow, M. (1987). Factors associated with work impairments in schizophrenic and nonschizophrenic patients. In R. R. Grinker (Ed.), *Clinical research in schizophrenia: A multidimensional approach* (pp. 280–298). Springfield, IL: Charles C. Thomas.

Wilder, J. F., Levin, G., & Zwerling, I. (1966). A two-year follow-up evaluation of acute psychotic patients treated in a day hospital. *American Journal of Psychiatry, 122*, 1095–1111.

Wolkon, G. H., Karmen, M., & Tanaka, H. T. (1971). Evaluation of a social rehabilitation program for recently released psychiatric patients. *Community Mental Health Journal, 7*, 312–322.

CHAPTER 12

PSYCHOGERIATRIC REHABILITATION

Roger L. Patterson

New developments in the application of learning theory and applied behavior analysis have created promising therapeutic approaches to the mentally ill elderly that combine medical, pharmacological, and psychosocial interventions. In two reviews of the literature including more than 100 studies, clear evidence was found for the efficacy of social learning techniques in reinstating activities of daily living, increasing social and leisure time participation, improving memory and cognition, overcoming depression and anxiety disorders, reducing incontinence, controlling wandering and dependence on caregivers, and improving the management of disabled elderly in their homes (Baltes & Werner-Wahl, 1987; Patterson, in press; Patterson & Jackson, 1980). Several problems, previously considered solely within the realm of biomedical intervention, have been shown to respond favorably to psychosocial and behavioral therapies—insomnia, headaches, lack of mobility, obesity, pain control, and sequelae of strokes.

The diagnostic classification of elderly mentally ill who have shown responsiveness to a biopsychosocial therapeutic approach includes those with dementias, schizophrenia, major depression and dysthymia, anxiety disorders, and substance abuse disorders. The associated physical and medical problems of the elderly have also been favorably affected by behavioral interventions; for example, the disabilities in self-care and mobility secondary to arthritis and joint problems, cardiovascular disease, and genitourinary and gastrointestinal disorders.

The advances now possible in the rehabilitation of elderly mentally ill persons are cogently illuminated by the following case study:

Mrs. S., a 63-year-old teacher and author, had gradually given up her occupation over a period of 2 years and lived an isolated and seclusive existence. She was hospitalized after suffering a venomous snake bite and, although medically cleared from the noxious effects of the snake toxin, refused to get out of bed, or to bathe or dress; she also became incontinent. Psychiatric consultation revealed a mute and uncooperative person who appeared regressed.

The patient was transferred from the general hospital to a psychiatric rehabilitation facility where she was found to respond to motivational interventions (social praise, token reinforcement) and skills training. Because of her excellent response to the behavior therapy, her diagnosis was changed to major depression from dementia and she was begun on antidepressant drug therapy. Further improvements were noted and she was able to return to living independently. At 1-year follow-up, she was no longer taking medication, but living an active life, maintaining her personal hygiene, reading voraciously, eating well, and exercising with long walks. (Patterson, 1985)

As this case illustrates, the practitioner may often find himself or herself confronted with elders who exhibit deficits in social and living skills or other functional abnormalities that may result from psychiatric and nonpsychiatric illnesses and environmental conditions. Often a combination of these factors is causative, and it may be poor treatment to try to eliminate any given deficit by treating only one presumptive cause.

Skills-training approaches, when applied concurrently with appropriate medical and social interventions, have demonstrated promise for improving the functioning and adaptation of many elderly persons with psychiatric and medical disorders. Advances in treatment and rehabilitation have occurred in remediating deficits in social and daily living skills, depression, memory deficits, dementia, and substance abuse. Together, these represent problems of public health magnitude and constitute the major causes of institutionalization of the elderly (Gallagher & Thompson, 1983; Health Care Financing Administration, 1981 cited in Pfeiffer, Johnson, & Chiofolo, 1981; Patterson, in press; Patterson & Jackson, 1980).

SOCIAL AND DAILY LIVING SKILLS

Prior to the initiation of skills-training approaches, performance of the elderly mentally ill in self-care and socialization was regarded as fixed. However, studies have shown that elderly psychiatric patients may be taught to overcome personal deficits readily. Elderly, state hospital female patients were taught in small groups to wash their hair, clean their rooms, and use the telephone with modeling and role-playing techniques in only six practice trials for each behavior (Rusin, 1978). Significantly, enhancement of performance on these tasks was noted when prizes were offered for improvements.

Behavior therapy techniques have been effective in improving participation in social and leisure events including arranging furniture appropriately (Peterson, Knapp, Rosen, & Pither, 1977), serving meals family-style in large bowls rather than individual servings (McClannahan & Risley, 1974), prompting people to use recreational materials, (Quattrochi-Tubin & Jasons, 1980), serving coffee and juice in a social area, (Blackman, Howe, & Pinkston, 1976), and opening a "store" for residents (McClannahan & Risley, 1973). Both primary (e.g., candy) and secondary (e.g., token) reinforcers have been shown to promote verbal interaction of elderly mental patients in several studies (Hoyer, Kafer, Simpson, & Hoyer, 1974; Mueller & Atlas, 1972). A criticism of such studies has been that the behaviors were not maintained after the prompts and reinforcers were removed; however, such generalization and maintenance was not taught as part of the studies. Also, this criticism has no relevance for situations such as institutions or other care homes in which maintenance programs may be continued indefinitely.

Social-skills training (Foxx, McMorrow,

Bittle, & Ness, 1986) employing a game format was successful in teaching 3 elderly retarded residents of an institution proper responses to a wide variety of social situations. Evidence of generalization of the newly acquired social skills beyond the classroom setting was demonstrated in the ward environment some weeks later. Also, the social interactions occurred among the trained residents, but not with other, untrained residents, indicating that proper social responses will persist only if reciprocated.

A recent innovation for remediating urinary incontinence generated by a National Institute on Aging Project (Burgio & Engel, 1987) used instrumented feedback of bladder pressures, sphincter activity, and intra-abdominal pressure to teach patients appropriate contraction and relaxation of relevant muscles to achieve controlled micturition. Similar methods have also been shown to be effective with fecal incontinence (Whitehead, Burgio, & Engel, 1985).

Methods for controlling wandering behavior among demented patients have used different colored signs to mark safe and dangerous areas (Hussian, 1982). By means of conditioning, three demented nursing home residents were taught to associate one color with positive reinforcement and a different color with noxious noise. Thereafter, the residents tended to go where the "safe" color was posted and to avoid areas marked by the other color. This technique was also used to teach people where to urinate.

Within the area of behavioral medicine, Bootzin and his associates (Bootzin & Engle-Friedman, 1987) have devised a multifaceted approach to overcome insomnia, including (a) information and support, (b) relaxation training, and (c) stimulus control instruction. This treatment approach was found to be effective, compared with no-treatment controls, in a group of 53 community residents aged 47 to 76 years. No sleeping medications were used during the study.

Other treatments within behavioral medicine have included presurgery relaxation training to reduce postsurgical pain and medication (Ceccio, 1984), the use of biofeedback to overcome foot drop after stroke (Burnside, Tobias, & Bursill, 1982), the use of training in self-control and the modification of nutritional habits to reduce obesity (Banders-van Halewijn, Choy, van Uitert, & deWaard, 1984), and teaching mute stroke victims to communicate by using sign language (Wisocki & Mosher, 1980).

Token economies (TE) were used early in the history of learning-based techniques as methods for improving the social and daily living skills of institutional residents (Atthowe & Krasner, 1968). In one well-designed study of the application of TE to the elderly, 80 elderly organic brain syndrome patients were randomly assigned to either a token economy or milieu therapy. Target behaviors in the TE included prosocial behavior, self-care, and housekeeping chores. Primary reinforcers that could be purchased with tokens included cigarettes, treats, and privileges. All primary reinforcers were available noncontingently on the milieu ward. The results revealed that in both groups one-third improved, and more improved overall than declined. However, there were important differences in both the nature of the improvements and in the type of resident who improved in each group. Self-care improved significantly in the TE while the milieu therapy produced improvements on bizarre and unusual behavior as well as incontinence. The residents who improved most in the milieu therapy were the less socially responsive, while those improving in the TE were actively psychotic, were in need of more care, and had been admitted more recently (Mishara, 1978).

Another TE program was compared with a control group of patients who had been discharged from the same ward the year before the TE was initiated. Using a cost-benefit analysis, the TE program consisted of four phases: In phase one, tokens were exchanged for primary reinforcers; in the next two phases privileges were also purchased with tokens. Phase four was a halfway house for those judged capable of independent living. The economic analysis included variables such as length of stay in the hospital, probability of recidivism, life expectancy of the resident, and projected hospital costs. Results revealed that $20 could be saved for every $1 invested in the program (Frank, Klein, & Jacobs, 1982).

In addition to professional and institutional programs, family management of skills deficits of elders has recently begun to receive attention. Pinkston and Linsk (1984) have published descriptions of assessments, intervention guidelines and examples of teaching families appropriate skills. Specifically, family members, with the assistance of behaviorally trained experts, have overcome problems of social isolation, dependency, self-care, and negative verbalizations. Hussian and Davis (1985) described several home-management modules that are given to families of elderly patients when they are discharged from a state hospital; the purpose of the modules is to help maintain appropriate behaviors at home.

Patterson (1987) reviewed these and other family-management techniques, and described an approach to intervention and prevention in the home using the concept of environmental supports. Environmental supports refer to reliably defined aspects of the normal environment which serve to prompt and maintain normal behavior, such as supportive relationships with spouse or spouse substitutes, pride in the home, and relationships with children. Based on the results of an assessment, elders and their families can be taught to make the home environment more supportive of elders' competent behaviors.

The Zarits and their associates have worked extensively to develop structured ways to help families manage victims of Alzheimer's disease (AD) and other senile dementias (Zarit, Orr, & Zarit, 1985). Most notably, they have developed ways of measuring the nature and magnitude of the burden of specific aspects of care. Using a stress-management model, they have developed ways of counseling families to solve problems and to make use of behavioral management skills and community supports to improve the quality of care and to reduce the stress of giving it. Individual, family, and group counseling with skills training is employed. An evaluative study of 100 AD caregivers assigned to either active or placebo controls did not support statistically the effectiveness of the treatments (Zarit, Anthony, & Boutsellis, in press). Surprisingly, both treatment and placebo groups improved.

In an ongoing 5-year study (in press), Gallagher and her associates at the Palo Alto Veterans Administration (VA) Hospital are extending previous work with cognitive-behavioral and psychoeducational skills-training approaches to work with caregivers and the victims of AD for whom they care. Earlier, Teri and Uomoto (1986) had found that the depression of both the caregiver and the AD victim for whom they cared had been reduced when the caregivers were taught cognitive–behavioral strategies to reduce depression. Based on this finding as well as others, the Palo Alto group designed and initiated a more extensive evaluation. Two separate active treatments involved (a) psychoeducational groups that were taught highly structured problem-solving skills, or (b) life-satisfaction classes which taught caretakers to increase pleasant events and decrease unpleasant events according to the behavioral approaches of Lewinsohn, Munoz, & Youngren (1986). Preliminary results on 65 caretakers indicated that both active therapies improved morale and decreased depression in caregivers significantly more than a group that did not receive immediate treatment, and which had identical measures of change taken while awaiting completion of treatment by the first group.

DEPRESSION AND ANXIETY

Within the last 10 years, some psychotherapies specifically designed to teach cognitive and behavioral skills to the elderly have been developed and subjected to empirical evaluation (Gallagher & Thompson, 1983).

One of these therapies is based on the assumption that depression may be increased by unpleasant events or decreased by pleasant events in one's life (Lewinsohn, Munoz, Youngren, & Zeiss, 1986; Lewinsohn, Antonuccio, Steinmetz, & Teri, 1984). Patients are taught to monitor their lives on a daily basis for the purpose of identifying specific events related to mood changes. Patients learn that their own activities and moods are, in fact, related to specific events. Problem solving follows so that elders may learn to increase pleasant events and decrease unpleasant ones in their normal environments. Training in (a) relaxation to reduce the aversiveness of some events, and (b) communication skills to improve the pleasantness of interactions with others are important parts of the process. All training is followed by homework in which the patient experiments with the newly learned methods in the natural environment. After the patient learns to improve his or her mood in this way, therapy ends with sessions devoted to specifying how the patient is to maintain the improvements after terminating the therapeutic relationship. Follow-up "booster" sessions are held at 6 and 12 weeks after therapy. These coping and problem-solving skills have been successfully taught to depressed persons in psychoeducational courses for groups of six to eight persons (Lewinsohn et al., 1984).

A related form of therapy developed for depression in the elderly is cognitive behavior therapy (Emery, Gallagher, & Thompson, 1985). This therapy also starts with the daily monitoring of mood and the events that affect it. However, the subsequent emphasis is to teach the patients to identify certain kinds of negative thoughts related to depression when they occur. Since such thoughts are usually gross exaggerations of unrealistic interpretations of events, patients can learn to change their views of events in their lives toward becoming more realistic and positive.

Thompson and Gallagher (1984) have reported on several studies comparing the effectiveness of these behavioral therapies with brief psychodynamic therapy and insight-oriented therapy. At the end of 6 weeks of treatment, all three therapy groups showed significant and approximately equal improvement, whereas the no-treatment control subjects had not improved. Overall, 70% of the treated subjects showed remission or significant improvement as measured by strict criteria. At a 1-year follow-up, only 11% of those treated with behavioral or cognitive therapy relapsed while 56% of an insight-oriented relational control group relapsed (Thompson, Gallagher, & Breckinridge, 1987).

One decided advantage of the skills-training approaches in that they may be taught successfully by paraprofessionals (Thompson, Gallagher, Nies, & Epstein, 1983) and can be disseminated widely. Moreover, these practical forms of skills training can be taught to caregivers of Alzheimer's patients for decreasing depression in both themselves and their wards (Teri & Uomoto, 1986).

In an area closely related to depression, elderly patients have also been taught to overcome fear and anxiety by using cognitive and behavioral skills. Hussian (1981) successfully dealt with the elevator phobia of 4 elderly state hospital residents by providing them with information about how an elevator works, teaching them how to make realistic coping statements, and how to relax their bodies. In this way they were able first to enter and then to ride the elevator comfortably. Similarly, Haley (1983) was able to help an elderly demented woman and her family to control her fearful crying out, which occurred whenever she was left alone in her room, despite assurances that someone was elsewhere in the house and would be back shortly. She was provided with relaxation training, a clock, and a clearly visible message board to indicate when someone would return. She learned to tolerate increasingly long periods of being left alone using these antecedents combined with reinforcement with ice cream for remaining alone quietly.

Medications have also been reported to be useful in the treatment of depression and anxiety in the elderly as with younger groups (Gerson, Poltkin, & Jarvik, 1988). While antidepressant drugs appear to be more effective than evocative, insight-oriented therapies (Jarvik, Mintz, Steuer, & Gerner, 1982), more structured and systematically applied behavior therapies achieve remission rates in mild to moderately depressed elders similar to those obtained by medication (Thompson, Gallagher, & Breckinridge, 1987). It is safe to conclude that both structured psychotherapies and antidepressant medications are effective with many, but not all, depressed elders. With regard to anxiety uncomplicated by depression, short-acting benzodiazepines administered in low doses have been recommended for elders (Baldessarini & Cole, 1988).

IMPROVING MEMORY

Unfortunately, there are no accepted medical treatments for memory losses related to aging—neither for the mild forgetfulness of normal aging nor for the severe forms seen in the cases of Alzheimer's disease, multi-infarct dementia, or other diseases. Experimentation with agents intended to elevate levels of cholinergic central nervous system (CNS) transmitters produced evidence of modest and brief improvement in some kinds of Alzheimer's patients, but the effect was not sufficient to constitute a therapy (Selzer, 1988).

Methods chiefly derived from experimental psychology have been found to improve cognitive functions of the elderly in laboratory studies but may have not been applied in practical rehabilitation programs (Yeasavage, 1985). Several memory-enhancing techniques have been empirically validated. Mnemonic strategies involve teaching elders to associate the words or images that need to be remembered with particular categories, other words, or other images, or a combination of these techniques. By means of such training, normal elderly can learn to perform nearly as well as untrained young people on selected tasks.

Another approach to improving memory in the elderly is to use relaxation techniques. The rationale for this method is that excessive emotionality may cause distraction, decreased attentiveness, and reduced recall. Training in anxiety reduction has been found as useful as training in the use of mnemonics and the orderly categorization of material to improve attentiveness and problem solving (Labouvie-Vief & Gonda, 1976).

Yeasavage (1984) studied the effectiveness of a combination of verbal association, visual association, and relaxation training by comparing improvements in face and name recall of an experimental group of normal elders given the combination treatment with those of a control group given solely mnemonic training combined with lectures on attitudes toward aging. The final performance of the experimental group was significantly better than that of the control. Furthermore, the amount of improvement was correlated with reduction in anxiety as measured by a standard scale. Evidently, relaxation training should be included as a component in a memory training program for the elderly, at least for those with elevated anxiety.

Training demented elders in verbal information is not a currently useful rehabilitation effort because of the limited capabilities of such individuals for long-term retention of this type of information. Only modest and short-term improvements can be expected. For example, 4 elderly community residents with dementia were trained to remember several types of verbal information for a limited time of up to 30 minutes. The training procedure used prompted practice and reinforcement of correct responses with praise and tokens. Two of the 4 who were available for follow-up retained only a small fraction of this information at 6- and 12-week posttreatment follow-ups (Johnson, Fralliciardi, & Patterson, 1977). Others have found only short-term retention following the use of mnemonics to teach verbal information and face-name association to demented subjects (Zarit, Zarit, & Reever, 1982).

In contrast, training the demented to remember how to find locations within their living areas is both more effective and more useful than teaching verbal information. McEvoy and Patterson (1987) were able to use a reverse chaining procedure to teach 12 demented elders to improve greatly their ability to find their bedroom, bed, dining room, and bathroom within their residential treatment facility.

MODULAR BEHAVIORAL REHABILITATION

The cumulative evidence documenting the efficacy of structured, skills-training methods of rehabilitation for elderly mentally disordered persons has attracted the interest of facility and program directors in applying these innovations to patients participating in residential and daycare programs. The most comprehensive effort in packaging behavioral rehabilitation for a large population of elderly mentally ill was carried out by Patterson and his associates at the Florida Mental Health Institute (1982). Methods of restoring personal and social functioning were organized in modules for both residential and daycare settings.

The residential component was unusual in that it did not focus on teaching people to conform to institutional requirements, but rather sought to teach skills required for community living. In contrast, most previous applications of learning-based approaches have occurred in institutions and have reinforced grooming, participating in ward activities, doing institution-based chores, and attending standard institutional therapies. The Day Treatment component selected people living in the local community who were regarded as being at risk of institutionalization due to failing abilities. The goal was to improve their community-living skills so that they could remain in the community.

The focus of the Modular Behavioral Program (MBP) was to provide relatively short-term rehabilitation to those state hospital patients aged 55 and older who could be rehabilitated (successfully returned to community living), regardless of diagnosis. A set of criteria was used to select patients who had at least a minimal chance of succeeding in a program designed to teach living skills for return to the community within a few months. Excluded were those who were (a) incontinent, (b) nonambulatory, (c) in need of hospital-based medical care, (d) unable to function in an open ward environment without one-to-one supervision, (e) dangerous to self or others. Of 275 patients in one evaluation of the MBP, 37% were psychotic. Their average age was 67.4, their mean of prior hospitalizations was 2.0, and their mean length of prior hospitalizations was 17.3 months.

The MBP was developed by pinpointing those functional deficits in the elderly that often resulted in institutionalization. Interventions to correct these functional deficits were then packaged into skills-training modules, each designed to address the needs of many individuals. Each module was made up of a manual containing the following:

1. A brief description of behavior modification techniques that were particularly relevant to teaching the designated skill area.
2. An assessment designed to measure the deficits of each individual within the skill area.
3. A description of the content to be taught and how to teach it incorporating the behavioral techniques.

All modular training incorporated verbal instructions, demonstrations of appropriate behavior, practice by the patients, and reinforcement in the form of positive feedback and tokens.

To make treatment truly programmatic and disseminable, an essential requirement was that all techniques and all manuals had to be readily usable by the lowest level of mental health direct-care staff. In this case, direct treatment personnel were those with a minimum of 1 or 2 years of post-high school training in human services, including an introduction to behavior modification.

Each module was used in a systematic sequence. First, each person to be treated was assessed for deficits within the subject area of each module during the first week in the program. Those identified as having deficits in any area were assigned for training in that module. After each 4 weeks of training, every patient was reassessed. When assessment results indicated that a particular area was mastered, the patient graduated from that area and was reassigned to other areas found deficient if warranted and available. When it was apparent that patients had either completed all necessary training or had reached their maximum level of performance, they were either returned to their own home, or a new home was found in the community that was suited to their level of abilities based upon the most recent assessments. With day-treatment patients, the goal was for them to adapt more successfully to their present homes although they could be also assisted with a move if assessment results indicated this to be necessary.

In addition to the modules, another program element targeted the alleviation of highly idiosyncratic behavior, such as hoarding, yelling, running water in the bathroom, and exhibiting aggression. A standard reporting form, which required the observer to describe the behavior, along with related antecedent and consequent events occurring each time the behavior was observed, was developed to assist in treatment. From a collection of these, the treatment team, including a behavioral psychologist, could decide how to alter either or both consequent and antecedent events in order to correct the behavior. This information also provided a data base for judging the necessity and effectiveness of the use of psychiatric medications. Continued data collection of the patient's problem behaviors after a plan was initiated revealed whether the plan was being followed and also whether it was effective or needed modification.

Another programmatic component was adequate utilization of leisure time. The staff scheduled and planned leisure time activities with the intent that patients learn new activities of three types: (a) things to do alone, (b) small-group activities, and (c) large-group activities. Training and reinforcement (social and token) were used in these areas as they were for the more formally structured program components. Among preferred activities were dancing, simple crafts, Bingo, card games, and leisurely walks. Television was of little interest to most.

Modules were first developed for activities of daily living (ADL). ADLs involve skills ranging from the basics of self-care (e.g., bathing, dressing) to more advanced skills such as obtaining health care, learning bus routes, and keeping budgets. Accordingly, ADLs were presented in three separate modules: ADL I included bathing, dressing, and eating safely; ADL II taught skills such as laundering, managing small amounts of money, and using a telephone; ADL III taught budgeting of time and money, housekeeping, and obtaining community resources.

Part of the rationale for this division of ADLs related to the types of community placements available. Obviously, if one could not master ADL I skills sufficiently, he or she would require continued personal care. However, there were some supervised homes suitable for people who could perform ADL I but not more complex activities. Still other people who mastered ADL II but not ADL III could generally live successfully in private boarding homes licensed by the state to provide room, board, cleaning, and minimal supervision. Those mastering ADL III could live independently with little or no supervision.

The social skills area may be divided into two parts (Liberman, DeRisi, & Mueser, 1989; Patterson, in press).

1. Efforts to improve the *quantity* of appropriate casual interactions.
2. Training for *more effective* interpersonal interactions.

Three modules helped to rebuild social skills: (a) Conversation Training taught people to sit and converse in pairs or small groups in a normal social setting: (b) Communication Effectiveness Training trained people to express basic affect to other individuals, concentrating on the expression of pleasure (I like that; thank you; you're a nice person) and displeasure (I don't like that; stop it): (c) Self-Esteem Training was addressed by getting people in groups to acknowledge publicly and privately their own desirable characteristics.

To deal with the relatively small percentage of the population who were disoriented, a Personal Information Training (PIT) module was developed to teach orientation to time, place, and person.

The MBP was subjected to a large-scale evaluation involving both experimental and quasi-experimental designs, including data from 275 residential and day-treatment patients. Evaluation questions included the following:

1. Did the patients learn the material taught in the modules?
2. Did they improve in their general condition as measured by the global behavioral rating scales?
3. Did treatment in the program result in successful community placement?

The evaluation results showed that overall improvements were made in each module. The quasi-experimental design was capable of demonstrating the unlikelihood that the improvements were due to such extraneous factors as biased sampling and coincidental, nonprogrammatic occurrences. Thus, it was very likely that changes observed in the modules were related to treatment in the program, although these changes could not, by this design, be said to be due to each specific module and not to some more general features of the program. For this reason, true experimental evaluations, using conventional statistical significance levels, were conducted on four modules: Conversation Training, Communication Effectiveness Training, Personal Information, and Self-Esteem Training. The findings demonstrated that the patients learned the behaviors as taught in these modules and that the learning was specific to the particular area taught.

The pretreatment scores on the Community Adjustment Potential Scale (CAP) (Hogarty & Ulrich, 1972) were significantly lower for the residential group than for the day-treatment group. By the time of discharge from the MBP (an average of about 4 months later) both groups showed improvement, but the residential group showed greater improvements so that the two groups were no longer significantly different. Significant improvements in Social Interest and Retardation on the Nurses Observation Scale for Inpatient Evaluation (Honigfeld, Gillis, & Klett, 1966) also were found for patients participating in the MBP. These results strongly support the effectiveness of the MBP.

The MBP evaluation included a comparison of rates of discharge to noninstitutional community settings of those who were transferred to the MBP from a state hospital with a matched group of these who remained. The comparison showed that at the end of 1 year from selection, 85% of the MBP group had been discharged to the community whereas only 37% of the residual state hospital patients had been similarly placed, a statistically significant difference. Furthermore, within 1 year of discharge, only 7% of the MBP group had been reinstitutionalized while 47% of the other group had been, also a significant difference. At the end of 1 year after discharge, 79% of those who entered the MBP were still in the community as compared with only 20% of the other group. An even greater testimonial to the effectiveness of the MBP was the fact that 2 years after discharge, 60% of the matched state hospital group, but only 9% of the MBP group, had been reinstitutionalized. This recidivism rate for the MBP is much lower than the overall rate of recidivism of 50.9% for all Florida state hospitals and recidivism rates from other studies.

The data from the day treatment program were much harder to interpret, as we could find no basis for comparison in the form of a group of high-risk elders with similar characteristics who were given other types of interventions. However, the results after 1 year found less than 10% of this group in psychiatric institutions and 13.2% in nursing homes. This was in spite of referring clinicians' predictions that all were in danger of institutionalization.

Of considerable interest in the MBP, though not crucial to the outcome, was the issue of whether progress during the behavioral treatment was directly related to long-term outcome. Obviously such a finding would further validate the treatment since it was possible that the impressive placement and recidivism rates could be accounted for by nontreatment variables, such as good placement work by social workers and accurate assessments permitting better matching of those discharged with the postdischarge environment. Thus, it was consistent with treatment-driven outcomes that actual improvements in community placement potential during participation in the MBP strongly predicted community tenure 1 year after discharge. A comparison between a group of recidivists and a group of nonrecidivists revealed that both groups had almost identical CAP scores at the time of admission. Although both groups improved on the CAP during treatment, the nonrecidivists improved more and were both clinically and statistically better on this measure at the time of discharge. The finding that clinically relevant within-treatment behavioral improvements of the elderly were related to long-term recidivism is probably unique in the psychogeriatric treatment literature.

Dementia and the MBP

With the wide acceptance of the more reliable definitions of and criteria for dementia in DSM-III, it became possible to determine the efficacy of the MBP for demented patients. To achieve this replication and extension of the earlier MBP evaluation, the progress of a clearly diagnosed group of dementia patients was compared with a matched group of nondemented as they were treated in the MBP. All patients were residential.

Comparable information was available regarding the progress of these groups in four modules (ADL I, ADL II, PIT, and Communications) as well as a new module, Spatial Orientation Training. The new module taught patients to find their way to the dining room, bathroom, and bedroom by a process of reverse chaining with correct responding accompanied by token and social reinforcement.

Evaluation of the MBP modules for demented patients revealed that even low-functioning demented patients were able to learn ADL I skills as well as the nondemented patients; however, training for the low-functioning demented patients required an average of over 15 weeks versus approximately $4\frac{1}{2}$ weeks for the nondemented and $7\frac{1}{2}$ weeks for the high-functioning demented (McEvoy & Patterson, 1987). Higher levels of daily living activities (e.g., laundry, money management) were not learned by the demented patients. Modest but significant improvements were found in the Personal Information Training module and substantial improvements in the Spatial Orientation module, equivalent to that found with the nondemented group. In Communication Effectiveness Training, the demented patients appeared to acquire skills readily (McEvoy & Patterson, 1987). These findings should encourage practitioners to mount restorative training programs for the demented elderly rather than viewing custodial care as the only option for them.

Alcohol Abuse and the MBP

Another diagnostic group for which the MBP developed a special program consisted of late-life onset alcohol abusers. Five specific modules were developed to teach information and skills thought to be needed to overcome elders' stress-related alcohol abuse and problem-drinking patterns (Dupree, Broskowski, & Schonfeld, 1984):

1. *Analysis of Drinking Behavior*, in which patients learned to define the antecedents of their own drinking, their pattern of drinking, and the consequences to them
2. *Self-Management in High-Risk Situations*, which instructed patients in skills necessary to deal with antecedents of drinking
3. *Alcohol Information and Education*, in which patients learned about the medical, psychological, statistical, and theoretical consequences of alcohol abuse
4. *General Problem-Solving Skills*, which taught practical methods of problem identification, solution generation, and decision making
5. *Social Support Network*, which instructed patients how to expand their social network and activities

In addition to these alcohol-specific modules, alcohol-abusing patients were also assessed for deficits in ADL, Self-Esteem, and all the other modules offered to the nonalcoholic patients of the full MBP and were given any training needed to overcome these deficits.

Using well-accepted measures, Dupree and his colleagues (1984) found that those who completed the program were able to change a pattern of regular abuse to no abuse, with these gains maintained for 12 months after treatment by all who "graduated." Furthermore, the program graduates showed highly significant improvement in community adjustment as rated by significant others and as measured by number and types of social contacts (Dupree et al., 1984). Despite the success of those who completed the program, this alcohol treatment program had a 50% dropout rate. Some significant differences between the dropouts and the graduates were that the dropouts drank more, were more depressed, felt less in control of their lives, and were less optimistic about success (Dupree, 1982). Closer integration of the MBP alcohol treatment component with psychiatric services that would provide indicated antidepressant drug therapy, antabuse, and medical monitoring (e.g., blood alcohol levels) might increase the response rates. In addition, the implementation of currently available cognitive behavior therapy modules for depression should counter the pessimism and helplessness found among the dropouts (Emery, Gallagher, & Thompson, 1985; Lewinsohn, Antonuccio, Steinmetz, & Teri, 1986).

CONCLUSIONS

Rehabilitation of the elderly must include skills-training components to be maximally effective. Traditional approaches using psychotherapy, pharmacotherapy, physical therapy, provisions of prostheses, social support, and external assistance are necessary and need to be improved. However, the effectiveness of all psychogeriatric services may be enhanced by the addition of skills-training components.

Drug and behavioral interventions can be combined to accomplish more than either approach alone. For example, in the treatment of depressive and psychotic symptoms of the elderly, drug therapy can ameliorate psychopathology and enable the affected individual to engage more effectively in psychosocial and skills-training activities. Assessment of the benefit/risk profile of pharmacological agents also can point in directions where behavioral rehabilitation can be harnessed to drug therapy to overcome side effects, improve patients' compliance with pharmacotherapy, and permit lower doses of drugs to be used (Medication Management Module, 1989; Liberman, 1987).

Psychoactive medications are generally more specifically keyed to particular diagnoses while skills training and other behavior therapy approaches in rehabilitation are nonspecific protective and strengthening factors that provide benefits for persons with a wide variety of diagnoses or diseases. Future treatment development will undoubtedly lead to advances in the crafting of joint drug and behavior therapies for targeted impairments within defined diagnostic groups. Much greater use of truly multidisciplinary approaches will be required for such efforts.

Rehabilitation work with the elderly is probably the most broadly interdisciplinary field of all human interventions. Therefore, professional chauvinism is highly destructive and is to be avoided. Unfortunately, the team approach has been trivialized by being interpreted as having members of several professions sit together to describe their *individual* approaches. This is not a team. A true team would agree as to the problems of the patient *independently* of any one profession; then each specialty would agree as to how the skills of each would be used to address each identified problem.

To participate effectively as a member of an interdisciplinary team working toward the rehabilitation of the psychogeriatric patient, clinicians must possess certain prerequisite attitudes and competencies:

- knowledge of human aging
- an optimistic, respectful, nonpatronizing approach to the elderly
- knowledge of the application of learning-based approaches
- willingness to work with, cooperate with, and respect the opinions of several disciplines, including medical specialists of several types, behavioral psychologists, social workers, nurses, rehabilitation therapists, and others who participate in caregiving (administrators, family members, attorneys, and social service workers)

Given these requirements, rehabilitation of the elderly may be an exciting and personally rewarding endeavor. Our society is in urgent need of multidisciplinary practitioners because of the rapidly increasing elderly population and the prohibitive human and economic costs of maintaining the elderly mentally ill at a less-than-optimal level of competence.

REFERENCES

Atthowe, J. M., & Krasner, L. (1968). A preliminary report on the application of contingent reinforcement procedure (token economy) on a "chronic" psychiatric ward. *Journal of Abnormal Psychology, 73*, 37.

Baldessarini, R. J., & Cole, J. O. (1988). Chemotherapy. In M. N. Armandi (Ed.), *The New Harvard Guide to Psychiatry* (p. 481). Cambridge, MA: The Belknap Press of Harvard University Press.

Banders-van Halewijn, E. A., Choy, Y. W., van Uitert, J., & de Waard, C. (1984). The Cordon study of weight reduction based on behavioral modification. *International Journal of Obesity, 8*, 161–170.

Baltes, M. M., & Werner-Wahl, H. (1987). Dependence in aging. In L. L. Carstensen & B. A. Edelstein (Eds.), *Handbook of clinical gerontology* (p. 204). Elmsford, NY: Pergamon Press.

Blackman, D. K., Howe, M., & Pinkston, E. M. (1976). Increasing participation in social interaction of the institutionalized elderly. *Gerontologist, 17*, 69–76.

Bootzin, R. R., & Engle-Friedman, M. (1987). Sleep disturbances. In L. D. Carstensen & B. A. Edelstein (Eds.), *Handbook of clinical gerontology* (p. 238). Elmsford, NY: Pergamon Press.

Burgio, K. L., & Engel, B. T. (1987). Urinary incontinence: Behavioral assessment and treatment. In L. L. Carstensen & B. A. Edelstein (Eds.), *Handbook of clinical gerontology* (p. 252). Elmsford, NY: Pergamon Press.

Burnside, I. G., Tobias, H. S., & Bursill, D. (1982). Electromyographic feedback in the remobilization of stroke patients: A controlled trial. *Archives of Physical Medical Rehabilitation, 63*, 217–222.

Ceccio, C. M. (1984). Postoperative pain relief through relaxation in elderly patients. *Orthopedic Nursing, 3*, 11–19.

Dupree, L. W. (1982). Gerontology alcohol project: Characteristics of treatment program graduates versus dropouts. *Gerontologist, 22*, 258–259.

Dupree, L. W., Broskowski, H., & Schonfeld, L. (1984). The gerontology project: A behavioral treatment program for elderly alcohol abusers. *Gerontologist, 24*, 510–516.

Emery, G., Gallagher, D., & Thompson, L. (1985). Cognitive therapy for depression in the elderly. New York: Guilford Press.

Foxx, R. M., McMorrow, M. J., Bittle, R. G., & Ness, W. (1986). An analysis of social skills generalization in two natural settings. *Journal of Applied Behavioral Analysis, 19*, 229–305.

Frank, P. J., Klein, S. K., & Jacobs, J. (1982). Cost-benefit analysis of behavioral program for geriatric inpatients. *Hospital & Community Psychiatry, 33*.

Gallagher, D., Lovett, S., & Zeiss, A. (in press). Interventions with caregivers of frail elderly persons. In M. Ory & K. Bond (Eds.), *Aging and health care: Social and policy perspectives*. New York: Tavistock Publications.

Gallagher, D., & Thompson, L. W. (1983). Depression. In P. M. Lewinsohn & L. Teri (Eds.), *Clinical geropsychology: New directions in treatment* (p. 7). Elmsford, NY: Pergamon Press.

Gerson, S. C., Poltkin, D. A., & Jarvik, L. F. (1988). Antidepressant drug studies 1964 to 1986: Empirical evidence for aging patients. *Journal of Clinical Psychopharmacology, 8*, 311–322.

Haley, W. E. (1983). A family-behavioral approach of the cognitively impaired elderly. *Gerontologist, 23*, 18–20.

Hogarty, G. E., & Ulrich, R. (1972). The discharge readiness inventory. *Archives of General Psychiatry, 26*, 414–426.

Honigfeld, G., Gillis, R. D., & Klett, J. (1966). *Cooperative studies in psychiatry*. Veteran's Administration Report No. 66. Perry Point, MD: Clinical Neurologic Research Laboratory.

Hoyer, W. J., Kafer, R. A., Simpson, S. C., & Hoyer, F. W. (1974). Reinstatement of verbal behavior in elderly mental patients using operant procedures. *Gerontologist, 14*, 149–152.

Hussian, R. A. (1981). *Geriatric psychology: A behavioral perspective*. New York: Van Nostrand Reinhold.

Hussian, R. A. (1982). Stimulus control in the modification of problematic behavior in elderly institutionalized patients. *International Journal of Behavioral Geriatrics, 1*, 33–46.

Hussian, R. A., & Davis, R. L. (1985). *Responsive care*. Champaign, IL: Research Press.

Jarvik, L. F., Mintz, J., Steuer, J., & Gerner, R. (1982). Treating geriatric depression: A 26-week interim analysis. *Journal of American Geriatric Sociology, 30*, 713–717.

Johnson, R., Fralliciardi, V., & Patterson, R. L. (1977, May). *A multiple baseline evaluation of a reality orientation procedure for disoriented geriatric clients*. Paper presented at the 23rd annual meeting of the Southeastern Psychological Association, Hollywood, FL.

Labouvie-Vief, G., & Gonda, J. N. (1976). Cognitive strategy training and intellectual performance in the elderly. *Journal of Gerontology, 31*, 327–332.

Lewinsohn, P. M., Antonuccio, D. O., Steinmetz, H., & Teri, L. (1984). *The coping with depression course: A psychoeducational intervention for unipolar depression*. Eugene, OR: Castalla Publishing.

Lewinsohn, P. M., Munoz, R., Youngren, M. A., & Zeiss, A. M. (1986). *Control your depression* (rev. ed.). New York: Prentice-Hall.

Liberman, R. P. (1987). Psychiatric rehabilitation of chronic mental patients. Washington, DC: American Psychiatric Press.

Liberman, R. P., DeRisi, W. J., & Mueser, K. T. (1989). *Social skills training for psychiatric patients*. Elmsford, NY: Pergamon Press.

McClannahan, L. E., & Risley, T. R. (1973). A store for nursing home residents. *Nursing Homes, 7*, 26–31.

McClannahan, L. E., & Risley, T. R. (1974). Design of living environments for nursing home resident. *Gerontologist, 14*, 236–240.

McEvoy, C. L., & Patterson, R. L. (1987). Behavioral treatment of deficit skills in dementia patients. *Gerontologist, 26*, 475–478.

Medication management module: A skills training program to improve responsible use of antipsychotic drugs. Trainer's manual, demonstration video, and patient's workbook available from Camarillo-UCLA Research Center, Box 6022, Camarillo, CA 93011, 1989.

Mishara, B. L. (1978). Geriatric patients who improve in token economy and general milieu treatment programs: A multivariate analysis. *Journal of Consulting Clinical Psychology, 46*, 1340–1348.

Mueller, D. J., & Atlas, L. (1972). Resocialization of regressed elderly residents: A behavioral management approach. *Journal of Gerontology, 3*, 390–392.

Patterson, R. L. (1985). Dementias arising in the senium and presenium. In R. Daitzman (Ed.), *Diagnosis and intervention in behavior therapy and behavioral medicine* (Vol. 4). New York: Springer.

Patterson, R. L. (1987). Family management of the elderly. In L. L. Carstensen & B. A. Edelstein (Eds.), *Handbook of clinical gerontology* (pp. 267–276). Elmsford, NY: Pergamon Press.

Patterson, R. L. (in press). Geriatric populations. In A. S. Bellak, M. Hersen, & A. E. Kazdin (Eds.), *International handbook of behavior modification and therapy* (2nd ed.). New York: Plenum Press.

Patterson, R. L., Dupree, L. W., Eberly, D. A., Jackson, G. M., O'Sullivan, M. J., Penner, L. A., & Dee-Kelly, C. (1982). *Overcoming deficits of aging: A behavioral approach*. New York: Plenum Press.

Patterson, R. L., & Jackson, G. M. (1980). Behavior modification with the elderly. In M. Hersen, R. M. Fisler, & P. Miller (Eds.), *Progress in behavior modification* (Vol. 9, pp. 206–241). New York: Academic Press.

Peterson, R. G., Knapp, T. J., Rosen, J. O., & Pither, B. F. (1977). The effects of furniture arrangement on the behavior of geriatric patients. *Behavior Therapy, 8*, 464–467.

Pfeiffer, E., Johnson, T. M., & Chiofolo, R. C. (1981). Functional assessment of elderly subjects in four service settings. *Journal of the American Geriatrics Association, 29*, 433–437.

Pinkston, E. M., & Linsk, N. L. (1984). *Care of the elderly: A family approach*. Elmsford, NY: Pergamon Press.

Quattrochi-Tubin, S., & Jasons, L. A. (1980). Enhancing social interactions and activity among the elderly through stimulus control. *Journal of Applied Behavior Analysis, 13*, 159–169.

Rusin, M. J. (1978). *Role play training of self-care skills with geriatric psychiatric patients*. Unpublished master's thesis, Florida State University.

Selzer, B. (1988). Organic mental disorders. In M. N. Armand (Ed.), *The new Harvard guide to psychiatry* (pp. 358–386). Cambridge, MA: Belknap Press of Harvard University Press.

Teri, L., & Uomoto, J. (August, 1986). *Treating depression in Alzheimer's disease: Teaching the caregivers behavioral strategies*. Paper presented at the annual meeting of the American Psychological Association. Submitted for publication.

Thompson, L. W., & Gallagher, D. (1984). Effectiveness of psychotherapy in the treatment of late-life depression. *Advances in Behavior Research Therapy, 6*, 127–139.

Thompson, L. W., Gallagher, D., & Breckinridge, J. S. (1987). Comparative effectiveness of psychotherapies for depressed elders. *Journal of Consulting Clinical Psychology, 55*, 385–390.

Thompson, L. W., Gallagher, D., Nies, G., & Epstein, D. (1983). Evaluation of the effectiveness of professionals and nonprofessionals as instructors of "Coping with Depression": Classes for elders. *Gerontologist, 23*, 390–396.

Whitehead, W. E., Burgio, K. L., & Engel, B. T. (1985). Biofeedback treatment of fecal incontinence in geriatric patients. *Journal of American Geriatric Sociology, 33*, 320–324.

Wisocki, P. A., & Mosher, P. M. (1980). Peer-facilitated sign language training for a geriatric stroke victim with chronic brain damage. *Journal Geriatric Psychiatry, 13*, 89–102.

Yeasavage, J. A. (1984). Relaxation and memory training in 39 elderly patients. *American Journal of Psychiatry*, 141.

Yeasavage, J. A. (1985). Nonpharmacologic treatment for memory losses with normal aging. *American Journal of Psychiatry*, 142.

Zarit, S. H., Anthony, C. R., & Boutsellis, M. (in press). Interventions with caregivers of dementia patients: A comparison of two approaches. *Psychology Aging*.

Zarit, S. H., Gallagher, D., & Kramer, N. (1981). Memory training in the community aged: Effects on depression, memory complaints and memory performance. *Educational Gerontology, 6*, 11–27.

Zarit, S. H., Orr, N. K., & Zarit, J. M. (1985). *The hidden victims of Alzheimer's disease: Families under stress*. New York: New York University Press.

Zarit, S. H., Zarit, J. M., & Reever, K. E. (1982). Memory training for severe memory loss: Effects on senile dementia patients and their families. *Gerontologist, 22*, 373–377.

CHAPTER 13

TREATMENTS OF MENTAL DISORDERS AND THE FUNCTIONAL CAPACITY TO WORK

Jim Mintz
Lois Imber Mintz
Catherine C. Phipps

It must be remembered that with adequate treatment some individuals suffering with chronic mental disorders not only have their symptoms and signs ameliorated but also return to a level of function close to that of their premorbid status (p. 71).

Social Security Regulations:
Rules for Determining Disability

According to the 1985 *Current Population Census* of the U.S. Bureau of the Census, more than 12 million people between the working ages of 16 and 64 are disabled (Bowe, 1986). This translates to about 1 American of working age in every 12, or 8% of the general population, having a work disability. It is estimated that approximately 1.7 million to 2.4 million persons, or between 14% and 20% of those with disabilities in the United States, have severe psychiatric impairments (Goldman, Gattozzi, & Taube, 1981). The Social Security Administration (SSA) operates the world's largest disability program, and mentally disabled individuals represent about 11% of those receiving Supplemental Security Income or Social Security Disability Income (Anderson, 1982).

Treatment of mental disorder might be expected to restore work capacity by addressing both sides of the vulnerability-stress balance. Treatments such as psychotropic medications modify basic biochemical vulnerabilities of the mentally disordered person, resulting not only in decreased symptoms but also in increased capacity in areas

This chapter is based on the final report for Research Grant No. 12-D-70272-9-01 from the Social Security Administration, *Treatments of Mental Disorders that Restore the Functional Capacity to Work* (Jim Mintz, PhD, Principal Investigator).

such as attention, information processing, and learning. Treatments such as psychotherapy or skills training may reduce stress by improving the family climate and providing the patient with increased coping skills and an increased sense of self-efficacy and confidence.

On the other hand, symptom remission will not always or even usually result in restoration of work capacity in the case of individuals with serious mental disorders. In some cases, residual impairments will continue to preclude employment. In other cases, recurrent symptom exacerbations may make stable gainful employment in the real competitive work market impossible, even though a person can work during periods of remission. A poor work history in itself becomes a barrier to employment. A simple listing of some of today's accepted psychiatric treatments—neuroleptic drugs, lithium, tricyclic antidepressants, benzodiazepines, exposure treatment for phobics, cognitive-behavioral treatment of depression, family therapy for schizophrenics—makes it clear that psychiatry has made considerable strides in the past 40 years in substantially relieving the symptoms of a variety of disorders, but does this imply that effective symptomatic treatment can be expected to restore work capacity?

There are surprisingly few hard data to answer this question. Psychiatric treatment studies characteristically focus exclusively on symptoms and ignore work outcomes, and even studies of symptom-oriented treatments may not draw detailed or sophisticated distinctions among psychiatric conditions (see, for example, Liberman & Phipps' review of behavioral treatments, 1987). Anthony and Jansen (1984) asserted strongly that "there is little or no correlation between a person's symptomatology and functional skills" (p. 540), but in support of this broad generalization they cite only evidence that mental hospitalization primarily affects symptoms rather than instrumental role functioning, hardly a surprising conclusion. In fact, no one has specifically reviewed the literature to evaluate the effects of psychiatric treatments on the capacity of individuals with well-specified particular mental disorders to return to work. The major reviews to date either do not focus on treatment at all (e.g., Avison & Speechley, 1987), allude to treatment findings only in general terms (e.g., Anthony & Liberman, 1986), or summarize findings across a diverse set of poorly done studies of mixed and unspecified diagnostic groups given varied rehabilitation treatments (e.g., Dion & Anthony, 1987). Thus, although there is a vast literature on psychiatric treatments, relatively little is known about the specific effects of treatments for specified conditions on the functional capacity to work.

The problem has significant implications for disability policy, psychiatric treatment and rehabilitation efforts, and the patients and their advocates. The lack of a secure knowledge base regarding effectiveness of treatments tied to specific disorders may affect the validity of disability determination. It seems obvious that a patient should not be classified as unable to work on the basis of having a mental disorder if effective treatments for that disorder exist which the individual has not tried. Successful identification of effective treatments would also pay off in obvious ways to rehabilitation agencies and clinicians, many of whom struggle with difficult patients whose problems are compounded by work insufficiency.

Mental health advocacy groups also have a keen interest in careful analyses of research findings regarding effective treatments of mental illness. Findings that certain treatments are clearly more effective than others in restoring the capacity of mentally disordered individuals to work should lead to increased pressures for appropriate research and treatment funding. A careful review of the literature may also identify areas in which research is simply lacking, and thus stimulate more productive fact finding.

Finally, consumers of mental health services—the patients, their families and advocates—need a secure foundation of knowledge as to which treatments are demonstrably effective, not only in terms of providing some measure of symptomatic relief but also in terms of restoring people to more fully functional lives in the work place. That knowledge base would provide a more informed and thus more rational basis on which patients and their advocates could rest their decisions about continued or alternative treatments. This review was designed to meet these needs. Its major objective is to summarize the current state of scientific knowledge of the effects of treatments on the capacity of mentally disordered people to work.

METHODS

Two complementary strategies were used to locate relevant publications—the computerized literature search of psychiatric, psychological, and rehabilitation data bases, and a detailed review of all articles published in nine leading scientific journals between 1983 and 1987.

Inclusion and Exclusion Criteria

To be included in this review, a study had to use samples of mentally disordered patients with diagnoses listed in the *Diagnostic and Statistical Manual of Mental Disorders*, 3rd ed. (DSM-III). However, studies of developmentally disabled persons (e.g., autistic, retarded) were excluded. Studies that included mixed diagnostic groups had to fulfill one of two conditions—either 50% or more of the patients came from one diagnostic group, or the results were listed separately for each diagnosis. The study had to involve evaluation of one or more specified psychiatric treatments, either psychiatric treatments aimed primarily at alleviating symptoms or vocational rehabilitation treatment focused directly on restoration of work capacity. The study had to include work-relevant measures as outcome variables. Studies were excluded if they included work functioning only in a composite measure in which the specific contribution of work was obscured, such as the Social Adjustment Scale (a composite measure that includes work along with measures of independent living skills, social skills, and family measures). In addition, studies that contained measures of prevocational skills or job-related skills or behaviors (e.g., social skills, job-seeking skills, anger management) were included only if they also contained reports of some measure of work functioning obtained in a work setting. Finally, articles that were not published in the English language were excluded.

Methods of Literature Search

Computerized searches of three data bases—REHABDATA, MEDLINE, and PsychINFO/PsychALERT—were conducted for the period covering 1983–1987. The starting date of 1983 was chosen because articles published prior to the introduction of DSM-III were considered likely to be diagnostically ambiguous. The search words covered each of three broad categories—mental disorders, treatment, and work. Each abstract was read by a licensed clinical psychologist who determined the potential relevance of the article to the project. All articles judged to be even potentially relevant on this basis were then read to determine if they met project criteria.

Computerized searches have definite limitations. They depend for their success on the appropriateness of the search key, on the publication abstract, and on the key words provided in the data base. Thus, if an article that included work outcome data did not refer to it in the title or the abstract, the computerized search would not identify it. To compensate for this characteristic, a second strategy was used to supplement the computerized search. All articles published in nine major journals from 1983 to 1987 were examined. The journals reviewed were the *Ar-*

chives of General Psychiatry, the *American Journal of Psychiatry*, the *Journal of Rehabilitation, Rehabilitation Counseling Bulletin, Hospital and Community Psychiatry*, the *Journal of Counseling Psychology*, and the *Journal of Consulting and Clinical Psychology*. In addition, two journals published in Great Britain were reviewed—*Psychological Medicine* and the *British Journal of Industrial Medicine*.

A licensed clinical psychologist examined each article carefully to determine whether it met the inclusion criteria listed above. In many cases, simply reading the title was sufficient, e.g., a study of brain chemistry or molecular biology. In others, careful reading of the abstract, methods section, tables and figures was necessary to identify relevant measures. In addition, the bibliographies of all relevant articles and of several important review articles in this area were carefully examined to identify other potentially relevant articles.

The Sample of Relevant Studies

The two methods of searching the literature turned out to be relatively independent, yielding few studies in common. On the one hand, the computerized searches covered many more publications than the nine that were individually examined. On the other hand, the review of journals turned up a number of articles that had relevant data but did not mention work in the abstract or key words and were missed by the computer search. The computer searches yielded approximately 800 abstracts for review. The journal review involved scanning of over 3,500 articles. From these, a total of 44 articles from 41 studies were judged to be appropriate for inclusion here. By diagnosis, they were classified as follows: schizophrenia or mixed population, mostly schizophrenic (16 articles), alcohol disorders (14), drug abuse (9), anxiety disorders (2), gamblers (2), and affective disorder (1).

Quality Ratings

The 41 studies vary widely in quality of design. To provide some objective basis for evaluation of the weight to be placed on each, a quality rating scheme developed by May (1974) and May and Van Putten (1974) was applied to each study. This is a complex and well thought out system for classifying studies in terms of design quality, using categories from I (Best) to VI (Worst).

In the May and Van Putten system, the experimental design used is the most important issue for evaluating the results obtained, and great weight is given to the presence of a control group and randomization. These emphases are appropriate for the purpose of this review—the evaluation of treatment effects. Without a control group, it is really impossible to determine whether any changes that occurred would not have occurred even without treatment for any number of possible reasons. Without randomization, it is impossible to determine whether differences between groups are due to experimental procedures or characteristics of the patients that would have led to group differences even if they had been exposed to identical treatments.

In fact, there is epidemiological evidence that patients may often be at a particularly low ebb at the time they enter treatment. If so, some degree of improvement or return to their more typical baseline level would be expected simply as time passes. The epidemiological study of Dohrenwend, Dohrenwend, Link, and Levav (1983) suggests strongly that mentally disordered *cases* may be functioning particularly poorly at the time they become *patients*, particularly in the area of work attainment. The authors suggest that a connection may exist between transient symptom exacerbations and work impairment.

Although they suggest that this association between social role functioning and symptoms may be less notable with severe chronic patients such as schizophrenics, at least one study of schizophrenics (Test, Knoedler, Allness, & Burke, 1985) indicates that work performance is unusually impaired at the time of admission even in that population. In that study, 54% of the patients had been their own primary financial support between age 18 and study admission, but only 8% were working at the time of admission.

Furthermore, over time, even chronic and severe patients may show substantial improvement that is not attributable to specific treatments. This is why controlled experimental designs are critical if one is to draw strong causal inferences in this area. For example, one long-term (Harding, Brooks, Ashikaga, Strauss, & Breier, 1987a) follow-up study of back ward patients found that many were working. In a companion study of schizophrenics from this sample (Harding, Brooks, Ashikaga, Strauss, & Breier, 1987b) (treatment is not specifically mentioned in this report), the authors state that "one-half to two-thirds of the sample had achieved considerable improvement or recovered" (p. 727).

Each of the studies in the sample was classified into one of May and Van Putten's six quality levels, with I being the highest and VI the lowest. The descriptive labels used below (from Excellent to Very Poor) were not part of May and Van Putten's original method but are provided simply to help the reader interpret the numerical system. Categories I-IV require that experimental and control subjects be treated at the same facility or that there is evidence of equivalence of treatment for subjects within treatment groups, a prospective design with at least 6 subjects either serving as their own control or assigned to a separate control or comparison group, and at least 50% of the sample drawn from the same diagnostic group. Category VI is reserved for articles that are uninterpretable for the purposes of this project, generally either because of the use of a diagnostically heterogeneous population or because no work data were presented separately. Studies in Category VI were not reviewed in this project.

RESULTS

All the studies reviewed below are summarized in Tables 13.1 through 13.5. Each table provides the first author and year of publication, sample size and diagnostic breakdown, quality rating, and a brief description of the setting, research design, employment measures and results.

Drug Addiction

Nine articles from six studies of the treatment of drug addicts were located (Table 13.1). These studies evaluated psychotherapy as a supplement to drug counseling in the context of a methadone maintenance program, tricyclic antidepressant treatment for depression in this population, methadone maintenance versus detoxification, residential therapeutic communities and vocational training.

Short-term Psychotherapy

There is conflicting evidence as to whether adding short-term individual psychotherapy to drug counseling in a conventional long-term methadone maintenance program results in meaningful gains in either vocational activity or drug rehabilitation. One study suggests that a cognitive-behavioral and a psychodynamically oriented psychotherapy were both equally useful adjuncts to drug counseling, particularly for patients with at least moderate levels of psychiatric impairment in addition to their addiction (Woody et al., 1983, 1984, 1985, 1987 [Quality Rating: III, Good]). However, a very similar study of a somewhat different dynamically oriented short-term psychotherapy (Rounsaville, Glazer, Wilber, Weissman, & Kleber, 1983 [Quality Rating: IV, Fair]) did not find any benefits in a similar treatment setting.

Antidepressant Medication

One placebo-controlled study of antidepressant medication (Kleber, Weissman, Rounsaville, Wilber, Prusoff, & Riordan, 1983 [Quality Rating: III, Good]) as an adjunct to methadone maintenance for depressed addicts found no specific benefits for active medication although work functioning did tend to improve as depressive symptoms waned in both treatment and control groups.

Vocational Rehabilitation

There was only one study of a vocational training program for this population. It suggested that although simply placing substance abusers in graduated supervised work settings may help them return to the work force, it probably does relatively little to help them establish long-term careers (Hammer, Ravndal, & Vaglum, 1985 [Quality Rating: IV, Fair]).

Residential Therapeutic Communities

A comparison of three quite different residential communities failed to find differences in symptom and work outcomes, but all of them were better than a simple short-term drug detoxification program (Bale et al., 1984 [Quality Rating: IV, Fair]).

Alcoholism

Fourteen studies involving treatment of alcoholics were located (Table 13.2). The topics included training in controlled drinking versus abstinence goals, lithium, comparisons of varying levels of treatment intensity and alcohol rehabilitation program evaluations.

Controlled Drinking

Three studies compared training in controlled drinking with a program based on abstinence goals (Foy, Nunn, & Rychtarik, 1984 [Quality Rating: I, Excellent]; Stimmel 1983 [Quality Rating, IV, Fair]; Sanchez-Craig, Annis, Bornet, & MacDonald, 1984 [Quality Rating: IV, Fair]). None of these studies found differences in work outcomes, and only one (Foy et al., 1984 [Quality Rating: I, Excellent]) reported differences in drinking outcomes. In that study, drinking outcomes were better with abstinence goals, at least for the first 6 months, but work outcomes were actually slightly better in the controlled drinking group.

Treatment Intensity

Several studies examined the question of whether *more* treatment or *more intense* treatment for alcoholics was better. These studies included controlled comparisons of inpatient with partial hospital treatment (McCrady et al., 1986 [Quality Rating: II, Very Good]), time limited versus unlimited treatment (Maisto, Sobell, Sobell, & Sanders, 1985 [Quality Rating: III, Good]), brief versus longer treatment (Walker, Donovan, Kivlahan, & O'Leary, 1983 [Quality Rating: IV, Fair]; Donovan, Kivlahan, & Walker, 1984 [Quality Rating: IV, Fair]), and of supportive therapy versus medication (Powell, Penick, Read, & Ludwig, 1985 [Quality Rating: I, Excellent]). None of these studies found differential effects on work outcomes. One study of inpatient versus outpatient treatment (Meyer, Berman, & Rivers, 1985 [Quality Rating: IV, Fair]) reported a significant interaction effect between socioeconomic status and treatment—lower status clients appeared to benefit more from outpatient treatment while higher status clients gained more as inpatients. This is the only study in this group that suggests any differential benefits as a function of treatment setting; the finding is complex and difficult to interpret. There are at least two reasons to discount this result somewhat, in addition to its inconsistency with the main thrust of the literature. First, patients were not randomly assigned to the two types of

Table 13.1. Summary of Studies on Drug Addiction

AUTHOR	N	QUALITY RATING	DESCRIPTION	DESIGN	EMPLOYMENT MEASURE	RESULTS
1. Bale et al. (1984)	562	IV: Fair	Three residential therapeutic communities versus drug withdrawal only	Four-group nonrandomized, pretest and posttest	Working or attending school, 2-year follow-up	Two of the residential programs were superior to withdrawal on the work measure, and all three were better on measures of illicit drug use
2. Hammer et al. (1985)	141	IV: Fair	Supervised graduated employment in a public vocational training program (Oslo, Norway)	Retrospective follow-up study of completers versus dropouts	Work activity at 5-year follow-up	Drug use decline after program participation. Patients who completed 3 months had better work performance
3. Kleber et al. (1983)	46	III: Good	Imipramine versus placebo in two public drug clinics	Two-group randomized double-blind clinical trial	Work ratings on Social Adjustment Scale at 8 weeks	Both groups showed significantly decreased depression and improved work ratings. No differences between treatments
4. Kosten et al. (1987)	204	IV: Fair	Methadone maintenance versus detoxification in a state mental health center	Two-group nonrandomized design with pre- and posttest stratified by primary source of income	Employment status at 30-month follow-up	Methadone maintenance was associated with better employment than detoxification except for patients on welfare, who did poorly regardless of treatment modality

5. Rounsaville et al. (1983)	72	IV: Fair	Interpersonal psychotherapy (IPT) added to methadone maintenance program versus maintenance alone	Two-group randomized clinical trial	Employment patterns at 12 and 24 months	No change in employment and no differences between treatments
6a. Woody et al. (1983)	110	III: Good	Two types of brief psychotherapy added to standard drug counseling in a methadone clinic	Three-group randomized clinical trial	Employment factor score, days worked, money earned at 1-month post-treatment	The Supportive-Expressive group had the most consistent significant improvements across all three work measures
6b. Woody et al. (1984)				Analysis with cases stratified by severity of psychiatric symptoms		No differences between treatments in employment outcomes across severity groups, but drug outcomes were better with psychotherapy for more severe cases
6c. Woody et al. (1985)				Analysis stratified by presence of personality or affective disorder		No significant differences in employment as a function of diagnostic subgroup
6d. Woody et al. (1987)					Analysis 5 months post-treatment (1 year after admission)	Overall, the dynamic psychotherapy group showed the most significant improvements over baseline on the three work measures

Table 13.2. Summary of Studies on Alcoholism

AUTHOR	N	QUALITY RATING	DESCRIPTION	DESIGN	EMPLOYMENT MEASURE	RESULTS
1. Donovan et al. (1984)	245	IV: Fair	Neuropsychological functioning as a prognostic indicator for inpatient alcoholism treatment	One-group pre- and post-treatment assessments	Hours worked weekly, 3-, 6-, and 9-month follow-up	Neuropsychological measures predicted work outcomes but were not related to drinking outcomes
2. Fagan & Mauss (1986)	123	V: Poor	Program evaluation of a rehabilitation program for skid row alcoholics	One-group pre- and post-treatment assessments	Employment status, monthly income with follow-up varying from 2 to 18 months	Employment and monthly income were higher at follow-up. Family contact (especially marriage) predicted good work outcomes
3. Fawcett et al. (1987)	105	I: Excellent	Lithium carbonate versus placebo in the treatment of alcoholics in two private medical centers	Two-group randomized clinical trial	Percent of work days missed with follow-up up to 12 months	Medication compliance was associated with better work attendance during the first 6 months of follow-up for both active medication and placebo groups
4. Foy et al. (1984)	62	I: Excellent	Controlled drinking skills training versus standard behavior treatment with abstinence goals in a VA Medical Center	Two-group randomized trial, pretest and posttest	Employment status at 12-month follow-up	Both groups significantly reduced their drinking, but the abstinence goals group had fewer abusive drinking days. Employment rates at 12 months were comparable in both treatment groups
5. Frances et al. (1984)	2215	V: Poor	Family history of alcoholism as a prognostic factor in Navy inpatient alcohol rehabilitation programs	Two-group nonrandomized retrospective study	Job performance ratings at 6, 12, and 24 months after treatment	Patients with more first-degree relatives with alcoholism had poorer job outcomes
6. Kolb et al. (1983)	749	V: Poor	Evaluation of Navy inpatient alcohol rehabilitation program	Retrospective follow-up of treated alcoholics, medical patients, and untreated controls	Job performance, unauthorized absences, and desertion	Job performance declined in all groups, but the decline was smaller for treated alcoholics than among the general Navy sample

7. Maisto et al. (1985)	48	III: Good	Time-limited versus open-ended outpatient alcohol rehabilitation treatment	Randomized clinical trial	Days employed over 18-month follow-up	Drinking behavior improved significantly, but employment decreased slightly (from 88% to 84% of possible days worked) with no group differences
8. McCardy et al. (1986)	174	II: Very Good	Partial hospitalization versus extended inpatient treatment in a private psychiatric hospital	Two-group randomized clinical trial	Employment rates and job losses due to drinking over a 12-month follow-up	Employment rates were unchanged from baseline. Almost one-third of the patients lost jobs, usually in the first 6 months
9. Meyer et al. (1985)	44	IV: Fair	Inpatient versus outpatient treatment in a general hospital alcohol rehabilitation program	Two-group nonrandomized design with posttest only	Employment, weeks missed with at least 3-month follow-up	Low socioeconomic status (SES) patients benefited more from outpatient treatment, and high SES patients did better with inpatient treatment
10. Powell et al. (1985)	148	I: Excellent	Medication only (Antabuse) versus medication plus support in a VA Medical Center outpatient clinic	Randomized controlled clinical trial	Job performance ratings with 12-month follow-up period	All groups, including minimally treated controls, were rated as slightly improved on job performance ratings with no difference among groups
11. Sanchez-Craig et al. (1984)	70	IV: Fair	Controlled drinking versus cognitive behavioral outpatient treatment with abstinence goals	Two-group nonrandomized design with pre- and posttest	Weeks worked full-time with 5-, 12-, 18- and 24-month follow-ups	Both groups reduced alcohol consumption. No differences in improvement in employment status, which tended to decline over the follow-up period
12. Stimmel et al. (1983)	105	IV: Fair	Controlled drinking versus abstinence goals for alcoholic opiate addicts being treated in an urban methadone maintenance program	Three-group randomized clinical trial with standard treatment control group	Employment status, days worked over a 30-month follow-up period	No differences in work outcomes among study groups
13. Waldo & Gardiner (1984)	77	V: Poor	Evaluation of a residential treatment program in a VA Medical Center	One-group evaluation study with pre- and posttest	Employment status at 1, 3, and 6 months	Employment rates were higher at discharge than at admission, with some decline during follow-up
14. Walker et al. (1983)	245	IV: Fair	Two week versus 7-week milieu-oriented inpatient treatment in a VA Medical Center	Two-group nonrandomized design with pre- and posttest	Employment status, hours worked weekly, monthly income at 3, 6, and 9 months	Both groups improved, with no differential treatment effects

treatment. Second, this finding was one of the few "significant" findings from a large number of exploratory analyses done and could well have been due to chance.

Lithium Carbonate

Fawcett et al., 1987 [Quality Rating: I, Excellent]; see also Fawcett et al., 1984, for an earlier interim report of this study) examined the efficacy of lithium carbonate. Compliance in taking medications—either lithium or placebo—was associated with better work attendance during the first 6 months only, but serum lithium levels were not associated with employment outcomes.

Alcohol Rehabilitation Program Evaluations

Finally, several program evaluation studies without control groups and follow-up studies of patients treated in alcohol rehabilitation programs were located. A study of an alcoholism reentry program (ARP) for skid row alcoholics (Fagan & Mauss, 1986 [Quality Rating: V, Poor]) reported gains in employment. A study in a VA residential treatment program (Waldo & Gardiner, 1984 [Quality Rating: V, Poor]) found that employment rates were higher at discharge with some decline over a 6-month follow-up period. Kolb, Baker, & Gunderson (1983 [Quality Rating: V, Poor]) found that alcoholics treated in a Navy rehabilitation program performed at least as well over time as other Navy men. Although the study was not a treatment evaluation, Frances, Bucky, & Alexopoulos (1984 [Quality Rating: V, Poor]) examined the relationship between treatment outcome and familial rates of alcoholism in male Navy alcoholic inpatients. Poorer job performance ratings were associated with a greater number of first-degree relatives with alcoholism, suggesting that alcohol rehabilitation programs may be less successful with more severely affected patients.

Anxiety, Panic and Affective Disorders

Only three studies reporting on work outcomes were found in this group of disorders (Table 13.3).

Behavioral Psychotherapy for Anxiety

Ginsberg, Marks, and Waters (1984 [Quality Rating: II, Very Good]) reported a randomized, controlled trial in England of behavioral psychotherapy provided by a nurse-therapist, compared with "routine management" provided by the patient's general practitioner. Roughly two-thirds of the patients had phobic disorders; the remainder had habit, obsessive-compulsive, and sexual disorders. At entry into the study, many of these patients indicated that their psychiatric disorder created difficulties for them in the work place by restricting their freedom of job choice, reducing efficiency, or impeding promotion. Both groups of patients appeared to derive some degree of symptomatic benefit over the course of the study, but at 1-year follow-up, the authors report that no significant changes in work functioning had occurred for either group. Behaviorally treated patients appeared to have somewhat better job attendance, but this was not statistically significant.

Benzodiazepine for Panic

Reich (1988 [Quality Rating: II, Very Good]) studied the effectiveness of treating 52 patients with panic disorder with benzodiazepine for 8 weeks. There was a significant reduction in panic attacks and anxiety for both treated groups compared to those who received placebo. Treated patients also showed a significant reduction in work disability scores. Presence of a DSM-III histrionic disorder was associated with poorer outcomes—both in terms of number of situational panic attacks and work disability.

Table 13.3. Summary of Studies on Pathological Gambling

AUTHOR	N	QUALITY RATING	DESCRIPTION	DESIGN	EMPLOYMENT MEASURE	RESULTS
1. Russo et al. (1984)	124	V: Poor	30-day inpatient program in a VA Medical Center	Uncontrolled evaluation study with posttest only	Employment status at 1 year	55% report no gambling activity at follow-up. 74% working daily, but no relationship between gambling status and work
2. Taber et al. (1987)	66	V: Poor	30-day inpatient program in a VA Medical Center	Uncontrolled evaluation study with pre- and posttest	Wage earner role on Psychiatric Status Schedule at 6-month follow-up	The patients showed significant reductions in gambling behavior and significant improvement on the employment measure at follow-up

A Single Case Study of Dysthymic Disorder

Mueser, Foy, and Carter (1986 [Quality Rating: V, Poor]) conducted a multiple baseline case study of a 28-year-old male with an Axis I diagnosis of dysthymic disorder and an Axis II diagnosis of schizoid personality. The patient had difficulty maintaining his job due to temper outbursts and sensitivity to criticism. Over a 4-month period, 13 sessions of behavioral treatment were conducted. The patient's performance improved, and these improvements were maintained at 1- and 3-month follow-ups. At 8 months, the patient was still employed and job performance was evaluated as good by his employer.

Pathological Gamblers

Two studies from the same research group reported on the effectiveness of an inpatient alcohol treatment program for pathological gamblers (Table 13.4). Six beds on an alcohol inpatient ward were reserved for the gamblers, who were treated together with alcoholic patients except for separate group psychotherapy and Gamblers Anonymous meetings. The first study (Russo, Taber, McCormick, & Ramirez, 1984 [Quality Rating: V, Poor]) was a weak retrospective follow-up study with no pretreatment measures. The second study (Taber, McCormick, Russo, Adkins, & Ramirez, 1987 [Quality Rating: V, Poor]) had a somewhat better prospective design in which pretreatment assessments were collected. In this study, there was a significant reduction in gambling behaviors, and patients showed significant improvement 6 months after treatment on the wage earner role dimension on the Psychiatric Status Scale. In the absence of a control group, the changes cannot be attributed to treatment unambiguously, but the report suggests that participants in the program did experience benefits in both symptoms and employment.

Schizophrenia

Sixteen studies of schizophrenic or mostly schizophrenic samples were located (Table 13.5). These are organized under four major headings—the effects of family therapy, of psychodynamic psychotherapy, of neuroleptic drugs, and of vocational rehabilitation programs.

Family Therapy

Two studies of family therapies were reviewed. Falloon, McGill, Boyd, and Pederson (1987 [Quality Rating: I, Excellent]) compared a behavioral family management approach with individual treatment. Key relatives appeared to be somewhat less dissatisfied with a patient's work functioning if they had participated in the family treatment, particularly at the end of the 9-month treatment period, but there was no statistical evidence of improvement in actual work functioning. Spencer et al. (1988 [Quality Rating: IV, Fair]) examined the effectiveness of adding a psychoeducational inpatient family intervention to standard care. There were no significant treatment effects at either 9- or 18-month follow-up points on work performance. In fact, it was not clear whether the treatment program was symptomatically effective, either.

Long-term Dynamic (Psychoanalytic) Psychotherapy

Sjostrom (1985 [Quality Rating: IV, Fair]) studied the effects of long-term psychotherapy based on psychodynamic theory. Patients also participated in social and rehabilitation activities and received neuroleptic treatment. The patients were chosen for inclusion in the study if someone on the health care team (e.g., doctor, nurse) judged that the patient was suitable for psychotherapy. A comparison group was selected from patients treated on other wards with conventional treatment, generally relying heavily on depot neuroleptics, and they were matched

Table 13.4. Summary of Studies on Anxiety and Affective Disorders

AUTHOR	N	QUALITY RATING	DESCRIPTION	DESIGN	EMPLOYMENT MEASURE	RESULTS
1. Ginsberg et al. (1984)	50	II: Very Good	Behavioral psychotherapy versus routine care from a general practitioner for anxiety disorders (mostly phobics) in mental health centers in Great Britain	Two-group randomized clinical trial	Work absences and patient ratings of work problems at 1 year follow-up	Clinical outcomes were significantly better for the behavior therapy group. Some work measures favored the behavioral treatment but these differences were not significant
2. Mueser et al. (1986)	1	V: Poor	Behavioral social-skills training in a VA Medical Center for a single case with dysthymia and personality disorder	Multiple baseline single-case design	Ratings of job performance at 1- and 3-month follow-up	Performance improved from baseline at the 3-month follow-up
3. Reich (1988)	52	II: Very Good	Diazepam versus alprazolam versus placebo in an outpatient mental health center and a VA Medical Center for panic disorder	Three-group randomized double-blind clinical trial	Ratings of work disability at 8 weeks	Both drug groups showed significant reductions in symptoms and work disability relative to the placebo group. Patients with histrionic personality disorders had poorer clinical outcomes and greater work disability

Table 13.5. Summary of Studies on Schizophrenia and Mixed Diagnoses (Mostly Schizophrenia)

AUTHOR	N	QUALITY RATING	DESCRIPTION	DESIGN	EMPLOYMENT MEASURE	RESULTS
1. Alanen et al. (1985a, 1985b)	100	V: Poor	Comparison of inpatient versus outpatient hospitalization in a community psychiatric hospital	Uncontrolled evaluation study with pre- and posttest	Employment rates at 5-year follow-up	Lower than average neuroleptic dose was significantly correlated with higher rates of employment
2. Bell & Ryan (1984)	**78** 32	IV: Fair	Comparison of inpatient psychosocial rehabilitation versus intensive psychotherapy versus standard milieu treatment in a VA Medical Center	Three-group nonrandomized study with posttest only	Employment rates at 6-, 12-, and 18-month follow-up	The rehabilitation program had nonsignificantly higher employment rates and nonsignificantly lower recidivism rates than the other two groups
3. Bond & Dincin (1986)	131	IV: Fair	Comparison of accelerated entry into transitional employment versus standard gradual employment in a psychosocial rehabilitation agency	Two-group randomized design, stratified by work experience	Employment rates and total earnings at 9 and 15 months	At 9 months, there were no differences in rehospitalization or competitive employment rates between the groups. However, significantly more accelerated patients were in some kind of paid employment, including transitional jobs, and they worked significantly more weeks. By 15 months, the trends were similar but all nonsignificant
4. Falloon et al. (1987)	36	I: Excellent	Comparison of an outpatient family management approach versus individual treatment in a public mental health center	Two-group randomized clinical trial	Work functioning at 9 and 24 months	Family informants in family treatment appeared to become somewhat more satisfied with the patients' work functioning at the end of treatment. There was no statistical evidence of actual gains in work activity over the 2-year study course

5. Gaebel & Pietzcker (1985)	72	IV: Fair	A comparison of inpatient versus outpatient treatment in a university psychiatric hospital	Four-group (medication compliers versus noncompliers, multiple versus first admissions) nonrandomized design with pretest and posttest	Work functioning on the Strauss-Carpenter Scale at 1-year follow-up	Medication compliers had fewer hospitalizations but poorer work outcomes. Chronic patients showed a significant worsening in work functioning during the follow-up period
6. Gaebel & Pietzcker (1985)	**86** 75	IV: Fair	A comparison of inpatient versus outpatient treatment in a university psychiatric hospital	Two-group nonrandomized (continuous versus noncontinuous neuroleptic treatment) with pretest and posttest	Work functioning on the Strauss-Carpenter Scale at 1-year follow-up	Continuously treated patients had better clinical outcomes but poorer work outcomes. Better work outcomes were associated with fewer symptoms. Prior work history accounted for 49% of the variance in work outcomes
7. Hogarty et al. (1988)	70	I: Excellent	Comparison of standard dose versus minimal dose fluphenazine in a psychiatric hospital and outpatient clinic	Two-group randomized double-blind clinical trial, patients stratified by familial expressed emotion	Employment rates, number of hours worked per week in the past month measured on the Major Role Adjustment Inventory at 1- and 2-year follow-up	No differences were found between the groups in relapse due to dose, expressed emotion, or their interaction. At 2-year follow-up, minimal dose patients had better work functioning than standard dose
8. Jacobs et al. (1984)	**52** 45	V: Poor	Evaluation of a job club program that provided training in job finding skills and assistance in locating employment located in a VA Medical Center	Uncontrolled evaluation with posttest only	Employment rates at 1, 2, 3, and 6 months	56% of the participants found jobs; of those, 67.5% were employed at 6-month follow-up
9. Johnson et al. (1983)	116	IV: Fair	Comparison of depot neuroleptics versus drug discontinuers in an outpatient clinic	Two-group nonrandomized design with pretest and posttest	Work function ratings at 12 and 18 months	Drug discontinuers had more relapses and poorer work functioning. Relapse-free drug discontinuers had similar work outcomes to drug continuers

Table 13.5. Continued

AUTHOR	N	QUALITY RATING	DESCRIPTION	DESIGN	EMPLOYMENT MEASURE	RESULTS
10. Katz et al. (1984)	69	IV: Fair	Evaluation of outpatient psychotherapy in a private psychiatric hospital	Two-group nonrandomized design (psychotherapy dropouts versus continuers) with pretest and posttest	Employment status at 2 years	No differences in overall employment rates or rates of full-time employment. Continuers had more part-time employment than discontinuers
11. Kecmanovic (1985)	58	IV: Fair	Comparison of day treatment versus inpatient treatment in a psychiatric hospital	Two-group nonrandomized design with posttest only	Working ability at 18 months	No differences were found between groups in ratings of symptoms or work
12. Ryan & Bell (1983)	**43** 7	V: Poor	Evaluation of an inpatient program emphasizing long-term psychoanalytically oriented psychotherapy in a VA Medical Center	Uncontrolled evaluation with posttest only	Employment rates and job ratings on the Strauss-Carpenter Level of Function Scale at 6 months	The rehospitalization rate was 34% with 84% at least mildly symptomatic. 20% of the patients were employed and they worked an average of $\frac{1}{4}$ of the possible working hours. Job quality was rated as only "moderately competent"
13. Sjostrom (1985)	57	IV: Fair	Evaluation of individual long-term psychoanalytically oriented psychotherapy versus conventional treatment in a psychiatric hospital in Sweden	Two-group nonrandomized design with posttest only	Work ratings on Strauss-Carpenter Scale at 6 and 8 years	Psychotherapy patients did significantly better on all measures including employment

14. Spencer et al. (1988)	**93** 76	IV: Fair	Comparison of inpatient family therapy versus standard hospital treatment in an acute psychiatric care inpatient unit	Two-group nonrandomized clinical trial	Ratings of primary work role at 18 months	No significant differences on clinical outcomes or work measures were found between the groups
15. Van Der Kolk & Goldberg (1983)	57	V: Poor	Comparison of depot fluphenazine versus oral medications in an urban mental health center	Retrospective follow-up study with two comparison groups	Employment status at 6 years	Both groups showed significant symptomatic improvement with the depot group showing a somewhat stronger trend. The oral medication group had better employment outcomes (61% versus 21%)
16. Wherley & Bisgaard (1987)	**370** 226	V: Poor	Comparison of 19 intensive, transitional, and supportive residential treatment programs	Retrospective follow-up study with three comparison groups	Vocational activity and rates of competitive employment at 6-month follow-up	All programs showed increases in vocational activity (18% to 48%) and competitive employment (3% to 25%). Competitive employment gains were highest for transitional program patients. No significance levels were provided

Note: When the sample includes mixed diagnoses, the number of schizophrenic subjects is displayed first in boldface, followed with the number of patients with other diagnoses.

for age and work in the year prior to treatment with the experimental group. The experimental group did significantly better on virtually all of the outcome variables, including employment.

Two nonexperimental studies done in the United States failed to replicate these positive findings. Ryan and Bell (1983 [Quality Rating: V, Poor]) examined the effectiveness of a psychoanalytically oriented long-term inpatient treatment environment. At a 6-month follow-up, the quantity and quality of work, as measured on the Strauss-Carpenter Scale, were at levels described by the authors as "indistinguishable from baseline rates" (p. 730). Katz, Frank, Gunderson, and Hamm (1984 [Quality Rating: IV, Fair]) compared 2-year outcomes of nonchronic schizophrenic patients who dropped out of a long-term psychotherapy research project with a self-selected group who had remained in psychotherapy for at least 6 months. The only significant difference between psychotherapy dropouts and continuers in the area of employment was that patients who remained in therapy had more part-time employment than discontinuers, a finding that was significant only in the second year of follow-up.

Neuroleptic Drugs

A surprising number of studies suggested that higher doses or more consistent neuroleptic treatment might be associated with poorer work outcomes. Gaebel and Pietzcker (1985a [Quality Rating: IV, Fair]) found that work functioning declined during a 1-year follow-up. It is interesting that this was true for medication-compliant patients, but not for noncompliant patients. In fact, one of the best discriminators between compliant and noncompliant patients was the quality of work functioning at follow-up, with compliant patients doing more poorly. In another study by Gaebel and Pietzcker (1985b [Quality Rating: IV, Fair]), schizophrenic patients who were continuously treated with neuroleptic medication had significantly shorter durations of employment ($p < .04$) than those treated noncontinuously. It is impossible in this study to determine cause and effect, but it is clear that continuously treated patients began treatment at lower employment levels, and then declined more during the follow-up year relative to patients who received medication intermittently. Finally, a significant interaction was found between chronicity, continuity of treatment, and employment outcome. As in the other study from these authors, continuous neuroleptic treatment was more strongly associated with poorer employment outcomes among chronic patients. Indeed, in that group, continuous medication predicted poor employment outcome even when pretreatment employment status was statistically controlled.

Johnson, Pasterski, Ludlow, Street, and Taylor (1983 [Quality Rating: IV: Fair]) compared chronic schizophrenic patients who made the decision on their own to discontinue neuroleptic therapy after remaining stable 12 to 48 months with a similar stabilized comparison group who did not express an interest in stopping their depot medication, and who continued to take their medication. Patients discontinued using the medications for two reasons: they stated that they felt cured, or they believed they would feel better without the medication. Relapse rates at 12 and 18 months were significantly higher among patients who discontinued medication. Work-role performance was somewhat impaired among patients who relapsed, but was not significantly affected by discontinuation of medication if the patient remained clinically stable. It should be noted that the definition of work-role effectiveness was apparently quite broad, encompassing competitive employment and rehabilitation activities.

Alanen, Rakkolainen, Rasimus, Laakso, and Kaljonen (1985a, 1985b [Quality Rating: V, Poor]) studied a group of patients described as "very similar to the criteria . . . in the DSM-III classification, although we did not adhere to the strict criterion of duration specified in DSM-III." The best predictor of working capacity at follow-up in this group was lower than average neuroleptic treatment. The authors note that the nonexperimental design does not permit causal conclusions, since amount of medication was related to the disappearance of psychotic symptoms. Patients whose symptoms disappeared received less medication, on average, during the follow-up. Nevertheless, the authors believe that their multivariate analytic models provide at least suggestive evidence that more neuroleptic treatment is associated with poorer employment outcomes for schizophrenics.

Van der Kolk and Goldberg (1983 [Quality Rating: V, Poor]) retrospectively grouped patients on the basis of whether the patient had been treated with depot fluphenazine or oral antipsychotic medication. Both medication groups showed significant symptomatic improvement, and the depot group did somewhat better ($p < .06$ for the comparison of depot versus oral medication on Brief Psychiatric Rating Scale (BPRS) improvement, with only the depot group changing significantly). In contrast, the oral medication group did significantly better ($p = .02$) on measures of employment, despite the fact that they had somewhat poorer pretreatment employment measures. However, overall, fewer than a quarter of the patients who participated in this study were gainfully employed at follow-up.

Finally, there is one well-designed controlled study that is consistent with the thrust of these relatively weak retrospective studies with regard to the effects of standard doses of neuroleptics on work functioning (Hogarty et al., 1988 [Quality Rating: I, Excellent]; see Hogarty et al., 1986, for a more detailed description of the study methodology). Patients were treated with a standard or a minimal dose of fluphenazine decanoate in a randomized double-blind study. Among the medication-compliant survivors at 1 year, patients in the minimal-dose condition who were living in households characterized as low in expressed emotion (EE) were more adequate in their role performance than those in high EE households. At the 2-year follow-up point, the minimal-dose recipients had far better work functioning than standard-dose patients. A measure of the hours employed among wage earners indicated that minimal-dose recipients were working approximately half-time, while standard-dose recipients worked only a few hours. Patients in the minimal-dose group, however, were slightly more symptomatic than the high-dose recipients.

Rehabilitation Programs

Kecmanovic (1985 [Quality Rating: IV, Fair]) compared post-release adjustment of schizophrenics treated during a 2-year period either in a day hospital or as inpatients. The same diagnostic and therapeutic procedures were used in both treatment conditions. All of the schizophrenic patients had been able to work prior to their last hospitalization, making this a very high-functioning sample. No significant differences were found between day- and full-time patients on any work outcome measure. Almost all the patients in both groups had returned to work. Only 10% of the sample was characterized as "unable to work" at follow-up, and no differences were found as a function of type of treatment.

Bell and Ryan (1984 [Quality Rating: IV, Fair]) compared the efficacy of a hospital-based psychosocial rehabilitation program which provided training in three primary areas (vocational, social, and community living) with a standard residential program and an intensive psychotherapy program. The rehabilitation program had less recidivism than the other two treatments, and somewhat higher employment rates, but neither of these differences was statistically significant.

Jacobs, Kardashian, Kreinbring, Ponder, and Simpson (1984 [Quality Rating: V, Poor]) evaluated the effectiveness of a job-seeking skills-training program (the job club) with psychiatric patients in a program evaluation study. At 6 months, about two-thirds of the patients were employed.

Bond and Dincin (1986 [Quality Rating: IV, Fair]) evaluated a transitional employment (TE) program in a psychosocial rehabilitation agency. Subjects in the study were randomly assigned to either a "gradual" condition in which they remained in the prevocational work crews for a minimum of 4 months, or to an "accelerated" condition in which they immediately began a paid group placement for a minimum of 2 days per week. Significantly more of the accelerated subjects (50%) were involved in some kind of paid employment, that is, competitive employment or rehabilitation program, than the gradual subjects (28%), but there was no difference when only competitive employment was analyzed (only 8% of the total sample was competitively employed). Analyses at 15 months used only those patients who were actively engaged at 9 months. Twenty percent of the accelerated patients were competitively employed as compared with 7% of the gradual patients ($p < .05$).

Wherley and Bisgaard (1987 [Quality Rating: V, Poor]) evaluated 19 residential treatment programs serving psychiatric clients. Four of the programs were termed *intensive*. These had a 1:5 staff-to-client ratio and offered substantial inhouse therapy. Six termed *transitional* had a 1:10 staff-to-client ratio and placed an emphasis on linking the clients with outside community services. Nine were termed *supportive*, having a 1:10 staff-to-client ratio designed to serve lower functioning clients that required a low-stress, longer term program. A 6-month sample of 596 clients was used for this study. At admission to the program 3.1% of the clients were competitively employed as compared to 12.8% at discharge and 25.2% at 6-month follow-up. All three programs showed increases in employment rates. The transitional program had the greatest number of clients competitively employed, but they also admitted the healthiest patient population. Vocational activity (job training, volunteer work, sheltered employment, and school) rose from 18.1% at admission to 35.5% at discharge and 47.7% at follow-up. No statistical significance figures are provided.

DISCUSSION

Substance Abuse Disorders

The most consistent attention to work outcomes appears in the literature on substance abusers. It is not clear why these groups of patients should invite attention to work restoration. Perhaps one reason is that between episodes of symptomatic exacerbation, many of these patients appear functionally well. In any event, specialized add-on or long-term treatments are probably of little value over and above standard regimens, and the evidence suggests that drug-free status is associated with good work outcomes. Whether this is because keeping people drug free improves the likelihood that they will return to work or because failure to find work increases the likelihood of relapse is not clear.

Drug Addiction

There is little convincing evidence that adding short-term psychotherapy or antidepressant medication to conventional long-term drug treatment programs, such as methadone maintenance or the residential community, leads to meaningful gains in vocational activity or drug rehabilitation. One study does suggest that short-term psychotherapy may be useful in some cases, but a very similar study failed to find any benefits for a very similar treatment. The one study of a vocational training program for this population suggested that simply placing substance abusers in graduated supervised work settings may help them return to the work force, but it probably does relatively little to help them establish long-term careers. Methadone maintenance has been the standard long-term therapy for opiate addiction in this country for over 15 years. Although no recent studies of its benefits were found for this review, the studies reviewed did suggest that long-term engagement in some form of drug treatment is associated with less illicit drug use, and that continued drug use and poor vocational outcomes are linked (Kosten, Rounsaville, & Kleber, 1987 [Quality Rating: IV, Fair]).

Alcoholism

On balance, these studies suggest that successful treatment of alcoholism that reduces the level of abusive drinking probably tends to increase productive work activity. However, this conclusion is offered only tentatively because the results of the studies are definitely mixed. Some studies found improved work functioning after treatment, but others found no real gains despite improvements in drinking behaviors. It is very clear, however, that variations in the goals, setting, type, or intensity of treatment make very little difference with respect to either symptomatic or vocational outcomes for alcoholics.

Anxiety and Depressive Disorders

Despite the prevalence of these disorders, there is almost no experimental literature on the relations between treatment and work in these groups. The few studies found—two from Great Britain and the other a single-case study—yield inconsistent results. One found no real benefits in the area of work for a mixed sample consisting primarily of phobic patients. Another suggested that anti-anxiety drugs may help restore work function in patients with panic disorders. The final study was a case report of an individual whose dysthymic and associated personality disorder was aggravating his work adjustment. That study suggested that a behavioral therapy program was effective in teaching more effective self-control. Obviously, these studies do not provide an adequate empirical base from which to draw substantive conclusions about treatments of anxiety or depression. This is ironic, since these are two areas in which contemporary pharmacology and psychotherapy have made particularly dramatic advances.

The almost complete lack of studies of anxiety and affective disorders is particularly striking because work impairment is acknowledged to be a common concomitant of many of those conditions. In fact, interference with occupational functioning satisfies one of the diagnostic criteria for social phobia in DSM-III-R (p. 243). Below are other examples from the DSM-III-R:

> In major depressive episodes the degree of impairment varies, but there is always some interference in social and occupational functioning (p. 221).
>
> [In cyclothymia] during periods of depression, social and occupational functioning are invariably impaired (p. 227).
>
> Impairment [in simple phobia] may be considered if the phobic object . . . cannot be avoided, such as a fear of elevators in someone living in a large city who must use elevators at work (p. 244).
>
> [In social phobia] fear of public speaking may interfere with professional advancement (p. 242).

Pathological Gambling

Only two relatively weak studies were reviewed in this area: one a retrospective follow-up with no pretreatment measures, and the other an uncontrolled prospective program evaluation. The results suggest that patients enrolled in the program did experience benefits in the 6 months following treatment, both with regard to gambling and employment. The design of these studies, however, does not permit any firm conclusions about the benefits of the treatment itself.

Schizophrenia

In the case of schizophrenic patients, there is little evidence that psychosocial treatments—even those that may be symptomatically beneficial such as family treatment (e.g., Falloon et al., 1987)—are of much benefit with regard to restoring work capacity. Dynamically oriented approaches to psychotherapy have not even demonstrated their capacity to benefit patients symptomatically. While family-oriented approaches do seem to have some symptomatic benefits for the schizophrenic patient, the evidence that they also lead to meaningful improvements in work functioning is weak at best. With regard to rehabilitation programs specifically designed to teach work-related skills, several studies suggest that schizophrenic patients can benefit from focused vocational intervention, but these studies tend to be methodologically weak and thus they are relatively unconvincing.

The most surprising results in the studies of schizophrenia are those bearing on the effects of neuroleptic drugs. A number of research projects converge on the finding that neuroleptic drugs have a negative impact on vocational functioning, all else being equal. All else is, of course, never equal. Neuroleptics have clearly demonstrated beneficial effects on schizophrenic symptoms, and there is at least one study suggesting that the relapses associated with unilateral neuroleptic withdrawal are also associated with relatively persisting social and vocational impairment. Neuroleptic drugs clearly attenuate symptoms and reduce relapse risk, but there is a striking consistency of findings that suggest that they may impair work capacity.

Unfortunately, almost all the studies are methodologically weak. Most are confounded, in that higher neuroleptic doses were characteristically prescribed or taken by patients who were more seriously ill. Indeed, the design flaws of this group of studies are considerable enough that the results, though consistent, would have to be almost completely discounted were it not for the recent report from Hogarty et al. (1988). Their randomized clinical trial is consistent with the notion that neuroleptic medications may have adverse effects on psychosocial aspects of outcome. That idea is not new. It was enunciated long ago by Gordon Paul (e.g., Paul & Lentz, 1977), who expressed concern that drugs may interfere with the learning process and thus impede full community restoration. More recently, psychopharmacologists have begun to express concerns about adverse side effects of excessive neuroleptics, such as sedation, akinesia, akathesia and dysphoria, that might well affect work function (e.g., Van Putten, Marder, Mintz, & Poland, 1988).

CONCLUSION

One of the most striking findings of this review was the widespread indifference of psychiatric treatment researchers to work outcomes. This is particularly apparent in the case of the affective and anxiety disorders. Although more than 4,000 research articles were reviewed, *not one* dealing with bipolar patients was found. Only one case study of a dysthymic individual with work impairment represented the depressive disorders. One study from England evaluated the effectiveness of a single nurse-therapist with a mixed, mostly phobic population, and one evaluated pharmacotherapy of panic. In view of the prevalence of these disorders and their acknowledged effects on work capacity, these holes in the literature are particularly disturbing.

A final note on methodology seems appropriate. Studies of psychiatric treatments fall broadly into one of two categories. First, there are the relatively well-controlled and well-designed clinical trials. These typically study a drug or well-defined psychosocial therapy. They focus solely on symptom outcomes. If work is presented at all in the analysis, it is part of some composite measure that reflects the thinking behind DSM-III-R's description of *impairment*, combining work, leisure, and social relations.

Second, there are evaluation studies of rehabilitation programs. Usually, some work-relevant measure is included in the assessment, although too often it is not clearly and directly relevant to work place performance (e.g., job interview skills, anger management). Usually the patient population will be mixed, and diagnostic distinctions will not be considered important. These studies usually conclude that the treatment program in question is of some benefit, but there is usually no control treatment or randomization, and if there is a comparison sample it is self-selected and thus hard to interpret.

As a result, we still know surprisingly little about the effects of psychiatric treatments—drugs, psychotherapies, and rehabilitation programs—on the capacity of various well-defined groups of patients to perform useful work. Obviously, this is a matter of great clinical and social significance. The two kinds of studies described above reflect an anachronistic division between *psychiatric treatment* and *rehabilitation program* research. Perhaps there are understandable historical and professional bases for that split. Clearly, however, if we are to begin to develop a substantial scientific data base regarding the effects of interventions on work capacity, rehabilitation researchers must significantly upgrade the methodological rigor of their work. Just as clearly, psychopharmacology and psychotherapy researchers must learn from their colleagues in rehabilitation that a symptomatically "effective" treatment is of questionable value if it fails to restore a patient's instrumental effectiveness.

REFERENCES

Alanen, Y. O., Rakkolainen, V., Rasimus, R., Laakso, J., & Kaljonen, A. (1985a). Developing a global psychotherapeutic approach to schizophrenia: Results of a five-year follow-up. *Yale Journal of Biology and Medicine, 58*, 383–402.

Alanen, Y. O., Rakkolainen, V., Rasimus, R., Laakso, J., & Kaljonen, A. (1985b). Psychotherapeutically oriented treatment of schizophrenia: Results of a five year follow-up. *Acta Psychiatrica Scandinavica, 71*, 31–49.

Anderson, J. R. (1982). Social Security and SSI benefits for the mentally disabled. *Hospital and Community Psychiatry, 33*, 295–298.

Anthony, W. A., & Jansen, M. (1984). Predicting the vocational capacity of the chronically mentally ill. *American Psychologist, 39*, 537–544.

Anthony, W. A., & Liberman, R. P. (1986). The practice of psychiatric rehabilitation: Historical, conceptual and research base. *Schizophrenia Bulletin, 12*, 542–559.

Avison, W. R., & Speechley, K. N. (1987, January). The discharged psychiatric patient: A review of social, social-psychological and psychiatric correlates of outcome. *American Journal of Psychiatry, 144*(1), 10–18.

Bale, R. N., Zarcone, V. P., Van Stone, W. W., Kuldau, J. M., Engelsing, T. M., & Elashoff, R. M. (1984). Three therapeutic communities: A prospective controlled study of narcotic addiction treatment: Process and two-year follow-up results. *Archives of General Psychiatry, 41*, 185–191.

Bell, M. D., & Ryan, E. R. (1984). Integrating psychosocial rehabilitation into the hospital psychiatric service. *Hospital and Community Psychiatry, 35*, 1017–1023.

Bond, G. R., & Dincin, J. (1986). Accelerating entry into transitional employment in a psychosocial rehabilitation agency. *Rehabilitation Psychology, 31*, 143–155.

Bowe, F. (1986). *Disabled in 1985: A portrait of American adults.* Hot Springs, AR: Arkansas Research and Training Center in Vocational Rehabilitation.

Dion, G. L., & Anthony, W. A. (1987, March). Research in psychiatric rehabilitation: A review of experimental and quasi-experimental studies. *Rehabilitation Counseling Bulletin*, 177–203.

Dohrenwend, B. S., Dohrenwend, B. P., Link, B., & Levav, I. (1983). Social functioning of psychiatric patients in contrast with community cases in the general populations. *Archives of General Psychiatry, 40*, 1174–1182.

Donovan, D. M., Kivlahan, D. R., & Walker, R. D. (1984). Clinical limitations of neuropsychological testing in predicting treatment outcome among alcoholics. *Alcoholism: Clinical and Experimental Research, 8*, 470–475.

Fagan, R. W., & Mauss, A. L. (1986). Social margin and social reentry: An evaluation of a rehabilitation program for skid row alcoholics. *Journal of Studies on Alcohol, 47*, 413–425.

Falloon, I. R. H., McGill, C. W., Boyd, J. L., & Pederson, J. (1987). Family management in the prevention of morbidity of schizophrenia: Social outcome of a two-year longitudinal study. *Psychological Medicine, 17*, 59–66.

Fawcett, J., Clark, D. C., Aagesen, C. A., Pisani, V. D., Tolkin, J. M., Sellers, D., McGuire, M., & Gibbons, R. D. (1987). A double-blind, placebo-controlled trial of lithium carbonate therapy for alcoholism. *Archives of General Psychiatry, 44*, 248–256.

Fawcett, J., Clark, D. C., Gibbons, R. D., Aagesen, C. A., Pisani, V. D., Tilkin, J. M., Sellers, D., & Stutzman, D. (1984). Evaluation of lithium therapy for alcoholism. *Journal of Clinical Psychiatry, 45*, 494–499.

Foy, D. W., Nunn, L. B., & Rychtarik, R. G. (1984). Broad-spectrum behavioral treatment for chronic alcoholics: Effects of training controlled drinking skills. *Journal of Consulting and Clinical Psychology, 52*, 218–230.

Frances, R. J., Bucky, S., & Alexopoulos, G. S. (1984). Outcome study of familial and nonfamilial alcoholism. *American Journal of Psychiatry, 141*, 1469–1471.

Gaebel, W., & Pietzcker, A. (1985a). Multidimensional study of the outcome of schizophrenic patients one year after clinic discharge: Predictors and influence of neuroleptic treatment. *European Archives of Psychiatry and Neurological Science, 235*, 45–52.

Gaebel, W., & Pietzcker, A. (1985b). One-year outcome of schizophrenic patients—the interaction of chronicity and neuroleptic treatment. *Pharmacopsychiatry, 18*, 235–239.

Ginsberg, G., Marks, I., & Waters, H. (1984). Cost-benefit analysis of a controlled trial of nurse therapy for neuroses in primary care. *Psychological Medicine, 14*, 683–690.

Goldman, H. H., Gattozzi, A. A., & Taube, C. A. (1981). Defining and counting the chronically mentally ill. *Hospital and Community Psychiatry, 32*, 21–27.

Hammer, T., Ravndal, E., & Vaglum, P. (1985). Work is not enough: A quasi-experimental study of a vocational training programme for young drug and alcohol abusers. *Journal of Drug Issues, 15*, 393–403.

Harding, C. M., Brooks, G. W., Ashikaga, T., Strauss, J. S., & Breier, A. (1987a). The Vermont longitudinal study of persons with severe mental illness, I: Methodology, study sample, and overall status 32 years later. *American Journal of Psychiatry, 144*, 718–726.

Harding, C. M., Brooks, G. W., Ashikaga, T., Strauss, J. S., & Breier, A. (1987b). The Vermont longitudinal study of persons with severe mental illness, II: Long-term outcome of subjects who retrospectively met DSM-III criteria for schizophrenia. *American Journal of Psychiatry, 144*, 727–735.

Hogarty, G. E., Anderson, C. M., Reiss, D. J., Kornblith, S. J., Greenwald, D. P., Javna, C. D., & Madonia, M. J. (1986). Family psychoeducation, social skills training, and maintenance chemotherapy in the aftercare treatment of schizophrenia. *Archives of General Psychiatry, 43*, 633–642.

Hogarty, G. E., McEvoy, J. P., Munetz, M., DiBarry, A. L., Bartone, P., Cather, R., Cooley, S. J., Ulrich, R. F., Carter, M., & Madonia, M. J. (1988). Dose of fluphenazine, familial expressed emotion, and outcome in schizophrenia: Results of a two-year controlled study. *Archives of General Psychiatry, 45*, 797–805.

Jacobs, H. E., Kardashian, S., Kreinbring, R. K., Ponder, R., & Simpson, A. S. (1984). A skills-oriented model for facilitating employment among psychiatrically disabled persons. *Rehabilitation Counseling Bulletin, 28*, 87–96.

Johnson, D. A., Pasterski, G., Ludlow, H. M., Street, K., & Taylor, R. D. (1983). The discontinuance of maintenance neuroleptic therapy in chronic schizophrenic patients: Drug and social consequences. *Acta Psychiatrica Scandinavica, 67*, 339–352.

Katz, H. M., Frank, A., Gunderson, J. G., & Hamm, D. (1984). Psychotherapy of schizophrenia: What happens to treatment dropouts. *Journal of Nervous and Mental Disease, 172*, 326–331.

Kecmanovic, D. (1985). Post release adjustment of day and inpatients. *International Journal of Social Psychiatry, 31*, 74–79.

Kleber, H. D., Weissman, M. M., Rounsaville, B. J., Wilber, C. H., Prusoff, B. A., & Riordan, C. E. (1983). Imipramine as treatment for depression in addicts. *Archives of General Psychiatry, 40*, 649–653.

Kolb, D., Baker, G. D., & Gunderson, E. K. (1983). Effects of alcohol rehabilitation treatment on health and performance of navy enlisted men. *Drug and Alcohol Dependence, 11*, 309–319.

Kosten, T. R., Rounsaville, B. J., & Kleber, H. D. (1987). Predictors of 2.5 year outcome in opiate addicts: Pretreatment source of income. *American Journal of Drug and Alcohol Abuse, 13*, 19–32.

Liberman, R. P., & Phipps, C. C. (1987). Innovative treatment and rehabilitation techniques for the chronically mentally ill. In W. W. Menninger & G. Hannah (Eds.), *The chronic mental patient: II* (ch. 5). Washington, DC: American Psychiatric Press.

Maisto, S. A., Sobell, L. C., Sobell, M. B., & Sanders, B. (1985). Effects of outpatient treatment for problem drinkers. *American Journal of Drug and Alcohol Abuse, 11*, 131–149.

May, P. R. A. (1974). Treatment of schizophrenia: A critique of reviews of the literature. *Comprehensive Psychiatry, 15*, 179–185.

May, P. R. A., & Van Putten, T. (1974). Treatment of schizophrenia: II. A proposed rating scale of design and outcome for use in literature surveys. *Comprehensive Psychiatry, 15*, 267–275.

McCrady, B., Longabaugh, R., Fink, E., Stout, R., Beattie, M., & Ruggieri-Authelet, A. (1986). Cost effectiveness of alcoholism treatment in partial hospital versus inpatient settings after brief inpatient treatment: 12-months outcome. *Journal of Consulting and Clinical Psychology, 54*, 708–713.

Meyer, J., Berman, J., & Rivers, P. C. (1985). Dispositional assessment with alcoholics. *International Journal of the Addictions, 20*, 1463–1478.

Mueser, K. T., Foy, D. W., & Carter, M. J. (1986). Social skills training for job maintenance in a psychiatric patient. *Journal of Counseling Psychology, 33*, 360–362.

Paul, G. L., & Lentz, R. (1977). *Psychosocial treatment of chronic mental patients*. Cambridge, MA: Harvard University Press.

Powell, B. J., Penick, E. C., Read, M. R., & Ludwig, A. M. (1985). Comparison of three outpatient treatment interventions: A twelve-month follow-up of men alcoholics. *Journal of Studies on Alcohol, 46*, 309–312.

Reich, J. H. (1988). DSM-III personality disorders and the outcome of treated panic disorder. *American Journal of Psychiatry, 145*, 1149–1152.

Rounsaville, B. J., Glazer, W., Wilber, C. H., Weissman, M. M., & Kleber, H. D. (1983). Short-term interpersonal psychotherapy in methadone-maintained opiate addicts. *Archives of General Psychiatry, 40*, 629–635.

Russo, A. M., Taber, J. I., McCormick, R. A., & Ramirez, L. F. (1984). An outcome study of an inpatient treatment program for pathological gamblers. *Hospital and Community Psychiatry, 35*, 823–827.

Ryan, E. R., & Bell, M. D. (1983). Follow-up of a psychoanalytically-oriented long-term treatment program for schizophrenic inpatients. *American Journal of Orthopsychiatry, 53*, 730–739.

Sanchez-Craig, M., Annis, H. M., Bornet, A. R., & MacDonald, K. R. (1984). Random assignment to abstinence and controlled drinking: Evaluation of a cognitive-behavioral program for problem drinkers. *Journal of Consulting and Clinical Psychology, 52*, 390–403.

Sjostrom, R. (1985). Effects of psychotherapy in schizophrenia. *Acta Psychiatrica Scandinavica, 71*, 513–522.

Spencer, J., Glick, I., Haas, G., Clarkin, J., Lewis, A., Peyser, J., DeMane, N., Good-Ellis, M., Harris, E., & Lestelle, V. (1988). A randomized clinical trial of inpatient family intervention III: Effects at 6-month and 18-month follow-ups. *American Journal of Psychiatry, 145*, 1115–1121.

Stimmel, B., Cohen, M., Sturiano, V., Hanbury, R., Korts, D., & Jackson, G. (1983). Is treatment for alcoholism effective in persons on methadone maintenance? *American Journal of Psychiatry, 140*, 862–866.

Taber, J. I., McCormick, R. A., Russo, A. M., Adkins, B. J., & Ramirez, L. F. (1987). Follow-up of pathological gamblers after treatment. *American Journal of Psychiatry, 144*, 757–761.

Test, M. A., Knoedler, W. H., Allness, D. J., & Burke, S. S. (1985). Characteristics of young adults with schizophrenic disorders treated in the community. *Hospital and Community Psychiatry, 36*, 853–858.

Van der Kolk, B. A., & Goldberg, H. L. (1983). Aftercare of schizophrenic patients: Pharmacotherapy and consistency of therapists. *Hospital and Community Psychiatry, 34*, 343–348.

Van Putten, T., Marder, S. R., Mintz, J., & Poland, R. E. (1988). Haloperidol plasma levels and clinical response: A therapeutic window relationship. *Psychopharmacology Bulletin, 24*, 172–175.

Waldo, M., & Gardiner, J. (1984). Vocational adjustment patterns of alcohol and drug misusers following treatment. *Journal of Studies on Alcohol, 45*, 547–549.

Walker, R. D., Donovan, D. M., Kivlahan, D. R., & O'Leary, M. R. (1983). Length of stay, neuropsychological performance, and aftercare: Influences on alcohol treatment outcome. *Journal of Consulting and Clinical Psychology, 51*, 900–911.

Wherley, M., & Bisgaard, S. (1987). Beyond model programs: Evaluation of a countrywide system of residential treatment programs. *Hospital and Community Psychiatry, 38*, 852–857.

Woody, G. E., Luborsky, L., McLellan, A. T., O'Brien, C. P., Beck, A. T., Blaine, J., Herman, I., & Hole, A. (1983). Psychotherapy for opiate addicts: Does it help? *Archives of General Psychiatry, 40*, 639–645.

Woody, G. E., McLellan, A. T., Luborsky, L., & O'Brien, C. P. (1985). Sociopathy and psychotherapy outcome. *Archives of General Psychiatry, 42*, 1081–1086.

Woody, G. E., McLellan, A. T., Luborsky, L., & O'Brien, C. P. (1987). Twelve-month follow-up of psychotherapy for opiate dependence. *American Journal of Psychiatry, 144*, 590–596.

Woody, G. E., McLellan, A. T., Luborsky, L., O'Brien, C. P., Blaine, J., Fox, S., Herman, I., & Beck, A. T. (1984). Severity of psychiatric symptoms as a predictor of benefits from psychotherapy: The Veterans Administration-Penn Study. *American Journal of Psychiatry, 141*, 1172–1182.

CHAPTER 14

FUTURE PROSPECTS FOR PSYCHIATRIC REHABILITATION

Robert Paul Liberman

The florid and negative symptoms and associated functional disabilities and social role handicaps of schizophrenia and other serious psychiatric disorders pose a major challenge to proponents of rehabilitation, be they practitioners, policy makers, program administrators, family members, or patients themselves. Cognitive dysfunctions that endure even during periods of symptom remission create learning disabilities that interfere with a patient's acquiring the coping skills required for more normalized adaptation to community life. Moreover, the volatile course of psychiatric disorders, with intercurrent and demoralizing relapses, frequently robs patients of the very social and family supports that can buffer stress and enhance quality of life.

The neurobiological and socioenvironmental determinants of disabling mental illnesses require a multifaceted approach to rehabilitation that must integrate pharmacological with psychosocial techniques. There is no place for unidimensional treatment and rehabilitation strategies, nor for single modalities that, in the past, have been trumpeted as remedies for the misery of mental illness. The intrusive symptoms of psychosis, anxiety, and depression devastate an individual's functioning and lead to protean handicaps in the roles of student, worker, family member, and friend. Judiciously prescribed, psychotropic drugs can diminish and relieve symptomatology; new generations of antipsychotic drugs promise even greater relief from hitherto refractory and disabling symptoms. Once control of an individual's symptoms permits responding to a learning environment, rehabilitation can compensate for social and vocational disabilities. Rehabilitation strategies assume two forms: (a) educational and skill-building techniques to strengthen and broaden a person's coping and relating, and (b) supportive environmental resources to buffer stress and provide social prostheses for overcoming disability.

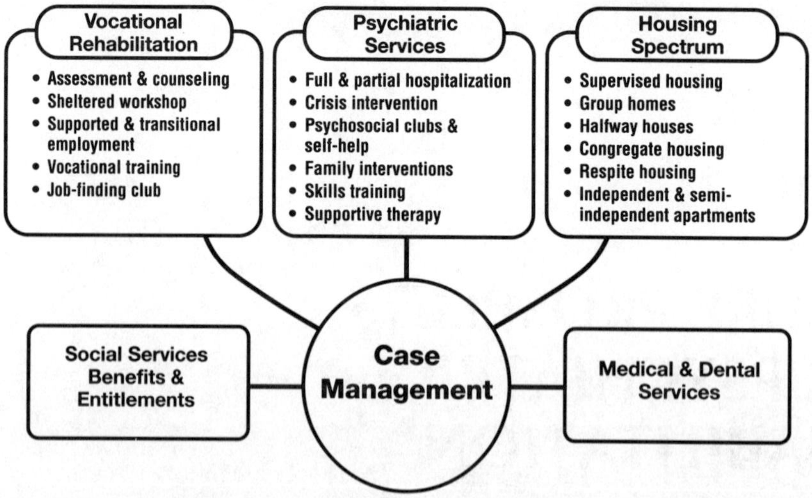

Figure 14.1. Comprehensive and coordinated services for the chronically mentally ill.

The biomedical and psychosocial interventions used in psychiatric rehabilitation must be provided within a service system that meets the diverse needs of persons with pervasive symptoms, disabilities, and handicaps; thus, comprehensive and continuous care should be available and accessible if rehabilitation is to optimize functioning. In Figure 14.1 is depicted a systems model for the delivery of comprehensive and coordinated services for the long-term mentally ill. In the arenas of vocational rehabilitation, psychiatric services, and housing, a continuum must exist to serve the changing needs of patients and clients properly. While the current zeitgeist of vocational rehabilitation has tilted toward supported employment strategies, it would be well not to throw out the "sheltered workshop baby" with the bath water. Many patients need and benefit from short or long periods of sheltered work before they are ready to face and cope with the stressors in the competitive workplace. Two vignettes will illustrate the value of sheltered work.

Linda had worked for 10 years as a high-paid executive in an advertising agency. She worked and lived on the "fast track" until she developed acute depression which responded poorly to medications. Her depression hung on and she was unable to return to work. Finally hospitalized, she asked to be assigned to the sheltered workshop to stuff envelopes and assemble toys. She said, "I needed to be able to accomplish something . . . anything. I couldn't concentrate on anything more complex than stuffing envelopes, but success with that improved my morale and gave me the confidence to plan for a return to my job."

Joe asked for help in getting a job. His symptoms had been under good control for more than 2 years and he had become a leader in his psychosocial clubhouse. Two attempts to place him in the clerical jobs for which he had interests and skills led to quick failures. Joe was unable to sustain the pace and productivity that the jobs required. He returned to a sheltered job in a hospital library where he got "work hardened" over a 1-year period. Then, he again tried a clerical job which was a success. He has held this job for 4 years and in the meanwhile got married.

If we are to improve on our track record in rehabilitation of the mentally ill, we must not only retain a continuum or spectrum of service options to meet the individual deficits and assets of patients, but we must also be alert to their changing needs. The concept of "flexible levels of intervention" must be employed by those clinicians responsible for orchestrating rehabilitation services. At times, this means increasing the frequency and intensity of intervention to avert or contain a relapse or decompensation—even if the intervention is as costly as a temporary hospitalization or daily home visits by a mobile treatment team. Assuming a flexible approach will mean that many anachronistic clinical practices will have to be abandoned, such as the tendency to see patients less often when they move from inpatient to outpatient status. When patients have become symptomatically stable and capable of independence is the very time when intensive training and rehabilitation are most useful. This, then, will require increasing the amount of services to our high functioning patients rather than simply maintaining them in what has been euphemistically termed *intermittent supportive therapy*. Algorithms can be constructed that connect the level of a patient's need for services at any stage of his or her illness with the specific form and intensity of clinical service that will meet the need as depicted in Chapter 5 of this handbook.

PRINCIPLES TO GUIDE REHABILITATION

We do not need fundamental breakthroughs in the causes and cures of schizophrenia and other mental disorders to make a significant difference in the social adaptation and quality of life of patients afflicted with these disorders. We do need to harness all of what we know about promoting and maintaining human functional capacities within the framework of a comprehensive and coordinated system of care. In addition to the principle of *flexible levels of intervention*, other imperatives can help to guide our work. These have only recently begun to penetrate our lexicon and consciousness. It will take decades before a new generation of practitioners and policy makers are imbued with these principles; however, this handbook and efforts at continuing professional education can short-circuit the otherwise generational lag in promoting change.

1. *Engage patients in accessible services through active outreach:* We must not wait for patients to present for treatment, nor delay our outreach efforts until they require rescue from jails or homeless existences on the streets and back alleys of our cities. By accepting the mentally disabled on their own terms and gradually shaping their engagement and participation in treatment and rehabilitation we can inseminate motivation and therapeutic alliances.

2. *Provide continuous and indefinite treatment and rehabilitation:* The future of rehabilitation lies in a lifelong approach toward gradually strengthening our patients' skills and adaptive capacities. We must recognize that patients require lengthy periods of consolidation of their therapeutic gains. Moratoria on moving ahead toward new patient goals should punctuate incremental progress that is measured in years and decades, not weeks and months.

3. *Engage the patient's and families' self-help and active participation in rehabilitation:* The days of viewing our patients as passive receptacles to fill with medications and therapy are long past. The consumer movement has touched the mentally ill as well as other groups of patients and we have begun to recognize the salutary effects of mobilizing and reinforcing the adaptive strivings of our patients and their relatives toward health and functioning. In addition, clinicians should expend time and effort in teaching patients and their families how to set realistic goals and to act as advocates for the treatment and social resources necessary for progress.

4. *Assist the patient and caregivers in the delicate balancing of risk taking with asylum:* It is well established that too much socioenvironmental stimulation (whether from physical substance abuse or tense social encounters) evokes relapses and too little

stimulation leads to apathy and withdrawal. The task for clinicians is to help patients and their caregivers to find that elusive therapeutic window of optimal environmental stimulation, recognizing that the window opens and closes differently for each person and at each phase of a person's illness. Clinicians will ply their craft by helping their patients learn from past experience and undertake new enterprises as "experiments" so that risk taking can be done without undue fear of failure and calamity.

5. *Develop long-term, reliable, and mutually respectful therapeutic relationships:* While it is not often practical to guarantee patients with long-term mental illnesses the same therapist or physician for many years, it is desirable to organize and deliver services through a team that buffers the stress associated with the inevitable staff turnover. Attachments to therapists and doctors do not by themselves create dependency; if the goals and methods of a long-term attachment aim toward self-help and graded steps toward autonomy, such attachments can inspire independence.

6. *Galvanize administrative and programmatic support for comprehensive and coordinated services:* Clinical activities never occur in an administrative vacuum; in fact, the most critical determinant of successful community support systems lies in the sanction and visible support for the spectrum of clinical services from the highest levels of local and state administration. The innovations described in this handbook will not take root unless program managers and policy makers mandate and support their use. This often requires administrators to have the courage of their convictions and insist that clinicians change their practices in line with demonstrated advances in the field.

WHAT INNOVATIONS ARE ON THE HORIZON?

The various chapters of this handbook have charted the state of the art for rehabilitation of persons with serious and long-term psychiatric disorders. What, then, does the future portend? A brief inventory of the domains of rehabilitation activity will offer a road map into the future.

1. *Illness self-management techniques,* such as the Medication and Symptom Management Modules (UCLA Social & Independent Living Skills Series, 1990), will permit patients to assume more of the responsibility for monitoring their psychopathology and seeking early and flexible levels of intervention. Just as diabetics monitor their own blood and urine sugar and hypertensives take their own blood pressures, the mentally ill will be taught how to identify their warning signs of relapse and to work collaboratively with their physicians in titrating their medications. Procedures for accomplishing symptom self-management are already being tested in research programs (Wirshing et al., 1990; UCLA Social & Independent Living Skills Series, 1990). With patients also more knowledgeable about the benefits and side effects of their medication, a true partnership in managing pharmacotherapy will yield improved compliance and reduced relapses (Eckman et al., 1990). The thoughtful blending of functional assessment and skills training with new low-dose neuroleptic drug strategies and the new generation of atypical antipsychotic drugs that will be coming onto the market promises to offer major advances in rehabilitation during the coming decade. It is essential to evaluate the residual deficits of individuals who have reached optimal benefit from pharmacotherapy and then design rehabilitative interventions that match and compensate for those deficits.

2. *Functional assessment* will become more individualized and better linked to prescriptions for rehabilitation. By specifying and targeting problems and goals in behavioral and operational terms, clinicians will have more success in engaging patients and their caregivers in a collaborative spirit for treatment. Functional analysis will supplement assessment such that the psychobiological and environmental antecedents and con-

sequences of problems and deficits will be highlighted and used for intervention programs. In addition to more exact methods for identifying motivation within patients through reinforcement surveys and observation of preferred and frequent behaviors, clinicians will amplify motivation for change by using "reinforcer sampling" and "exposure in vivo" techniques.

3. *Social learning and assertive community treatment* proponents will consolidate their techniques and procedures so that behavior therapy can be placed in the service of training patients in community living. A humanistic blending of the TCL or PACT framework for delivering continuous clinical services (Test, Chapter 7, in this handbook) with the social learning and social skills training techniques that have been developed primarily in hospital settings (Corrigan, Schade, & Liberman, Chapter 5; Glynn & Mueser, Chapter 6, in this handbook). Life adjustment teams will employ structured skills-training techniques while engaging the patient in naturalistic settings in the community; for example, patients will learn dating and friendship skills directly in their homes and in recreational sites.

4. *Social skills training will receive an infusion of new principles and techniques from research on cognitive sciences.* Linguistic analysis will decipher the deficits responsible for incoherence and other forms of thought disorder, making it possible to design conversational skills-training programs that will overcome or compensate for these communication obstacles. Studies on cognitive schemas and dissection of the critical cognitive markers of vulnerability to psychosis will permit more focused, laboratory-based training and remediation techniques. Advances in interactive, laser-disc and computerized video will result in less labor-intensive skills-training approaches that capitalize on patients' self-directed learning to improve durability and generality of skills acquired through over-practice and frequent booster sessions. As laboratory studies reveal more about the pathophysiology of schizophrenia and other disabling psychiatric disorders, skills-training techniques can be constructed to remediate directly patients' problems in information processing and other intervening cognitive, behavioral, and psychophysiological processes that are dysfunctional. It is important, in this regard, to insist on individualization of rehabilitation so that treatment techniques are keyed to the stage or phase of illness currently affecting the individual patient.

5. *Normalization of the lives of the long-term mentally ill will improve with a wider array of supported employment, housing options, and access to educational opportunities that promote community adaptation.* Chapter 8 in this handbook, by Lukoff, Sullivan, and Goisman, reporting educational programs about AIDS prevention and sex for persons with schizophrenia, represents the increasing recognition that the mentally ill no longer live cloistered existences and have left the asylums for community life with all its attendant dangers, temptations, and stressors.

Even more important for normalization will be expansion of work opportunities for the mentally ill and the vocational rehabilitation services that will accompany such expansion. With the anticipated contraction in the work force because of lowered birth rates and a continuing robust growth in the economy, jobs will become more accessible to disabled persons. It will be the challenge of the 1990s and beyond to harness supportive psychiatric services—including ready access to psychiatrists for medication titration and crisis intervention—to job sites. The outcome data from vocational rehabilitation suggest that follow-along psychiatric services are more critical to the long-term vocational success of the chronic mentally ill than is job coaching per se.

The type and frequency of follow-along psychiatric services need to be tailored to the individual's symptom patterns, work tolerance, stress vulnerability, and social disabilities. We are moving toward that day in the future when we will be able to create clinical decision trees that guide us in connecting the appropriate psychiatric services to the individual needs of our patients who are likewise participating in individually tailored vocational rehabilitation programs. One such decision tree is presented in Chapter 5 of this handbook.

Skills-training modalities may be uniquely adaptable to the arena of vocational rehabilitation. It is possible to use currently available technology for skills training to teach patients to improve their coping ability with the challenges that occur on the job—criticism from supervisors, ambiguities in the work expectations, small talk with coworkers at lunch breaks, asking for time off to attend psychiatric appointments. One might ask, "Would training patients in job maintenance skills reduce the duration and intensity of supported employment services and enable faster and more enduring placement in competitive employment?"

The best available conceptual models for understanding the rehabilitation process—stress-vulnerability-coping-competence and impairment-disability-handicap—which were sketched in Chapter 1 of this handbook can permit us to grasp the sensitivity of certain psychiatric patients to high-expectancy rehabilitation programs. Those patients with a high psychobiological vulnerability to stress will be more exquisitely sensitive to high-demand rehabilitation settings. One way of identifying these sensitive patients is to assess their symptom status: Persons with continuing psychotic symptoms and cognitive impairments have been shown to respond more poorly to high demand treatment situations. Data from studies at the UCLA Clinical Research Center for Schizophrenia and Psychiatric Rehabilitation indicate clearly that having a diagnosis of schizophrenia or bipolar disorder and suffering from persisting psychotic symptoms reduces work capacity and employability. Future progress in vocational rehabilitation will require a much closer working relationship between the psychiatrist who determines the diagnosis and monitors the symptoms, and the rehabilitation worker who monitors and reinforces job performance.

6. *Case management has been both maligned and ballyhooed as a modality for the seriously mentally ill.* However, case management is not so much a modality as a means of organizing services and ensuring that the pervasive needs of the mentally ill are met. Already, community-based systems of care are reorganizing their staffing resources in accord with the use of case management to bolster strained support networks and to provide fixed and continuous points of responsibility for professional caregiving. In years to come, case managers will increasingly use skills-training techniques to aid patients in their course through the red tape of various agencies, coordinating and orchestrating the broad spectrum of medical-psychiatric treatment, social services, and rehabilitation modalities. The big question mark, however, is whether society—through its legislative and governing bodies—will prioritize the funding of the needed resources for the seriously mentally ill. Given the concerns over cost containment in health services across the United States, the voices of the mentally ill and their advocates requesting a sufficient piece of the health dollar "pie" will have to be heard over the pleas of those with cancer, heart disease, and neuromuscular diseases. Case management will be as effective as there are resources to coordinate. If there are insufficient psychiatrists to diagnose and prescribe medications for the seriously mentally ill because the reimbursement and third party payment mechanisms are paltry, then case managers will spin their wheels.

7. *Family involvement and participation* in the advocacy for services and research will continue to spread. Already, the National Alliance for the Mentally Ill has become the single most vocal and effective advocate for enhanced research funding in psychiatry. Family support groups abound throughout the country and the consciousness of psychiatrists and other mental health and rehabilitation professionals has been raised to

include family members in diagnosis, education about mental illnesses, prognosis, treatment planning, and rehabilitation.

Strategies have been developed to improve the families' interactions with their seriously mentally ill relatives, thereby decreasing family burden and enhancing the social support required by patients. The effective methods described by Strachan in Chapter 9 of this handbook are only the beginnings of a growing partnership among patients, parents, and professionals. In the coming decade, we shall see an array of behavioral and educational techniques developed and validated for improving the communication, problem solving, and stress management of families harboring a mentally ill relative. These techniques will empower both patients and relatives, enabling them to set and achieve goals that will promote patient autonomy and reduce disability.

NEW CHALLENGES

There are three major challenges to the continued growth and maturity of psychiatric rehabilitation. These are reckoning with new disability groups, disseminating new rehabilitation approaches from researchers and innovators to practice settings, and defining professional boundaries and resolving turf battles over which discipline should serve which group of patients or clients.

There are no well-documented, effective approaches for dealing with the seriously mentally ill who are homeless or who suffer from dual diagnoses of substance abuse or dependence superimposed upon schizophrenia or other major mental disorder. Research demonstration projects are just beginning to address these difficult to treat populations who more often than not are willing to be rescued but refuse to accept treatment. Before significant advances can be made in offering rehabilitation to these groups, more will have to be known about the biobehavioral and social determinants and consequences of homelessness and the mentally ill, chemical abusers. One avenue to improve insight into the nature of these problems is ethnography, in which the adaptive strivings of the homeless mentally ill or the dually diagnosed can be charted as well as their predicaments.

Two other disability groups who are underserved are the head injured and the elderly. Head-injured individuals share many of the symptomatic and functional impairments and disabilities of persons with schizophrenia and affective disorders. They suffer from the same types of cognitive and memory deficits as those with serious mental disorders. Psychiatry has not addressed this population as much as neurologists and rehabilitation and behavioral psychologists. Similarly, the needs of those with geropsychiatric disorders—Alzheimer's disease, other dementias, chronic depressions—are rarely met. The burden of care has fallen disproportionately to custodial types of nursing homes or to family members. In both of these types of disorders, it is not clear which disciplines have what special expertise to offer. Neurology, psychiatry, family practice and general medicine, psychology, and rehabilitation medicine will increasingly struggle over the responsibilities for serving these disabled persons.

Once developed and validated, effective methods of rehabilitation face many obstacles to organization and widespread dissemination. There is incredible inertia in social services and it often requires a full generation before new methods are brought into professional schools where the next generation of practitioners are prepared. Another set of obstacles to the adoption of innovations derives from failure of administrative leadership and top management to endorse and tangibly support innovations. Indifference to innovation or, worse, opposition to anything that might "rock the boat," must be contended with by even the most enthusiastic practitioner and innovator.

Beyond demonstrating the credibility of an innovation through empirical validations and replications, interpersonal contact is an essential component in promoting utilization by practitioners. One way to use interpersonal influence is to have individuals with the requisite technical skills serve as linkage agents or technology brokers with mental health and rehabilitation workers in the field. By serving as role models, clinicians functioning in the linkage capacity can leverage change by trading on their own credibility.

Also important in promoting change and renewal is organizational consultation for administrators as well as technology transfer for clinicians. The resource requirements, the staffing issues, and the organizational parameters of the change process can be pinpointed by consultants who are sensitive to service delivery settings and their constraints. In one review of change in human service organizations, technical assistance on the very process of change itself and how to overcome the psychological resistance of staff was found to be critical to the success of innovation (Backer, Liberman, & Kuehnel, 1986). If administrative consultation, including needs assessments and anticipation of unintended side effects of innovation, is provided, it is more likely that the key element of leadership and support from within the organization will emerge. Particularly helpful in fostering change is the use by administrators of incentives for staff to adopt innovations. This can be done through rewriting job descriptions, annual performance appraisals and awards, quality assurance mechanisms, inservice training, and through visible endorsement, encouragement, and praise for those courageous enough to embark on new techniques.

Persistent championship of innovations by one or more staff members from within the agency or institution considering change is often a critical factor in motivating peers to accept the innovations. The most effective champions are those who are viewed by their peers as informal or formal clinical leaders and who are able to develop successful therapeutic alliances with their patients or clients. Active and directive training methods can be used to amplify the impact of champions through "hands-on" inservice learning experiences. These are described in another publication in the context of training mental health and rehabilitation practitioners in psychiatric rehabilitation techniques (Kuehnel & Liberman, 1990).

A major constraint to the adoption of innovations and model programs has been the uniqueness of the staff, facilities, and patient population in which the innovation or model program was developed. What works in one setting does not necessarily fit another setting or environment. One way to overcome this problem is to increase the adaptability of an innovation by modularizing it; that is, breaking it up into its components and introducing the components in a selective manner. Recent advances in social-skills training—as outlined in Chapter 5, "Social-Skills Training," in this book—have emphasized establishing specific curricula for training mentally disabled persons. These curricula, organized into modules with skill areas and learning activities, are readily disseminable because they are packaged into trainer's manuals, demonstration videos, and patient's workbooks (UCLA, 1990). The modules are portable and can be used by almost any professional or paraprofessional who possesses good interpersonal and relationship skills (Eckman, Liberman, Phipps, & Blair, 1990; Liberman & Eckman, 1989). The packaging of a wide range of psychosocial rehabilitation programs into "user friendly" modules holds much promise for the rapid dissemination and adoption of novel and efficacious services.

REFERENCES

Backer, T. E., Liberman, R. P., & Kuehnel, T. G. (1986). Dissemination and adoption of innovative psychosocial interventions. *Journal of Consulting and Clinical Psychology, 54*, 111–118.

Eckman, T. A., Liberman, R. P., Phipps, C. C., & Blair, K. (1990). Teaching medication self-management skills to schizophrenics. *Jour-*

nal of Clinical Psychopharmacology, 10, 33–38.

Kuehnel, T. G., & Liberman, R. P. (1990). Competency-based training of psychiatric practitioners in the rehabilitation of chronic mental disorders. In H. Lefley & D. Johnson (Eds.), *Mental health professionals and families of the mentally ill*. Washington, DC: American Psychiatric Press.

Liberman, R. P., & Eckman, T. A. (1989). Dissemination of skills training modules to psychiatric facilities. *British Journal of Psychiatry, 155* (suppl 5), 117–122.

Liberman, R. P., Corrigan, P., & Schade, M. (1989). Drug and psychosocial treatment interactions in schizophrenia. *International Review of Psychiatry, 1*, 283–294.

UCLA Social & Independent Living Skills Series. (1990). Available from Dissemination Coordinator, Camarillo-UCLA Research Center, PO Box 6022, Camarillo, CA 93011-6022.

Wirshing, W., Eckman, T. A., Liberman, R. P., & Marder, S. (1990). Management of risk of relapse in schizophrenia through training chronic patients in self-management skills. In C. Tamminga & S. C. Schulz (Eds.), *Schizophrenia research*. New York: Raven Press.

AUTHOR INDEX

SUBJECT INDEX

ABOUT THE EDITOR AND CONTRIBUTORS

ABOUT THE EDITOR

Robert Paul Liberman, M.D. is Professor of Psychiatry at the UCLA School of Medicine and Chief of the Rehabilitation Service at the Brentwood (Psychiatric) Division of the West Los Angeles Veterans Affairs Medical Center. He heads a national demonstration program for vocational restoration and social and independent living skills at the largest Veterans Affairs Medical Center in the United States. Closely linked to these psychiatric rehabilitation programs is a Clinical Research Center for Schizophrenia, directed by Liberman and funded since 1977 by the National Institute of Mental Health. A large number of interdisciplinary research studies are undertaken under the aegis of the Clinical Research Center, all spirited by a conceptualization of major mental disorders that incorporates factors such as stress, vulnerability, coping, and competence. Liberman is also the Director of the Camarillo/UCLA Clinical Research Unit at Camarillo State Hospital where treatment studies are carried out using pharmacological and behavioral methods for refractory and chronic schizophrenics. He has published over 200 articles, books, and chapters in the areas of psychiatric rehabilitation, treatment of schizophrenia, social skills training, behavioral and family therapy and education and training in public psychiatry. His most recent books are *Psychiatric Rehabilitation of Chronic Mental Patients, Social Skills Training for Psychiatric Patients,* and *Resource Book for Psychiatric Rehabilitation*. He is on the Board of Directors of the American Association of Community Psychiatrists, the Executive Council of the Association for Clinical Psychosocial Research, and the American Psychiatric Association Committees on Rehabilitation and Veterans Affairs.

ABOUT THE CONTRIBUTORS

William A. Anthony, Ph.D. is a Professor and Executive Director of the Center for Psychiatric Rehabilitation at Boston University. The center conducts research and technical assistance projects throughout North America and Europe, and also provides clinical psychiatric rehabilitation services to persons disabled by severe mental illness. Dr. Anthony is the author of over 100 articles, books, and book chapters, the majority on psychiatric rehabilitation. His most recent books include *Psychiatric Rehabilitation*, authored with Mikal Cohen and Marianne Farkas, and *Psychiatric Rehabilitation Programs: Putting Theory into Practice*, edited with Marianne Farkas. Dr. Anthony is co-editor of the *Psychosocial Rehabilitation Journal*.

Frank Baker, Ph.D. is Professor and Director of Health Psychology in the Department of Environmental Health Sciences at The Johns Hopkins School of Hygiene and Public Health. Before joining the faculty at Johns Hopkins in 1985, Dr. Baker had served for 10 years as the Director of the Division of Community Psychiatry and Professor of Psychology and Preventive Medicine at the Medical School of the State University of New York at Buffalo. During this period, he directed several large evaluation studies of case management and community support services for the New York State Office of Mental Health. From 1965 to 1974 Dr. Baker was a member of the faculty of the Harvard Medical School Laboratory of Community Psychiatry. Dr. Baker received his Ph.D. in psychology from Northwestern University in 1964. He is a fellow of the American Psychological Association and the American Orthopsychiatric Association. He is the author of 12 books and 79 book chapters and journal articles.

Gary R. Bond, Ph.D. is Professor of Psychology and Director of the Doctoral Program in Rehabilitation Psychology at Indiana University–Purdue University at Indianapolis. His research awards include a Research Scientist Development Award from the National Institute of Mental Health and awards from the American Psychological Association and the American Rehabilitation Counseling Association. Formerly, Director of Research at Thresholds in Chicago, Dr. Bond has over 40 journal articles and book chapters, mainly on psychiatric rehabilitation and self-help groups.

Patrick W. Corrigan, Psy.D. is Assistant Professor of Clinical Psychiatry and Director of the Partial Hospitalization Program at the University of Chicago Dr. Corrigan has published more than 20 papers on behavioral and cognitive rehabilitation.

Shirley M. Glynn, Ph.D. is an Assistant Research Psychologist in the Department of Psychiatry and Behavioral Science at the UCLA Neuropsychiatric Institute and a Research Psychologist at the West Los Angeles Veterans Affairs Medical Center (Brentwood Division), Los Angeles, California. Previously, she was the psychologist on the Clinical Research Unit at Camarillo State Hospital, Camarillo, California where she conducted research and developed social learning programs for the seriously mentally ill. She has published articles, primarily on the behavioral treatment of patients with schizophrenia and other psychotic disorders. Her current clinical research is focused on behavioral family therapy and behavioral interventions for medical problems and health-risk behaviors among psychiatric patients.

Robert M. Goisman, M.D. is a Staff Psychiatrist in the Continuing Care Service and Director of the Phobia Clinic at the Massachusetts Mental Health Center, Boston. Recently he was also Clinic Director at the Brighton–Allston Mental Health Clinic, Brighton, Massachusetts. An Instructor in Psychiatry at Harvard Medical School, his publications and research interests are in the areas of psychiatric rehabilitation, anxiety disorders, behavior therapy, and psychiatric education in public sector settings. He is Massachusetts States Representative for the American Association of Community Psychiatrists and a member of the Public Sector Committee of the Massachusetts Psychiatric Society.

James Intagliata, Ph.D. is presently a Senior Consultant with the Chicago office of RHR International, a management consulting firm. Prior to joining RHR in 1985 he served 2 years as Director of Research for the Institute of Human Development at the University of Missouri in Kansas City. From 1976 to 1983, Dr. Intagliata was on the faculty of the Division of Community Psychiatry at the State University of New York at Buffalo. During his academic career, his research focused primarily on evaluating the community-based care systems designed to serve developmentally disabled individuals as well as the chronic mentally ill. Particular research interests included the evaluation of community residential care environments, case management systems, community support service programs, and family support services including respite care. Dr. Intagliata received his Ph.D. in Psychology from the State University of New York at Buffalo in 1976. He is the author of two books and 50 journal articles and book chapters.

David Lukoff, Ph.D. is a Professor of Psychology at Saybrook Institute Graduate School in San Francisco and a part-time staff psychologist at the San Francisco Veterans Affairs Day Treatment Center. He has authored articles on holistic health treatment and on AIDS and sex education for schizophrenic patients as well as articles on transpersonal approaches for working with psychotic patients. He is a member of the California Task Force on Families and Serious Mental Illness.

Jim Mintz, Ph.D. is a Professor in the Department of Psychiatry and Biobehavioral Sciences (Division of Medical Psychology) at the University of California, Los Angeles. He is past President of the Society for Psychotherapy Research. He has published over 100 journal articles and book chapters in the areas of psychotherapy, drug abuse, depression, schizophrenia, and research methods in psychiatry. He is currently Chief of the Methodology and Statistical Services Unit of the UCLA Clinical Research Center for Schizophrenia and Psychiatric Rehabilitation.

Lois Imber Mintz, Ph.D. is an Assistant Research Psychologist in the Department of Psychiatry and Biobehavioral Sciences. Her primary research interest has been in the interface of social and clinical psychology, particularly person perception, and she has published research findings on perception of psychiatric deviance, movement and hyperactivity in children, and family attitudes and perceptions in schizophrenia.

Kim T. Mueser, Ph.D. is Associate Professor of Psychiatry and Director of Psychology Training at Medical College of Pennsylvania at Eastern Pennsylvania Psychiatric Institute. Dr. Mueser has coauthored over 80 journal articles, treatment manuals, and book chapters. His clinical research interests involve social learning treatment of psychiatric patients and behavioral family therapy.

Keith Nuechterlein, Ph.D. is Professor of Medical Psychology and Director of the Aftercare Clinic at the University of California, Los Angeles, Department of Psychiatry and Biobehavioral Sciences. He also serves as Chief of the Cognition, Psychophysiology, and Neuropsychology Laboratory of the UCLA Clinical Research Center for the Study of Schizophrenia. He is currently on the Editorial Boards of the *Schizophrenia Bulletin* and *International Journal of Methods in Psychiatric Research* and is one of the editors of *Current Psychology: Research & Reviews*. His primary research interests involve information-processing and neuropsychological factors in vulnerability to schizophrenia and environmental triggers for schizophrenic psychotic episodes. Dr. Nuechterlein is the principal investigator of a large, interdisciplinary, longitudinal study of the initial phase of schizophrenia currently underway at UCLA.

Roger L. Patterson, Ph.D. is a Staff Psychologist and Coordinator of Day Treatment, W. V. Chappell, Jr. Veterans Affairs

Outpatient Clinic, Daytona Beach, Florida. Previously, he was Chairperson of the Department of Aging and Mental Health, Florida Mental Health Institute, University of South Florida. In this capacity, he was responsible for the design, development, implementation, and evaluation of a large-scale behavioral rehabilitation program for elderly mental health patients as applied both in residential care and day treatment. He is first author of the book, *Overcoming Deficits of Aging: A Behavioral Approach*, and has authored and coauthored many other articles. He has also been invited to speak on rehabilitation of the elderly at numerous major universities, both in the United States and Europe.

Catherine C. Phipps, M.A. was a Staff Research Associate in the Department of Psychiatry and Biobehavioral Sciences at the time this research was completed. She has participated in a number of research projects in the areas of rehabilitation medicine and is currently working for a private practice corporation providing services in the area of supported work for developmentally and psychiatrically disabled individuals in the Los Angeles area.

Deborah B. Pitts, O.T.R., M.B.A. is Coordinator of Rehabilitation Medicine Services at the Brentwood Veterans Affairs Medical Center in Los Angeles, California. Prior to coming to the West Los Angeles Veterans Affairs Medical Center, Ms. Pitts was instrumental in the transitioning of a traditional day treatment program to a psychosocial rehabilitation clubhouse, known as Arden House. During her 10 years as program director, she also actively promoted the integration of psychiatric rehabilitation principles into the mental health system of Los Angeles County. She is presently working with the San Diego County Department of Mental Health Services in their efforts to integrate psychiatric rehabilitation principles.

Mark L. Schade, M.L. is Implementation Coordinator and Program Director of the Social Learning Program at Austin State Hospital, Austin, Texas. As such, he is responsible for implementing a comprehensive, research-based psychosocial rehabilitation program for severely disabled adult psychiatric patients, including ongoing standardized observational assessment of staff and patient behavior. He has coauthored several articles and book chapters on skills training and psychosocial rehabilitation with schizophrenic patients.

Will Spaulding, Ph.D. is Associate Professor, Department of Psychology, University of Nebraska–Lincoln, Coordinator of the Schizophrenia and Psychiatric Rehabilitation Specialization in the University of Nebraska–Lincoln Doctoral Clinical Psychology Program, and Chief Psychologist of the Extended Care Psychiatric Rehabilitation Program, Lincoln Regional Center. He has published on the psychopathology, clinical assessments, and treatment of schizophrenia and related disorders, and on training and education in psychiatric rehabilitation. He was an editor of the 1984 Nebraska Symposium on Motivation, *Theories of Schizophrenia and Psychosis*. He is currently Principal Investigator of a National Institute of Mental Health-funded research project on the effectiveness of cognitive therapy in psychiatric rehabilitation of schizophrenia.

Angus Strachan, Ph.D. is an Associate Clinical Professor of Psychology in the Psychology and Psychiatry Departments at UCLA. Previously, he was Co-Chief of the Family Treatment and Assessment Laboratory in the UCLA Clinical Research Center for the Study of Schizophrenia. He has written numerous articles on schizophrenia and family therapy. Currently, he is in independent practice in Santa Monica, California, with a focus on family therapy and has recently founded Strachan Associates, an organizational consulting firm.

J. Greer Sullivan, M.D. is Assistant Research Psychiatrist at the UCLA School of Medicine, Staff Psychiatrist for the Rehabilitation Medicine Service at the Brentwood Veterans Affairs Medical Center Los Angeles, and Senior Natural Scientist at

RAND Corporation in Santa Monica, California. Her research activities include health services studies of seriously mentally ill populations. Her clinical interests include side effects of antipsychotic medication, especially sexual side effects.

Mary Sullivan, M.S.W. is Director of the Extended Care Psychiatric Rehabilitation Program, Lincoln Regional Center, and Adjunct Clinical Assistant Professor, Department of Psychology, University of Nebraska–Lincoln. She has 10 years' experience in the development and administration of psychiatric rehabilitation services and is currently a coinvestigator and senior therapist in a National Institute of Mental Health-funded research project on the effectiveness of cognitive therapy in psychiatric rehabilitation.

Mary Ann Test, Ph.D. is Professor, School of Social Work, and Affiliate Professor, Department of Psychiatry, at the University of Wisconsin, Madison. She was codeveloper of the Training in Community Living model of community treatment; her 20-year long research program has involved the development and evaluation of more effective community care models. She is the author of one book and numerous papers on topics related to the community treatment of persons with severe mental illness. Her current research involves a 12-year prospective study of the long-term community treatment of young adults with schizophrenic disorders.

Jerome V. Vaccaro, M.D. is Assistant Professor of Psychiatry at the UCLA School of Medicine and Assistant Chief of Rehabilitation Services at the Brentwood Veterans Affairs Medical Center in Los Angeles, California. He is a founding member of the Board of Directors of the American Association of Community Psychiatrists, edited their publication, *Community Psychiatrist*, from 1985–1989, and will edit their new journal, *Community Psychiatric Practice*. Dr. Vaccaro is a 1983–1984 Public Psychiatry Fellow of the American Psychiatric Association. He received his medical school and psychiatric residency training at the Albert Einstein College of Medicine, where he was chief resident in social and community psychiatry from 1984–1985. Dr. Vaccaro directed a community mental health center and taught at the University of Hawaii for 4 years prior to joining the faculty at UCLA. He has edited one book and published articles and book chapters in the areas of community psychiatry, psychiatric rehabilitation, treatment of schizophrenia, and education and training in public psychiatry. His current research and clinical work involves developing and testing new psychosocial treatments and treatment systems for the seriously mentally ill.

Joseph Ventura, M.A. is Co-Director of the Diagnosis and Psychopathology Assessment Unit of the UCLA Clinical Research Center for Schizophrenia and Psychiatric Rehabilitation in Los Angeles, California. He is also a Staff Research Associate for the UCLA School of Medicine.

Charles J. Wallace, Ph.D. is Associate Research Psychologist at the UCLA Department of Psychiatry and Chief of the Behavioral Assessment and Social Skills Laboratory of the Clinical Research Center for Schizophrenia. He has been on the faculty of the Fuller Graduate School of Psychology and the Cambridge Professional School of Psychology and has lectured throughout the United States on psychological testing, research methods, and statistics. For 8 years he was Clinical and Research Director of the Camarillo–UCLA Clinical Research Unit where he conducted research on behavior therapy in schizophrenia. He has been the creative force behind the design, development, and field testing of the "user friendly" modules for training social and independent living skills and has developed and validated the Independent Living Skills Survey, an instrument for functional assessment of the seriously mentally ill. Dr. Wallace is currently Principal Investigator of a public-academic liaison research grant from the National Institute of Mental Health that will determine the impact of the social and independent living skills training modules on the symptomatic and social outcomes of persons with chronic mental disorders served by a community mental health program.

Louis Jolyon West, M.D. was Professor and Chairman of Psychiatry at the University of Oklahoma for 15 years (1954–1969) and for the next 20 years (1969–1989) held the same position at the University of California, Los Angeles where he was also Director of the UCLA Neuropsychiatric Institute and Psychiatrist-in-Chief of the UCLA Medical Center. He now serves as Director of the UCLA Preventive Psychiatry Program. He has been an active consultant to Veterans Administration Hospitals for more than 35 years. He has also served as National Consultant in Psychiatry to the Surgeon General, United States Air Force; and on many advisory bodies including the Special Medical Advisory Group of the Veterans Administration; the National Advisory Mental Health Council (National Institute of Mental Health); and the National Advisory Committee on Alcoholism to the Secretary of Health, Education, and Welfare; the Board of Trustees of the American Psychiatric Association; the American Psychiatric Association Council on Research and Development (as Chairman) and many others. He has contributed to literature on alcoholism, drug abuse, pain, sleep, dissociation, hypnosis, hallucinations, methods of psychiatric treatment, racism, terrorism, cults and violence.

General Psychology Series

Editors: **Arnold P. Goldstein,** Syracuse University
Leonard Krasner, Stanford University &
SUNY at Stony Brook

Vol. 44. EVANS & CLAIBORN—*Mental Health Issues and the Urban Poor*
Vol. 46. BARBER, SPANOS & CHAVES—*Hypnosis, Imagination and Human Potentialities*
Vol. 47. POPE—*The Mental Health Interview: Research and Application*
Vol. 48. PELTON—*The Psychology of Nonviolence**
Vol. 49. COLBY—*Artificial Paranoia—A Computer Simulation of Paranoid Processes*
Vol. 50. GELFAND & HARTMANN—*Child Behavior Analysis and Therapy, Second Edition*
Vol. 51. WOLPE—*Theme and Variations: A Behavior Therapy Casebook**
Vol. 52. KANFER & GOLDSTEIN—*Helping People Change: A Textbook of Methods, Fourth Edition*
Vol. 53. DANZIGER—*Interpersonal Communication**
Vol. 55. GOLDSTEIN & STEIN—*Prescriptive Psychotherapies*
Vol. 56. BARLOW & HERSEN—*Single-Case Experimental Designs: Strategies for Studying Behavior Changes, Second Edition*
Vol. 57 MONAHAN—*Community Mental Health and the Criminal Justice System*
Vol. 58 WAHLER, HOUSE & STAMBAUGH—*Ecological Assessment of Child Problem Behavior: A Clinical Package for Home, School and Institutional Settings*
Vol. 59 MAGARO—*The Construction of Madness: Emerging Conceptions and Interventions into the Psychotic Process*
Vol. 60 MILLER—*Behavioral Treatment of Alcoholism**
Vol. 61 FOREYT—*Behavioral Treatments of Obesity*
Vol. 62 WANDERSMAN, POPPEN & RICKS—*Humanism and Behaviorism: Dialogue and Growth*
Vol. 63 NIETZEL, WINETT, MACDONALD & DAVIDSON—*Behavioral Approaches to Community Psychology*
Vol. 64 FISHER & GOCHROS—*Handbook of Behavior Therapy with Sexual Problems.* Vol. I: General Procedures. Vol. II: Approaches to Specific Problems*
Vol. 65 BELLACK & HERSEN—*Behavioral Assessment: A Practical Handbook, Third Edition*
Vol. 66 LEFKOWITZ, ERON, WALDER & HUESMANN—*Growing Up to Be Violent: A Longitudinal Study of the Development of Aggression*
Vol. 67 BARBER—*Pitfalls in Human Research: Ten Pivotal Points*
Vol. 68 SILVERMAN—*The Human Subject in the Psychological Laboratory*
Vol. 69 FAIRWEATHER & TORNATZKY—*Experimental Methods for Social Policy Research**
Vol. 70 GURMAN & RAZIN—*Effective Psychotherapy: A Handbook of Research**
Vol. 71 MOSES & BYHAM—*Applying the Assessment Center Method*
Vol. 72 GOLDSTEIN—*Prescriptions for Child Mental Health and Education*
Vol. 73 KEAT—*Multimodal Therapy with Children*
Vol. 74 SHERMAN—*Personality: Inquiry & Application*
Vol. 75 GATCHEL & PRICE—*Clinical Applications of Biofeedback: Appraisal and Status*
Vol. 76 CATALANO—*Health, Behavior and the Community: An Ecological Perspective*
Vol. 77 NIETZEL—*Crime and Its Modification: A Social Learning Perspective*
Vol. 78 GOLDSTEIN, HOYER & MONTI—*Police and the Elderly*
Vol. 79 MIRON & GOLDSTEIN—*Hostage*
Vol. 80 GOLDSTEIN et al.—*Police Crisis Intervention*
Vol. 81 UPPER & CAUTELA—*Covert Conditioning*

Vol. 82 MORELL—*Program Evaluation in Social Research*
Vol. 83 TEGER—*Too Much Invested to Quit*
Vol. 84 MONJAN & GASSNER—*Critical Issues in Competency-Based Education*
Vol. 85 KRASNER—*Environmental Design and Human Behavior: A Psychology of the Individual in Society*
Vol. 86 TAMIR—*Communication and the Aging Process: Interaction Throughout the Life Cycle*
Vol. 87 WEBSTER, KONSTANTAREAS, OXMAN & MACK—*Autism: New Directions in Research and Education*
Vol. 89 CARTLEDGE & MILBURN—*Teaching Social Skills to Children: Innovative Approaches, Second Edition*
Vol. 90 SARBIN & MANCUSO—*Schizophrenia—Medical Diagnosis or Moral Verdict?**
Vol. 91 RATHJEN & FOREYT—*Social Competence: Interventions for Children and Adults*
Vol. 92 VAN DE RIET, KORB & GORRELL—*Gestalt Therapy: An Introduction**
Vol. 93 MARSELLA & PEDERSEN—*Cross-Cultural Counseling and Psychotherapy*
Vol. 94 BRISLIN—*Cross-Cultural Encounters: Face-to-Face Interaction*
Vol. 95 SCHWARTZ & JOHNSON—*Psychopathology of Childhood: A Clinical-Experimental Approach, Second Edition*
Vol. 96 HEILBRUN—*Human Sex-Role Behavior*
Vol. 97 DAVIDSON, KOCH, LEWIS & WRESINSKI—*Evaluation Strategies in Criminal Justice*
Vol. 98 GOLDSTEIN, CARR, DAVIDSON & WEHR—*In Response to Aggression: Methods of Control and Prosocial Alternatives*
Vol. 99 GOLDSTEIN—*Psychological Skill Training: The Structured Learning Technique*
Vol. 100 WALKER—*Clinical Practice of Psychology: A Guide for Mental Health Professionals*
Vol. 101 ANCHIN & KIESLER—*Handbook of Interpersonal Psychotherapy*
Vol. 102 GELLER, WINETT & EVERETT—*Preserving the Environment: New Strategies for Behavior Change*
Vol. 103 JENKINS—*The Psychology of the Afro-American: A Humanistic Approach*
Vol. 104 APTER—*Troubled Children/Troubled Systems*
Vol. 105 BRENNER—*The Effective Psychotherapist: Conclusions from Practice and Research*
Vol. 106 KAROLY & KANFER—*Self-Management and Behavior Change: From Theory to Practice**
Vol. 107 O'BRIEN, DICKINSON & ROSOW—*Industrial Behavior Modification: A Management Handbook*
Vol. 108 AMABILE & STUBBS—*Psychological Research in the Classroom: Issues for Educators and Researchers**
Vol. 109 WARREN—*Auditory Perception: A New Synthesis**
Vol. 110 DiMATTEO & DiNICOLA—*Achieving Patient Compliance: The Psychology of the Medical Practitioner's Role*
Vol. 111 CONOLEY & CONOLEY—*School Consultation: A Guide to Practice and Training*
Vol. 112 PAPAJOHN—*Intensive Behavior Therapy: The Behavioral Treatment of Complex Emotional Disorders*
Vol. 113 KAROLY, STEFFEN & O'GRADY—*Child Health Psychology: Concepts and Issues*

Vol. 114 MORRIS & KRATOCHWILL—*Treating Children's Fears and Phobias: A Behavioral Approach*
Vol. 115 GOLDSTEIN & SEGALL—*Aggression in Global Perspective*
Vol. 116 LANDIS & BRISLIN—*Handbook of Intercultural Training*
Vol. 117 FARBER—*Stress and Burnout in the Human Service Professions*
Vol. 118 BEUTLER—*Eclectic Psychotherapy: A Systematic Approach*
Vol. 119 HARRIS—*Families of the Developmentally Disabled: A Guide to Behavioral Interventions*
Vol. 120 HERSEN, KAZDIN & BELLACK—*The Clinical Psychology Handbook, Second Edition*
Vol. 121 MATSON & MULICK—*Handbook of Mental Retardation, Second Edition*
Vol. 122 FELNER, JASON, MORITSUGU & FARBER—*Preventive Psychology: Theory, Research and Practice*
Vol. 123 CENTER FOR RESEARCH ON AGGRESSION—*Prevention and Control of Aggression*
Vol. 124 KRATOCHWILL & MORRIS—*The Practice of Child Therapy, Second Edition*
Vol. 125 VARNI—*Clinical Behavioral Pediatrics: An Interdisciplinary Biobehavioral Approach*
Vol. 126 RAMIREZ—*Psychology of the Americas: Mestizo Perspectives on Personality and Mental Health*
Vol. 127 LEWINSOHN & TERI—*Clinical Geropsychology: New Directions in Assessment and Treatment*
Vol. 128 BARLOW, HAYES & NELSON—*The Scientist Practitioner: Research and Accountability in Clinical and Educational Settings*
Vol. 129 OLLENDICK & HERSEN—*Child Behavioral Assessment: Principles and Procedures*
Vol. 130 BELLACK & HERSEN—*Research Methods in Clinical Psychology*
Vol. 131 GOLDSTEIN & HERSEN—*Handbook of Psychological Assessment, Second Edition*
Vol. 132 BELLACK & HERSEN—*Dictionary of Behavior Therapy Techniques*
Vol. 133 COOK—*Psychological Androgyny*
Vol. 134 DREW & HARDMAN—*Designing and Conducting Behavioral Research*
Vol. 135 APTER & GOLDSTEIN—*Youth Violence: Programs and Prospects*
Vol. 136 HOLZMAN & TURK—*Pain Management: A Handbook of Psychological Treatment Approaches*
Vol. 137 MORRIS & BLATT—*Special Education: Research and Trends*
Vol. 138 JOHNSON, RASBURY & SIEGEL—*Approaches to Child Treatment: Introduction to Theory, Research and Practice*
Vol. 139 RYBASH, HOYER & ROODIN—*Adult Cognition and Aging: Developmental Changes in Processing, Knowing and Thinking*
Vol. 140 WIELKIEWICZ—*Behavior Management in the Schools: Principles and Procedures*
Vol. 141 PLAS—*Systems Psychology in the Schools*
Vol. 142 VAN HASSELT & HERSEN—*Handbook of Adolescent Psychology*
Vol. 143 BRASSARD, GERMAIN & HART—*Psychological Maltreatment of Children and Youth*
Vol. 144 HERSHENSON & POWER—*Mental Health Counseling: Theory and Practice*
Vol. 145 GOLDSTEIN & KRASNER—*Modern Applied Psychology*
Vol. 146 CARSTENSEN & EDELSTEIN—*Handbook of Clinical Gerontology*
Vol. 147 HERSEN & BELLACK—*Dictionary of Behavioral Assessment Techniques*

Vol. 148. VAN HASSELT, STRAIN & HERSEN—*Handbook of Developmental and Physical Disabilities*
Vol. 149. BLECHMAN & BROWNELL—*Handbook of Behavioral Medicine for Women*
Vol. 150. MAHER & ZINS—*Psychoeducational Interventions in Schools: Methods and Procedures for Enhancing Student Competence*
Vol. 151. LAST & HERSEN—*Handbook of Anxiety Disorders*
Vol. 152. KAZDIN—*Child Psychotherapy: Developing and Identifying Effective Treatments*
Vol. 153. RUSSELL—*Stress Management for Chronic Disease*
Vol. 154. HUGHES—*Cognitive Behavior Therapy with Children in Schools*
Vol. 155. HIGGINBOTHAM, WEST & FORSYTH—*Psychotherapy and Behavior Change: Social, Cultural and Methodological Perspectives*
Vol. 156. WINETT, KING & ALTMAN—*Health Psychology and Public Health: An Integrative Approach*
Vol. 157. HESTER & MILLER—*Handbook of Alcoholism Treatment Approaches: Effective Alternatives*
Vol. 158. WHITE—*The Troubled Adolescent*
Vol. 159. HOWES—*The Psychology of Human Cognition: Mainstream and Genevan Traditions*
Vol. 160. SEGALL, DASEN, BERRY & POORTINGA—*Human Behavior in Global Perspective: An Introduction to Cross-Cultural Psychology*
Vol. 161. HERSEN & LAST—*Handbook of Child and Adult Psychology: A Longitudinal Perspective*
Vol. 162. SNYDER & FORSYTH—*Handbook of Social and Clinical Psychology: The Health Perspective*
Vol. 163. JOHNSON & GOLDMAN—*Developmental Assessment in Clinical Child Psychology: A Handbook*
Vol. 164. MARTIN—*Handbook of Behavior Therapy and Psychological Science: An Integrative Approach*
Vol. 165. WINIARSKI—*Aids-Related Psychotherapy*
Vol. 166. LIBERMAN—*Handbook of Psychiatric Rehabilitation*
Vol. 167. OLLENDICK & HERSEN—*Handbook of Child and Adolescent Assessment*
Vol. 168. HAYNES—*Models of Causality in Psychopathology: Toward Dynamic, Synthetic and Nonlinear Models of Behavior Disorders*

*Out of print in original format. Available in custom reprint edition.